Nutrition for the Primary Care Provider

Supported by an unrestricted educational grant from the Nestlé Nutrition Institute.

World Review of Nutrition and Dietetics

Vol. 111

Series Editor

Berthold Koletzko Munich

Nutrition for the Primary Care Provider

Volume Editor

Dennis M. Bier Houston, Tex.

Co-Editors

Jim Mann Dunedin
David H. Alpers St. Louis, Mo.
H.H. Este Vorster Potchesfstroom
Michael J. Gibney Dublin

20 figures, 8 in color and 50 tables, 2015

KARGER Basel · Freiburg · Paris · London · New York · Chennai · New Delhi · Bangkok · Beijing · Shanghai · Tokyo · Kuala Lumpur · Singapore · Sydney

Dennis M. Bier
USDA/ARS Children's Nutrition Research Center
Baylor College of Medicine
1100 Bates Street
Houston, TX 77030-2600 (USA)

Jim Mann
Medicine and Human Nutrition
University of Otago
PO Box 56
Dunedin 9054 (New Zealand)

David H. Alpers
Washington University School of Medicine
660 S. Euclid Ave.
St. Louis, MO 63110 (USA)

H.H. Este Vorster
Faculty of Health Sciences
Centre of Excellence for Nutrition
North-West University
Potchefstroom 2531 (South Africa)

Michael J. Gibney
School of Agriculture and Food Science
University College Dublin
Science Centre – South Belfield
Dublin 4 (Ireland)

Library of Congress Cataloging-in-Publication Data

Nutrition for the primary care provider / volume editor, Dennis M. Bier ;
co-editors, Jim Mann, David H. Alpers, H.H. Este Vorster, Michael J. Gibney.
p. ; cm. -- (World review of nutrition and dietetics, ISSN 1660-2242
; vol. 111)
Includes bibliographical references and index.
ISBN 978-3-318-02666-5 (hard cover : alk. paper) -- ISBN 978-3-318-02667-2
(e-book)
I. Bier, Dennis M., editor. II. Mann, Jim, editor. III. Alpers, David H.,
editor. IV. Vorster, H. H., editor. V. Gibney, Michael J., editor. VI.
Series: World review of nutrition and dietetics ; v. 111. 0084-2230
[DNLM: 1. Nutritional Physiological Phenomena. 2. Physicians, Primary
Care. 3. Nutrition Policy. 4. Nutrition Therapy. W1 WO898 v.111 2014 / QU
145]
RM216
615.8'54--dc23
2014030004

Bibliographic Indices. This publication is listed in bibliographic services, including Current Contents® and PubMed/MEDLINE.

www.karger.com
Printed in Germany on acid-free and non-aging paper (ISO 9706) by Kraft Druck, Ettlingen
ISSN 1660–2242
e-ISSN 1662–2898
ISBN 978–3–318–02666–5
e-ISBN 978–3–318–02667–2

KARGER 125 YEARS

Contents

List of Contributors

Saira Adeel
Division of Endocrinology, Metabolism and Lipids
Department of Medicine
Emory University School of Medicine
101 Woodruff Circle, NE-WMRB1301
Atlanta, GA 30322 (USA)
E-Mail saira.adeel@emory.edu

Denis Barclay
Nestec SA
Avenue Nestlé 55
CH–1800 Vevey (Switzerland)
E-Mail denis.barclay@outlook.com

Susan I. Barr
Food, Nutrition & Health
The University of British Columbia
2205 East Mall
Vancouver, BC V6T 1Z4 (Canada)
E-Mail susan.barr@ubc.ca

Swati Bhardwaj
Nutrition and Fatty Acid Research
National Diabetes, Obesity and
Cholesterol Foundation (N-DOC)
D 16/8, 2nd Floor, Ardee City, Sector 52
Gurgaon, Haryana, 122011 (India)
E-Mail swati7681@gmail.com

Zulfiqar A. Bhutta
Center of Excellence in Women and Child Health
Aga Khan University
Stadium Road
PO Box 3500
Karachi 74800 (Pakistan)
E-Mail zulfiqar.bhutta@aku.edu

Bruce R. Bistrian
Clinical Nutrition
Beth Israel Deaconess Medical Center
1 Deaconess Road
Boston, MA 02215 (USA)
E-Mail bbistria@bidmc.harvard.edu

Nancy F. Butte
USDA/ARS Children's Nutrition Research Center
Department of Pediatrics
Baylor College of Medicine
1100 Bates Street
Houston, TX 77030-2600 (USA)
E-Mail nbutte@bcm.edu

Kevin D. Cashman
School of Food and Nutritional Sciences and
Department of Medicine
Room 242, Food Science Building
Cork (Ireland)
E-Mail k.cashman@ucc.ie

Ian D. Caterson
The Boden Institute of Obesity, Nutrition, Exercise
and Eating Disorders
The University of Sydney
Medical Foundation Bldg (K25)
92–94 Parramatta Road
Camperdown, NSW 2050 (Australia)
E-Mail ian.caterson@sydney.edu.au

Matt Cave
University of Louisville and Robley Rex VAMC
505 S. Hancock Street, CTR512
Louisville, KY 40202 (USA)
E-Mail m0cave01@louisville.edu

Mei Chung
Nutrition/Infection Unit
Department of Public Health and Community Medicine
School of Medicine
Tufts University
136 Harrison Avenue, M&V Wing 1st Floor
Boston, MA 02111 (USA)
E-Mail mei_chun.chung@tufts.edu

Sheila E. Crowe
Division of Gastroenterology
Department of Medicine
University of California at San Diego
9500 Gilman Drive #0063
La Jolla, CA 92093-0063 (USA)
E-Mail secrowe@ucsd.edu

Paul M. Coates
Office of Dietary Supplements
National Institutes of Health
6100 Executive Boulevard
Room 3B01, MSC 7517
Bethesda, MD 20892-7517 (USA)
E-Mail coatesp@od.nih.gov

Adam Drewnowski
Center for Public Health Nutrition
University of Washington
355 Raitt Hall #353410
Seattle, WA 98195-3410 (USA)
E-Mail adamdrew@uw.edu

Susan J. Fairweather-Tait
Norwich Medical School
University of East Anglia
Bio-Medical Research Centre (BMRC) 0.04
Norwich NR4 7TJ (UK)
E-Mail s.fairweather-tait@uea.ac.uk

Alice A. Gibson
The Boden Institute of Obesity, Nutrition, Exercise
and Eating Disorders
The University of Sydney
Medical Foundation Bldg (K25)
92–94 Parramatta Road
Camperdown, NSW 2050 (Australia)
E-Mail alice.gibson@sydney.edu.au

Susanna Magrietha Hanekom
Center of Excellence for Nutrition
North-West University
Private Bag X6001
Potchefstroom 2520 (South Africa)
E-Mail grieta.hanekom@nwu.ac.za

Ferdinand Haschke
Department of Pediatrics
Paracelsus Medical University
Müllner Hauptstrasse 48
AT–5020 Salzburg (Austria)
E-Mail fhaschk@gmail.com

L. John Hoffer
Lady Davis Institute for Medical Research
Jewish General Hospital
3755 Cote-Ste.-Catherine Road
Montreal, QC H3T 1E2 (Canada)
E-Mail l.hoffer@mcgill.ca

Elizabeth J. Johnson
Jean Mayer USDA Human Nutrition Center on Aging
Tufts University
711 Washington Street
Boston, MA 02111 (USA)
E-Mail elizabeth.johnson@tufts.edu

Walter H. Kaye
UCSD Eating Disorder Research and Treatment Program
UCSD Department of Psychiatry
Chancellor Park
4510 Executive Dr., Suite 315
San Diego, CA 92121 (USA)
E-Mail wkaye@ucsd.edu

Timothy Key
Cancer Epidemiology Unit
Nuffield Department of Population Health
University of Oxford
Richard Doll Building, Roosevelt Drive
Oxford OX3 7LF (UK)
E-Mail tim.key@ceu.ox.ac.uk

H. Salome Kruger
Centre of Excellence for Nutrition
North-West University
PO Box 20333
Noordbrug
Esselen Street
Potchefstroom 2522 (South Africa)
E-Mail salome.kruger@nwu.ac.za

Neeraj Kumar
Department of Neurology
Mayo Clinic
E8A, Mayo Building, 200 First St. SW
Rochester, MN 55905 (USA)
E-Mail kumar.neeraj@mayo.edu

Joseph Lau
Center for Evidence-Based Medicine
Public Health Program
Brown University
121 S. Main Street, 8th floor
Providence, RI 02912 (USA)
E-Mail joseph_lau@brown.edu

John Leung
Food Allergy Center at Tufts Medical Center and Floating Hospital for Children
Departments of Gastroenterology, Pediatric Gastroenterology, and Allergy and Immunology
Tufts Medical Center
800 Washington Street
Boston, MA 02111 (USA)
E-Mail jleung3@tuftsmedicalcenter.org

Luis Marsano
University of Louisville and Robley Rex VAMC
505 S. Hancock Street, CTR512
Louisville, KY 40202 (USA)
E-Mail luis.marsano@louisville.edu

Jim Mann
Department of Human Nutrition
University of Otago
PO Box 56
Dunedin 9054 (New Zealand)
Email jim.mann@otago.ac.nz

Enrica Marzola
Department of Neuroscience
University of Turin
Via Cherasco 11
IT–10126 Turin (Italy)
E-Mail enrica.marzola@gmail.com

Richard D. Mattes
Department of Nutrition Science
Purdue University
212 Stone Hall, 700 W. State Street
West Lafayette, IN 47907-2059 (USA)
E-Mail mattes@purdue.edu

Ronald J. Maughan
School of Sport, Exercise and Health Sciences
Loughborough University
Ashby Road
Loughborough LE11 3TU (UK)
E-Mail r.maughan@lboro.ac.uk

Rachael McLean
Departments of Preventive and Social Medicine and Human Nutrition
University of Otago
PO Box 56
Dunedin 9054 (New Zealand)
E-Mail rachael.mclean@otago.ac.nz

Anoop Misra
Fortis C-DOC Center of Excellence for Diabetes, Metabolic Diseases and Endocrinology
B16 Chirag Enclave
New Delhi 110016 (India)
E-Mail anoopmisra@metabolicresearchindia.com

Emily S. Mohn
Jean Mayer USDA Human Nutrition Center on Aging
Tufts University
711 Washington Street
Boston, MA 02111 (USA)
E-Mail emily.mohn@tufts.edu

Jonathan Obert
University of Louisville and Robley Rex VAMC
505 S. Hancock Street, CTR512
Louisville, KY 40202 (USA)
E-Mail jonathan.obert@louisville.edu

Ulf Risérus
Clinical Nutrition and Metabolism
Department of Public Health and Caring Sciences
Uppsala Science Park
SE–75185 Uppsala (Sweden)
E-Mail ulf.riserus@pubcare.uu.se

Hamid M. Said
University of California/VA Medical Program-151
5901 E. 7th St
Long Beach, CA 90822 (USA)
E-Mail hmsaid@uci.edu

Rehana A. Salam
Division of Women and Child Health
Aga Khan University
Stadium Road
PO Box 3500
Karachi 74800 (Pakistan)
E-Mail rehana.salam@aku.edu

Dale A. Schoeller
Nutritional Sciences
University of Wisconsin
1415 Linden Dr.
Madison, WI 53706 (USA)
E-Mail dschoell@nutrisci.wisc.edu

James S. Scolapio
Division of Gastroenterology
University of Florida, Jacksonville Campus
4555 Emerson Street, Suite 300
Jacksonville, FL 32207 (USA)
E-Mail james.scolapio@jax.ufl.edu

Susan M. Shirreffs
New Product Research
GlaxoSmithKline
980 Great West Road
Brentford, TW8 9GS (UK)
E-Mail susan.m.shirreffs@gsk.com

Kyra A. Sim
The Boden Institute of Obesity, Nutrition, Exercise and Eating Disorders
The University of Sydney
Medical Foundation Bldg (K25)
92–94 Parramatta Road
Camperdown, NSW 2050 (Australia)
E-Mail kyra.sim@sydney.edu.au

Donna J. Smith
Division of Gastroenterology
University of Florida, Jacksonville Campus
4555 Emerson Street, Suite 300
Jacksonville, FL 32207 (USA)
E-Mail donna.smith@jax.ufl.edu

Sally P. Stabler
Division of Hematology
School of Medicine
University of Colorado
12700 E. 19th Avenue, Room 9122
RC2, Campus Box B170
Aurora, CO 80045 (USA)
E-Mail Sally.Stabler@ucdenver.edu

Vin Tangpricha
Division of Endocrinology, Metabolism and Lipids
Department of Medicine
Emory University School of Medicine
101 Woodruff Circle, NE-WMRB1301
Atlanta, GA 30322 (USA)
E-Mail vin.tangpricha@emory.edu

Diana Thomas
Mathematical Sciences
Montclair State University
Richardson Hall 205
1 Normal Ave
Montclair, NJ 07043 (USA)
E-Mail thomasdia@mail.montclair.edu

Paul R. Thomas
Office of Dietary Supplements
National Institutes of Health
6100 Executive Boulevard
Room 3B01, MSC 7517
Bethesda, MD 20892-7517 (USA)
thomaspaul@od.nih.gov

Averalda E. van Graan
Centre of Excellence for Nutrition
North-West University
Potchefstroom Campus
Private Bag X6001
Potchefstroom 2520 (South Africa)
E-Mail averalda.vangraan@nwu.ac.za

H.H. Este Vorster
Centre of Excellence for Nutrition
North-West University
Potchefstroom Campus
Private Bag X129
Potchefstroom 2520 (South Africa)
E-mail este.vorster@nwu.ac.za

Foreword

Nutrition takes center stage amongst all the lifestyle-related players which contribute to health or disease. Indeed, nutrition underlies the prevention and management of the most prevalent conditions faced by today's primary care providers. In developed countries, the erosion of our dietary habits is a major contributor to conditions such as type 2 diabetes, cardiovascular diseases and obesity. A large proportion of the health care budget of developed countries is consumed by the management of these increasingly widespread disorders. In addition to these well-known conditions, physicians also face a plethora of the more subtle manifestations of inadequate nutrition, such as liver disease, neurological disorders or anemia. And the problem of nutrition-related conditions is not only confined to the borders of the developed world. In developing countries, the specter of malnutrition is two-headed: on the one hand, a large percentage of the population is afflicted by malnutrition, but on the other hand, there is a rising trend in the same noncommunicable diseases that afflict the 'westernized' nations, such as metabolic conditions, obesity and cardiovascular disease.

Nutrition for the Primary Care Provider is aimed at physicians around the world who treat patients from all walks of life. The first section of the book is devoted to the basic principles of nutrition, covering the fundamentals of body composition, energy balance and appetite as well as the importance of the different macro- and micronutrients. The following section builds on the principles of the first by focusing on the special needs for specific circumstances including pregnancy, exercise, food allergies and religion. The third section, Nutrition for Disease States, provides an overview of our latest understanding of various disease states and how they are influenced by nutrition. The final section on Food Policy takes a bird's eye view, offering perspectives on global sustainability, the rapidly changing face of malnutrition and the role played by the food industry in consumer health.

We hope that this book will not only serve as a practical reference source but also shape the way physicians use nutrition as a tool to prevent and cure disease.

Karen Yeow, Medical Writer

Bier D, et al. (eds): Nutrition for the Primary Care Provider. World Rev Nutr Diet. Basel, Karger, 2015, vol 111, pp 1–6
DOI: 10.1159/000362289

Evidence-Based Approach to Inform Clinical Nutrition Practice

Mei Chung[a] Joseph Lau[b]

[a]Nutrition/Infection Unit, Department of Public Health and Community Medicine, School of Medicine, Tufts University, Boston, Mass., and [b]Center for Evidence-Based Medicine, School of Public Health, Brown University, Providence, R.I., USA

Key Words

Evidence-based practice · Systematic reviews · Nutrition recommendations · Nutrition guidelines · Clinical practice

Key Messages

- Nutrition is an important factor that underlies many chronic diseases, and dietary modification plays an important role in the management of established disease states. There is thus an expectation for nutrition recommendations and clinical practice guidelines to be evidence based.
- The systematic review is a comprehensive synthesis of available evidence for addressing a specific clinical question. Evidence-based clinical practice guidelines are formulated statements aimed at facilitating clinical decision-making for specific clinical circumstances.
- Systematic reviews and evidence-based guidelines are the two best sources of information to assist clinical decision-making, and are important tools for addressing clinical questions.
- The practitioner should be aware of unique nutrition-specific parameters that must be taken into consideration before applying the findings of systematic reviews or evidence-based guidelines to daily practice.
- In the clinic, it is necessary to integrate the best available evidence with clinical expertise, patient values and preferences, and cultural beliefs.

Introduction

The ultimate goal of evidence-based practice is to improve health outcomes and quality of care by applying valid up-to-date research findings to clinical practice. Although evidence-based practice began in medicine, over the past 20 years this approach for informing clinical decision-making has been embraced by other fields, including nutrition. There is now an appreciable body of evidence to suggest that nutrition is an important determinant of many chronic diseases and that dietary modification has a role in the management of established disease states. Thus, there is an expectation that nutrition recommendations and nutrition clinical practice guidelines should be evidence based. The systematic review, an integral component of the evidence-based approach, is a comprehensive synthesis of available evidence that meets predefined eligibility criteria to address a specific clinical question or range of questions. It uses rigorous processes to minimize bias [1], and can provide busy primary care providers with a 'quick and easy way' to the best synthesized scientific evidence for informing clinical practice. Evidence-based guidelines are systematically developed statements based on scientific

Table 1. Example of research questions formulated based on the PI(E)CO components

Clinical nutrition care process	Example research question structure
Nutrition assessment	What is the ***O*** *accuracy, reliability, or agreement* of ***E*** *calculated energy expenditure* (assessment) versus ***C*** *measured energy expenditure by indirect calorimetry* (assessment) among ***P*** *obese children*?
Nutrition diagnosis	What is the ***O*** *sensitivity and specificity* of ***E*** *nutrition assessment tools* (assessment) to diagnose ***C*** *vitamin deficiency* (nutrition diagnosis by a reference standard) among ***P*** *adult men and women*?
Nutrition intervention	Among ***P*** *pregnant or breastfeeding women*, what are effects of ***I*** *maternal dietary supplementation of omega-3 fatty acids* versus ***C*** *placebo or no supplementation* on ***O*** *infant health outcomes*?

P = Population of interest; I/E = intervention/exposure of interest; C = control or comparator of interest; O = outcome of interest.

evidence to assist practitioner and patient decisions about appropriate health care for specific clinical circumstances.

While sharing the same principles with evidence-based medicine, the application of evidence-based methods to nutrition needs to incorporate unique nutrition-related considerations [2]. This chapter focuses on examples of these issues and how they should be considered when evaluating evidence to inform clinical nutrition practice.

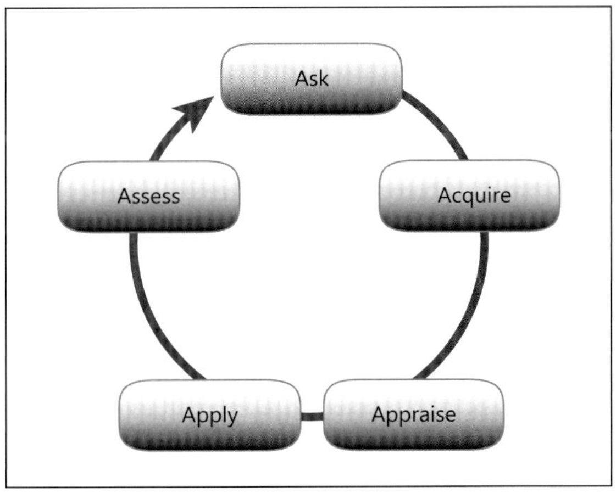

Fig. 1. Basic steps of evidence-based clinical nutrition practice.

Basic Steps of Evidence-Based Clinical Nutrition Practice

Basic steps of evidence-based clinical nutrition practice are presented in figure 1.

Step 1: Ask a Clinical Question

Important clinical questions may not be directly answerable from the literature. For example, 'Should dietary supplements be recommended to my patients?' is an important clinical question but needs to be specifically focused in order to seek for research evidence. A well-constructed research question will help to identify the correct information, or evidence. One useful way of defining a research question is to use the PI(E)CO approach:

- Population or patient: Who is the target population?
- Intervention or Exposure: What intervention or exposure are you interested in?
- Control or comparison: What are you comparing the intervention or exposure with?

- Outcome: What outcomes are you interested in measuring?

The PI(E)CO approach is most suitable for formulating a research question on the comparative efficacy of two alternative clinical nutrition interventions, but can also be used to define research questions on nutrition assessment or diagnosis (table 1).

Step 2: Acquire the Best Evidence for Informing Clinical Nutrition Decision-Making

In everyday clinical nutrition practice, many questions arise, such as what nutrition information or advice should be discussed with patients, and the benefits and harms of performing a particular nutritional assessment, diagnosis, intervention, or monitoring and evaluation [3]. With more than 1,900 new articles being added to Medline® each day[1], clinicians have a daunting task to keep up with the rapidly expanding knowledge base related to health. An evidence-based approach to clinical decision-making is time-consuming and requires considerable skill. Systematic reviews and evidence-based clinical practice guidelines are the two best sources of information to assist clinical decision-making. Many organizations have produced systematic reviews on nutrition-disease relationships or nutritional interventions (table 2). Many of these systematic reviews have also been used to support evidence-based nutrition guidelines or practice recommendations.

Searching and Evaluating Evidence-Based Practice Guidelines

Evidence-based practice guidelines can be identified by searching National Guideline Clearinghouse (http://www.guidelines.gov) and limiting the searches to guidelines that used systematic reviews as part of their methods for analyzing the evidence. Other important aspects of guideline development, such as conflict of interest disclosure and grading of body of evidence, should also be evaluated. A high quality, trustworthy, evidence-based practice guideline should be based on a systematic review of the existing evidence and apply an explicit and transparent process that minimizes distortions, biases, and conflicts of interest [4].

Searching and Evaluating Systematic Reviews

Published systematic reviews can be identified through PubMed® Clinical Queries search for 'Systematic Reviews'. The PI(E)CO components of your clinical question can also be used to effectively find relevant systematic reviews. For a systematic review, the PI(E)CO components define much of the eligibility criteria for selecting the studies, and thus define the relevance of the systematic reviews to inform clinical practice. Unique nutrition-related considerations [2] for evaluating the relevance of a systematic review to inform clinical nutrition practice include: baseline nutrient exposure, nutrient status (e.g. nutrient deficient vs. sufficient, or malnutrition vs. overnutrition/obesity), bioequivalence of bioactive compounds, bioavailability, multiple and interrelated biological functions, undefined nature of some nutritional interventions (e.g. food preparation methods and the formulation of dietary supplements), and uncertainties in dietary intake assessment.

Step 3: Appraise the Evidence for Its Validity and Usefulness

Systematic reviews vary in their quality [5], which can affect their usefulness in clinical nutrition practice [6]. Poor-quality systematic reviews can lead clinicians to the wrong conclusions and ultimately to inappropriate clinical decisions. The Institute of Medicine has published a report that included 21 standards to ensure objective, transparent, and scientifically valid systematic reviews [7].

[1] Over 1,900 indexed per day was based on 724,831 indexed citations added to Medline® in 2011 divided by 365 days (http://www.nlm.nih.gov/bsd/stats/cit_added.html).

Table 2. Organizations producing systematic reviews or evidence-based guidelines on nutrition-disease relationships or nutritional interventions

Sources	Clinical nutrition topics
3ie International Initiative for Impact Evaluation (http://www.3ieimpact.org/)	3ie aims to generate new evidence of what works, synthesize and disseminate this evidence, build a culture of evidence-based policy-making, and develop a capacity to produce and use impact evaluations. 3ie's Systematic Review Programme provides a range of research synthesis products and services include a database of systematic reviews of the effectiveness of social and economic interventions in low- and middle-income countries, such as the following topics related to food and nutrition: – Community-based interventions for improving perinatal and neonatal health outcomes in developing countries: a review of the evidence. – Impact of maternal education about complementary feeding and provision of complementary foods on child growth in developing countries.
Academy of Nutrition and Dietetics, Evidence Analysis Library (http://www.adaevidencelibrary.com)	The Evidence Analysis Library aims to promote evidence-based dietetics practice through an online library of systematic reviews on important dietetic practice questions and evidence-based guidelines and toolkits. Topics are organized according to diseases/health conditions, nutrients, foods, life cycle and nutrition, and the nutrition care process. Topics under the nutrition care process include: – Screening and referral system – Health disparities nutrition assessment – Nutrition assessment – Nutrition diagnosis – Nutrition intervention – Nutrition monitoring and evaluation – Outcomes management system
Agency for Healthcare Research and Quality Effective Health Care Program (http://www.effectivehealthcare.ahrq.gov/)	The Effective Health Care Program develops a wide array of products for researchers and others interested in the systematic study of evidence and research methods. Selected evidence reports on clinical nutrition topics include: – Dietary supplements in adults taking cardiovascular drugs – Adjuvant treatment for phenylketonuria – Vitamin D and calcium: a systematic review of health outcomes – Comparative effectiveness of treatments to prevention fractures in men and women with low bone density or osteoporosis
Community Preventive Services Task Force The Community Guide – Promoting Good Nutrition (http://www.thecommunityguide.org/nutrition/index.html)	The Guide to Community Preventive Services is a free resource to help you choose programs and policies to improve health and prevent disease in your community. Systematic reviews are used to answer these questions: – School-based programs promoting nutrition and physical activity – Provider-oriented intervention (e.g. education, reminders) – Interventions in community settings (e.g. reducing screening time, technology-based interventions, specific settings)
The Cochrane Collaboration The Cochrane Library (http://www.thecochranelibrary.com)	The Cochrane Library consists of over 5,000 Cochrane systematic reviews that aim to help health care providers, policy-makers, patients, their advocates and carers, make well-informed decisions about health care. Selected Cochrane reviews on clinical nutrition topics include the following: – Enteral nutritional therapy for induction of remission in Crohn's disease – Protein restriction for children with chronic kidney disease – Nutrition support for bone marrow transplant patients – Protein and energy supplementation in elderly people at risk of malnutrition

Table 2 (continued)

Sources	Clinical nutrition topics
United Sates Department of Agriculture Center for Nutrition Policy and Promotion Nutrition Evidence Library (http://www.nel.gov/) Dietary Guidelines for Americans (http://www.cnpp.usda.gov/ DietaryGuidelines.htm)	The Nutrition Evidence Library provides a detailed evidence portfolio for each of the 2010 Dietary Guidelines Advisory Committee's systematic reviews, which form the bases for the Dietary Guidelines for Americans. Topics are organized into the following categories: – Alcohol – Carbohydrates – Energy balance and weight management – Fatty acids and cholesterol – Food safety and technology – Nutrient adequacy – Protein – Sodium, potassium, and water
World Cancer Research Fund & American Institute for Cancer Research (WCRF/AICR) Food, Nutrition, Physical Activity, and the Prevention of Cancer: A Global Perspective (http://www.dietandcancerreport.org/)	The WCRF/AICR Continuous Update Project (CUP) is an ongoing review of cancer prevention research that provides up-to-date evidence on how people can reduce their cancer risk through diet and physical activity. They provide cancer site systematic reviews, and separate reviews on cancer survivorship, the determinants of weight gain, overweight and obesity.

A critical step in evidence synthesis is the quality assessment of the primary studies included in the systematic review. Quality assessment helps to determine the validity of the study findings and to interpret the effects of methodological and clinical/biological heterogeneity on the study results. The readers of any systematic review, however, should be aware that there are intrinsic subjective components in any quality appraisal tool, and there is no true reference standard for quality. Thus, it is important to have transparent reporting of quality assessment indicators in order to minimize subjectivity and errors in quality appraisal. Quality appraisal is important because the strength of a body of evidence that underlies the answers to a particular research question is primarily determined by the validity of the primary studies relevant to that research question. Several nutrition-specific issues may need to be considered as part of quality assessment indicators, such as uncertainty in measuring nutrient exposures (e.g. validity of dietary assessment methods or nutrient biomarkers) and controlling for potential confounding by other lifestyle factors.

Steps 4 and 5: Apply the Evidence to Clinical Nutrition Practice and Assess the Impacts of the Evidence-Based Practice

In the clinical decision-making process, it is necessary to integrate the best available evidence with clinical expertise, patient values and preferences, and cultural beliefs. Clinical nutrition practice ideally should be based on high strength of evidence (incorporating quality, quantity, and consistency of the evidence) and high applicability to the clinical setting. When applying the evidence to clinical practice, clinicians should also account for the constraints of clinical decision-making, such as policies, community standards, time, and resources. After the evidence-based practice is applied, changes to quality of care should be assessed and analyzed to inform future adjustments [8] to the evidence-based clinical nutrition practice.

Conclusions

- Systematic reviews and evidence-based clinical practice guidelines can provide an objective summary and critical appraisal of the available evidence and can increase transparency in the clinical decision-making process. However, they are not free of limitations [9].
- To use these evidence-based resources effectively, an understanding of the strengths and limitations of the systematic reviews and clinical practice guidelines is needed.
- Many unique nutrition considerations have been identified and need to be incorporated into the clinical nutrition decision-making process.
- Further research on how to integrate and analyze these unique nutrition considerations in systematic reviews [10] is needed to promote and inform evidence-based clinical nutrition practice.

References

1 Cook DJ, Mulrow CD, Haynes RB: Systematic reviews: synthesis of best evidence for clinical decisions. Ann Intern Med 1997;126:376–380.
2 Lichtenstein AH, Yetley EA, Lau J: Application of systematic review methodology to the field of nutrition. J Nutr 2008;138:2297–306.
3 Lacey K, Pritchett E: Nutrition Care Process and Model: ADA adopts road map to quality care and outcomes management. J Am Diet Assoc 2003;103:1061–1072.
4 Institute of Medicine: Clinical Practice Guidelines We Can Trust. Washington, The National Academies Press, 2011.
5 Chung M, Balk EM, Ip S, et al: Reporting of systematic reviews of micronutrients and health: a critical appraisal. Am J Clin Nutr 2009;89:1099–1113.
6 Wolfenden L, Wiggers J, Tursan d'Espaignet E, Bell AC: How useful are systematic reviews of child obesity interventions? Obes Rev 2010;11:159–165.
7 Institute of Medicine: Finding What Works in Health Care: Standards for Systematic Reviews. Washington, The National Academies Press, 2011.
8 Langley GL, Nolan KM, Nolan TW, et al: The Improvement Guide: A Practical Approach to Enhancing Organizational Performance, ed 2. San Francisco, Jossey-Bass Publishers, 2009.
9 Egger M, Dickersin K, Smith GD: Problems and limitations in conducting systematic reviews; in Egger M, Smith GD, Altman DG (eds): Systematic Reviews in Health Care: Meta-Analysis in Context, ed 2. London, BMJ Publishing Group, 2008.
10 Chung M, Balk EM, Ip S, et al: Systematic review to support the development of nutrient reference intake values: challenges and solutions. Am J Clin Nutr 2010;92:273–276.

Bier D, et al. (eds): Nutrition for the Primary Care Provider. World Rev Nutr Diet. Basel, Karger, 2015, vol 111, pp 7–12
DOI: 10.1159/000362290

Nutrient Adequacy

H.H. Vorster

Centre of Excellence for Nutrition, North-West University, Potchefstroom Campus, Potchefstroom, South Africa

Key Words

Nutrient adequacy · Nutritional assessment · Nutritional status · Nutrient recommendations · Nutrient goals · Food-based dietary guidelines

Key Messages

- Nutrient adequacy, a result of consumption of sufficient amounts of all essential nutrients and energy to meet individual requirements, is a prerequisite for normal growth, development and health.
- Two thirds or more of hospital patients suffer from malnutrition at initial presentation.
- A variety of standardized methodological tools to assess, restore and maintain nutritional status are available.
- A holistic approach is advised, including processes of screening for malnutrition, assessing nutritional status, diagnosing specific deficiencies, and designing and implementing an appropriate medical nutrition therapy plan.
- Health professionals should be aware of and use available methodological and interpretive tools to assist them in this important task.

Introduction

Human growth, development and health throughout the life course, from preconception until death, are dependent upon adequate nutrition. Nutrient adequacy means being nutrition secure through the appropriate consumption of energy and all essential nutrients in sufficient amounts over time. Nutrient adequacy leads to 'optimal' nutritional status in which both under- and over-nutrition are avoided.

Many 'apparently' healthy individuals may suffer from some form of malnutrition, and up to two thirds or more of hospitalized patients may be malnourished, often because of the multiple effects of disease on the intake, absorption, metabolism, storage and excretion of nutrients [1]. It is therefore important for health professionals (HPs) to screen patients for risk of nutritional inadequacies [1, 2], to assess nutritional status, and to implement and evaluate appropriate medical nutrition therapy (MNT) when necessary. These processes are complex and need specialized skills.

Table 1. Steps to follow for restoring and maintaining nutrient adequacy

Sequence of steps	Measurement and evaluation tools
1. Nutritional screening: To identify those at risk and vulnerable (e.g. children, pregnant women, the elderly, the poor, and the ill).	Routine medical history information when admitted to hospital/clinic. Standardized, simple, brief, generic and flexible hospital questionnaires, screening forms and checklists to be used by all HPs. Nutritional scores are available.
2. Nutritional status assessment: To identify those that need nutrition support to restore and maintain optimal nutrition status and to design appropriate MNT interventions.	Methods include standardized ecological, dietary intake, anthropometric, biochemical and clinical (physical) examinations. For each type, appropriate tables, charts, growth curves, etc. with recommended values available.
3. Diagnosis: Classification of malnutrition for planning of an appropriate MNT plan.	Integrate the information obtained in 1 and 2, and design an appropriate plan to address the specific nutrition problem, either by counselling, diversification of diets, supplementation or specialized medical intervention.
4. Designing and implementation of MNT plan.	The MNT plan must define the nutrition problem, therapeutic goals, appropriate intervention, educational needs of patients, including an evaluation plan. After evaluation (by reassessing) and adjustments to care if necessary, the discharge documents of the hospital/clinic should be completed (for follow-up care).

A variety of methodological tools have been developed to assist HPs to restore and maintain the nutritional status of individuals, each with appropriate recommendations, standards, charts and cut-points indicating 'normal' ranges and values for optimal, under- and overnutrition. Comprehensive descriptions of these can be found in most nutrition texts, especially those for clinical dietetic and nutrition practice [1].

This chapter shows how these processes and tools are interlinked, and highlights some new developments in nutritional assessment methodology.

A Holistic Approach to Achieving and Maintaining Nutrient Adequacy

The steps to be taken to achieve nutrient adequacy are summarized in table 1. They often form part of established protocols and algorithms in hospitals and clinics. The same steps can be followed for patients outside clinical settings.

Nutritional Status Assessment

A summary of available methods and tools to assess nutritional status is given in table 2. In clinical settings, it is often not possible to obtain accurate nutrient intakes, and HPs must rely on indices calculated from anthropometric measurements, using standardized tables and charts [1] for evaluation of assessment results.

Different levels or stages of depletion/repletion should be considered because they may need different assessment methodologies. Blood values of a micronutrient will not necessarily reflect intakes or status, because the body has well-coordinated, tightly controlled regulatory systems to maintain blood levels of nutrients within narrow ranges, as well as different storage mechanisms for different nutrients. The stages of depletion and repletion and the suggested assessment methods are briefly summarized in table 3.

Table 2. Summary of general nutritional assessment methods

Nutrition status assessment methods	Application and interpretation
Ecological methods: Documentation of all factors known to influence nutrition intakes: medical, social, health (e.g. allergies, dental problems), medication use, and nutrition history, cultural factors, recent weight changes, etc.	Noninvasive, suitable for all settings, nonspecific. Also used for screening purposes. Use standardized hospital forms and checklists.
Dietary and nutrient intake measurement: Use of validated questionnaires, interviews and recording methods to assess dietary patterns, food and nutrient intake over specified times: 24-hour recalls, weighed food records, diet histories (diaries), qualitative and quantitative food frequency questionnaires, or short questionnaires. Translate dietary data to nutrients with computer programs based on food composition tables.	Use validated questionnaires; food composition and nutrient recommendation tables necessary for calculations, interpretation and comparisons. Most noninvasive method. Low cost, high throughput. Suitable for all settings. Have many limitations: under- and overreporting, impaired memory, etc. Verify intakes by using biomarkers: metabolomic finger-printing of the food metabolome, in spot urine samples; may identify new biomarkers.
Anthropometry: Measurement of physical dimensions and gross body composition; usually weight and height (for age), body circumferences (head in children, waist, hip, mid-arm, etc.) and 7 skin folds (to calculate fat percent). Several indices and ratios are calculated from these measurements, including weight-for-age, height-for-age, and weight-for-height z-scores in children, body mass index (BMI), waist-hip ratio etc. Impedance, dual-energy X-ray absorptiometry and other methods used to determine body fat percentage.	Noninvasive and reliable. Growth charts, tables with cut-points and standards available in nutrition texts. Low-cost, high throughput. Suitable in all settings, especially to monitor growth of children and assess hospital patients. Indicative of past nutritional history. Standardized equipment should be used.
Laboratory methods: Static and functional tests, using capillary blood, dried blood spots, venous blood, serum, plasma, spot urine, 24-hour urine or saliva. Tests can be behavioral, physiological, biochemical, nutrient challenge tests, or using genomics and/or a metabolomics approach to identify dietary intake markers and/or markers of nutritional status.	Provide 'unbiased' scientific data. Invasive. For some nutrients, cut-points and normal ranges are available, but may be nonspecific (other contributing and confounding factors influence results). May be difficult to interpret because of a lack of standards and cut-points. Often expensive equipment and 'sophisticated' expertise needed.
Clinical (physical) methods: Medical history and physical (clinical) examinations looking for well-established signs and symptoms of nutrient deficiencies (skin, hair, tongue, eyes, etc.), by using systematic inspection, palpitation, percussion and auscultation techniques. Handgrip dynamometry used to assess muscle strength.	Suitable for all settings, but HPs must be specially trained to recognize symptoms of specific deficiencies. Use a holistic approach in which observations are integrated with other assessment results for correct diagnosis. Specific texts and illustrations of signs of malnutrition, especially micronutrients, are available.

Table 3. Measurement of stages of depletion/repletion of nutrient status

Depletion/repletion stage	Suggested assessment method
1. Dietary inadequacy	Dietary intakes
2. Decreased level in reserve tissue store	Biochemical laboratory
3. Decreased level in body fluids	Biochemical laboratory
4. Decreased functional level in tissues	Anthropometry and/or biochemical
5. Decreased concentration and activity of nutrient-dependent enzymes or messenger RNA for relevant protein synthesis	Biochemical and molecular laboratory methods; metabolic and functional challenge tests
6. Functional change	Physiological and behavioral assessments
7. Clinical symptoms	Clinical: anthropometry (growth), clinical signs
8. Anatomical signs	Clinical: anthropometry (growth), clinical signs

New Developments in Nutrient Assessment Tools

Nutrient Recommendations

Nutrient recommendations (NRs) are evidence-based recommendations designed by authoritative bodies, such as the United Nations (WHO, FAO) Agencies or the USA Institute of Medicine [3] for defining adequate nutrient intakes. Although the ranges of optimal intake for specified age, sex and activity groups given in different sets of NRs are remarkably similar, the terminology used is varied and confusing. UN agencies recently harmonized the terminology and suggest the following terms [4]:

- Nutrient intake values (NIVs): An umbrella term. It includes the average nutrient requirement (ANR) and upper nutrient level (UNL) and terms derived from these. It is synonymous with the term 'daily reference values' (DRVs) or 'dietary reference intakes' (DRIs) used in many countries and 'nutrient reference values' (NRVs) used by the food industry to label products.
- Average nutrient requirement: The ANR is estimated based on distributions of nutrient intakes required to achieve a specific outcome in a specified population. If those intakes are distributed normally, the population's mean requirement is its ANR. If not normally distributed, data must be transformed and the resulting median is the ANR. ANRs are established for all essential nutrients, but also for those of public health relevance, such as dietary fiber. The ANR is similar to the estimated average requirement (EAR) used in the USA, Canada and the UK, and the average requirement (AR) used in Europe.
- Upper nutrient level: The highest level of habitual nutrient intake that is likely to pose no risk of adverse health effects in almost all individuals in the general population. It is determined by using the 'no observed adverse effect level' (NOAEL) and the 'lowest observed effect level' (LOAEL) with an appropriate uncertainty factor. It is similar to the 'upper tolerable nutrient intake level' (UL) used in the USA and Canada, and the 'upper end of safe intake range' used in the UK and Europe.
- Individual nutrient level$_x$ (INL$_x$): The INL is derived from the ANR where x is a percentile of the mean chosen to guide individual intakes. It is similar to the Recommended Dietary Allowance (RDA) used in the US and Canada, the 'reference nutrient intake' (RNI) used in the UK, and the 'population reference intake' (PRI) used in Europe. An INL$_{98}$ would be the level that, based on scientific evidence, would meet the need of 98% of individuals in a particular age and sex group.

NRs are used for assessment of nutritional status (by comparing reported intakes with NRs), for the planning of nutrition policies, strategies, programs and regulatory frameworks, for implementing nutrition programs, and also for surveillance and for evaluating the outcomes of interventions. Most nutrition textbooks include tables of NRs, often still called the RDAs. They can also be found on the websites of several UN Agencies (such as the WHO or FAO) that provide scientific advice for member countries on achieving nutrition security.

Dietary Goals

Dietary goals, such as those of the WHO [5], are recommendations from authoritative bodies to lower the risk of overweight, obesity and many noncommunicable diseases (NCDs) and often include recommendations for nutrients and/or foods that are not essential but of public health importance, or that should be limited or avoided (e.g. added sugars or salt). Planning interventions in patients suffering from nutrition-related NCDs will rely on both NRs and dietary goals. Some scientific and/or professional societies have their own regularly updated dietary goals [6].

Food-Based Dietary Guidelines

A set of food-based dietary guidelines (FBDGs) is a tool to educate individuals and groups on

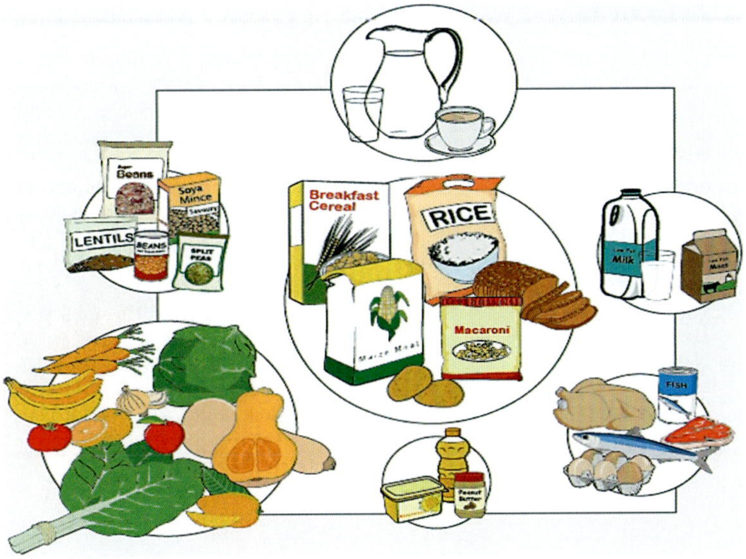

Fig. 1. The South African Food Guide: indicating only those groups of foods (with examples from traditional foods) that should be eaten regularly. The size of the circles is in proportion to the amounts that should be eaten. Used with permission from the SA Department of Health, Directorate Nutrition, 2013.

healthy eating. FBDGs are based on foods and eating patterns, and consist of short, positive, and 'marketable' science-based messages that aim to change eating behavior towards more optimal diets. People eat foods and not nutrients. Nutrition scientists have therefore 'translated' NRs into guidelines that consumers can understand and relate to [7]. FBDGs should be country specific, based on existing eating patterns, traditional foods and foods and beverages that are available, accessible and affordable. FBDGs are supported by a food guide (see fig. 1) and other relevant educational materials that may help with targeted implementation. Any set of FBDGs should lead to adequate nutrition, but also to diets that will help to protect against development of NCDs. More than 50 countries have developed FBDGs for their own populations [8]. Most have messages on the basic food groups: cereals and grains, vegetables and fruit, legumes or pulses, milk and dairy, animal-derived foods (meat, fish, chicken and eggs), and fats and oils, to advise that people should eat and enjoy a variety of foods. Some also advise on alcohol consumption, food hygiene, breastfeeding and physical activity.

Growth Standards

An essential tool to evaluate the growth of children is growth reference data. Many nutrition texts still give growth charts based on the growth of children that have been formula fed. The WHO [9] recently published physical growth curves based on a multicenter study in which the growth of breastfed children was monitored. These charts provide growth reference data for children of 0–60 months, and 5–19 years. Their website [9] also includes application tools for use of these charts in assessing growth and nutritional status.

Conclusions

- Nutrient adequacy of individuals can be achieved by following a systematic, integrated approach of screening, assessment, diagnosis and implementation of appropriate MNT plans.
- HPs should be aware that there are many methodological as well as interpretation, evaluation, and education tools available to assist them in this important task.

References

1 Mahan LK, Escott-Stump S (eds): Krause's Food, Nutrition & Diet Therapy, ed 10. Philadelphia, WB Saunders, 2000, p 1194.
2 Pablo AMR, Izaga MA, Alday LA: Assessment of nutritional status on hospital admission: nutritional scores. Eur J Clin Nutr 2003;57:824–831.
3 Institute of Medicine, Food and Nutrition Board, RDA subcommittee on the tenth edition of the recommended dietary allowances, ed 10. Washington, National Academy Press, 1989.
4 King JC, Vorster HH, Tome DG: Nutrient intake values (NIVs): a recommended terminology and framework for the derivation of values. Food Nutr Bull 2007;28:S16–S26.
5 WHO: Diet, nutrition and the prevention of chronic diseases. Report of a joint FAO/WHO consultation. WHO Technical Support Series No. 916. Geneva, WHO, 2003.
6 Krauss RM, Eckel RH, Howard B, et al: AHA Dietary Guidelines: Revision 2000. A statement for health professionals from the Nutrition Committee of the American Heart Association. Circulation 2000;102:2284–2299.
7 FAO/WHO: Preparation and use of food-based dietary guidelines. Report of a joint FAO/WHO consultation. WHO Technical Support Series No. 880. Geneva, WHO, 1998, pp 1–108.
8 http://www.fao.org/aghumannutrition/nutritioneducation/49741/en/, updated 2013 (accessed February 2013).
9 http://www.who.int/childgrowth/en/, 2006 and 2007 (accessed February 2013).

Nutrition for Health

Bier D, et al. (eds): Nutrition for the Primary Care Provider. World Rev Nutr Diet. Basel, Karger, 2015, vol 111, pp 13–18
DOI: 10.1159/000362291

Energy Balance and Body Composition

Dale A. Schoeller[a] Diana Thomas[b]

[a]Nutritional Sciences, University of Wisconsin, Madison, Wisc., and [b]Mathematical Sciences, Montclair State University, Montclair, N.J., USA

Key Words

Adiposity · Body mass index · Body fat · Body composition · Energy balance

Key Messages

- Changes in weight and height over time are critical parameters for detecting health-related energy imbalances.
- Current adult adiposity can be evaluated using body mass index (BMI). The healthy BMI range is between 18.5 and 25. Though medically useful, BMI is an imperfect measure of excess fat.
- Other clinical methods for assessment of fat percentage (such as skin-fold measurement, bioelectrical impedance analysis, or dual X-ray absorptiometry) should be used to determine an individual's overall health status.
- It is difficult to assess energy intake or energy expenditure with sufficient accuracy to predict an individual's weight change. The application of weight change models can be useful for summarizing the components of energy metabolism as they capture weight-dependent alterations in energy balance.
- The evolution of an individual's weight over time can indicate potential energy imbalances, highlighting trends towards obesity and increased risk of related illnesses.

Introduction

In the last 30 years, global health concerns have shifted focus from malnutrition to obesity. Despite the serious health consequences of both directions of energy imbalance, most physicians do not respond with equal concern with regard to obesity. Indeed, weight status is frequently not recorded in a patient's chart. Yet changes in weight and height over time are critical statistics for detecting health-related energy imbalances. Current weight status is a summary of energy balance over time and, when tracked, can indicate the risk of existing or future chronic disease. These trends, however, can only be identified by frequent recording in the patients' chart.

Interpreting Weight Status

Current adult adiposity is easily evaluated using the body mass index (BMI), which is weight (kg)/height (m)^2 [705 × weight (lbs)/height (in)^2]. The healthy BMI range falls in between 18.5 and 25. Individuals with BMI below the healthy range are classified as underweight and those with BMI ex-

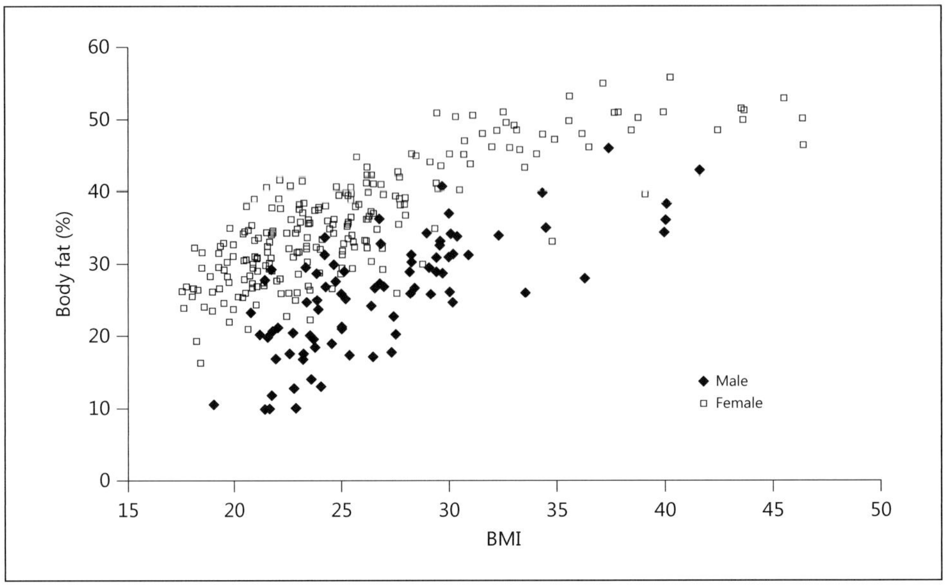

Fig. 1. Percent body fat increases with BMI, but is highly variable for a given BMI. At the same BMI, percent body fat is about 10 percentage points greater in women than in men. Values are for adults between 18 and 60 years of age.

ceeding the healthy range are classified as overweight (BMI between 25 and 30) or obese (BMI 30 or greater). Childhood adiposity cannot be as easily classified using BMI, largely because classification cut-points vary with age. Instead, classification of adiposity in children is based on the percentile of weight-for-height as a function of age and sex using the CDC growth charts, or BMI z-scores (the number of standard deviations away from the 50th percentile). Online calculators have been developed to determine percentile and z-scores for children; these are available on the CDC website (http://www.cdc.gov/healthyweight/assessing/bmi/childrens_bmi/about_childrens_bmi.html).

Adult BMI cut-points were developed from epidemiological evidence that individuals classified as underweight are more at risk for contracting infectious diseases. Moreover, unintentional weight loss is an indicator of limited access to food, gastrointestinal disease, wasting diseases, or eating disorders. Individuals classified as obese have increased risk for prediabetes, diabetes, cardiovascular disease, hypertension, stroke, certain cancers, and all-cause mortality. Children not classified at a healthy weight are also at risk for these comorbidities. The rise in pediatric obesity from 5 to 20% over the past 35 years has been followed by a concomitant increase in chronic disease (e.g. type 2 diabetes), raising concerns regarding excess weight in children.

Body Composition

BMI is an anthropomorphic indicator of body composition and though medically useful, it is an imperfect measure of excess fat [1]. A high BMI can result from either excess body fat or, less frequently, elevated muscularity. This is evidenced by the high variance in percent fat versus BMI (fig. 1). Waist circumference provides an addi-

Table 1. Classification of weight and waist circumference status

Children <18 years, weight-for-height percentile	
<5th percentile for age and sex	undernourished
≥5th percentile for age and <85th for sex	healthy weight
≥85th percentile for age and <95th for sex	overweight
≥95th percentile for age and sex	obese
Adults, BMI	
<18.5	undernourished
≥18.5 and <25	healthy weight
≥25 and <30	overweight
≥30 and <35	class I obesity
≥35 and <40	class II obesity
≥40	class III obesity
Adults, waist circumference	
Male >102 cm (>40 in)	high metabolic risk
Female >88 cm (>35 in)	high metabolic risk

tional clinical measurement to distinguish between body types (table 1). Waist circumference is an excellent indicator of abdominal fat, which is the fat depot most highly associated with chronic disease [2].

Numerous methods exist for body composition assessment [3]. The most common body composition model is the two-compartment model, which divides the body into fat (neutral lipids) and fat-free mass (water, protein, mineral, structural lipid and carbohydrate) and generally expresses adiposity as a percent of body mass (table 1). Clinically feasible methods of determining percent body fat are skin-fold measurement or bioelectrical impedance analysis (BIA), but the accuracy varies widely depending on the methodology and instrument. Additionally, skin-fold and BIA-assessed body fat are less accurate especially among obese populations. The most common clinically applicable three-compartment assessment of body composition (fat, nonosseous fat-free tissue, and bone mineral) is dual X-ray absorptiometry (DXA).The bone mineral measure, expressed either as bone mineral mass or bone mineral density, includes risk assessment of osteoporosis, along with body composition estimates of prior energy balance status (DXA measurement protocols for these two outcomes differ). While the expense and/or increased burden on the patient make other methods of body composition assessment less accessible, some methods such as magnetic resonance imaging (MRI) provide highly accurate estimates. Other measurements include ultrasound, isotope dilution for total body water, and underwater weighing. MRI, ultrasound, and isotope dilution require expensive equipment and trained operators, while underwater weighing also requires patients to be submerged in a water tank. The recent development of air displacement plethysmography, however, offers a somewhat more practical alternative to underwater weighing.

Clinical assessment of percent fat can be applied to determine health status. Young and middle-aged adult percent fat values of <6% in males and <12% in females may indicate undernutrition. Obesity as classified by BMI corresponds to body fat percentages above 25% fat in males and 35% in females (percentages vary slightly with age and race) [1]. As a total mass, body fat in healthy adults averages 12 kg and provides thermal and mechanical insulation and a valuable energy store. Body fat has an energy density of 9.5 kcal/g (39.7 kJ/g) and can provide 114,000 kcal (476 MJ) of energy during starvation. Lipid energy stores can vary, however, from 33,000 kcal (140 MJ) in athletes, to over 500,000 kcal (2,010 MJ) in class III obese individuals, compared to a carbohydrate store of only about 2,000 kcal.

Energy Balance

Since energy can neither be created nor destroyed, energy intake must equal the summed energy output and changed body energy stores. Energy intake can be defined as either gross energy (total chemical energy of foods that can be released by combustion), digestible energy (total chemical energy of foods minus fecal energy loss), or metabolizable energy (total chemical energy of foods minus fecal and urinary energy loss). Metabolizable energy represents food energy available to the body for use in all metabolic processes and ranges from 93 to 97% of gross energy. Increased fecal loss in response to high fiber diets is factored into nutrient databases. However, disease states including malabsorptive diseases, ketoses, and uncontrolled diabetes reduce database accuracy.

When an individual is in energy balance, metabolizable energy intake equals total energy expenditure (TEE), and body weight is relatively constant over a given time frame. TEE has three major components: resting metabolic rate (RMR), physical activity energy expenditure (PAEE) and thermic effects of meals (TEM). RMR, the rate of energy expenditure at rest, after an overnight (12- to 15-hour) fast, and in a thermal neutral environment, is the largest component and comprises between 50 and 65% of TEE. PAEE is the most variable component both between and within individuals and comprises between 25 and 40% of TEE. TEM is the energy associated with the metabolism and storage of the macronutrients from meals and comprises 6–12% of TEE. Because RMR is the most easily measured or formulaically predictable component of TEE, TEE is usually expressed as a multiple of RMR. This multiplier (TEE/RMR) is referred to as PAL and averages between 1.7 and 1.9 [4] but can vary from 1.4 (very sedentary) to over 2.0 (elite athletes or heavy manual laborers) [5].

Energy balance is rarely achieved on a day to day basis. Daily energy intake varies with a standard deviation of 25%, and TEE varies with a standard deviation of about 10%. When time averaged over a few weeks, however, energy balance is usually observed in weight-stable individuals. In individuals who are not weight stable, the discrepancy between energy intake and energy expenditure, referred to as the energy gap, is best calculated from changes in body composition. Because measurement of body composition is complex, body weight is typically used as a proxy to compute the energy gap. The average adult gains about 1 kg/year of body weight in the United States, and studies have shown that this weight gain is largely fat. The fraction of this gain as fat varies with BMI, but a 1-kg change in weight corresponds to an increase in energy stores of 7,600 kcal/year (31 MJ/year), or only 20 kcal/day (90 kJ/day); an imbalance of <1%. Studies indicate, however, that the estimated energy gap is not a result of daily imbalance, but rather an accumulation of a few larger imbalances occurring on a limited number of days [6, 7]. Nevertheless, an annual gain of 1 kg continued for over 15–20 years will result in an increased BMI of 5.

A common misconception based on overly simplified energy balance calculations is that a small (on the order of 20 kcal/day) change in either energy intake or expenditure will lead to obesity or a medically significant weight loss. This calculation, however, does not account for the passive energy regulatory system. Energy expenditure varies with body size (fig. 2). While continued imbalance will lead to weight gain, greater weight will simultaneously increase energy expenditure. Therefore for continued weight gain, energy intake must increase to offset the energy expenditure associated with higher weight. As such, there are two energy gaps associated with the difference between an individual who is

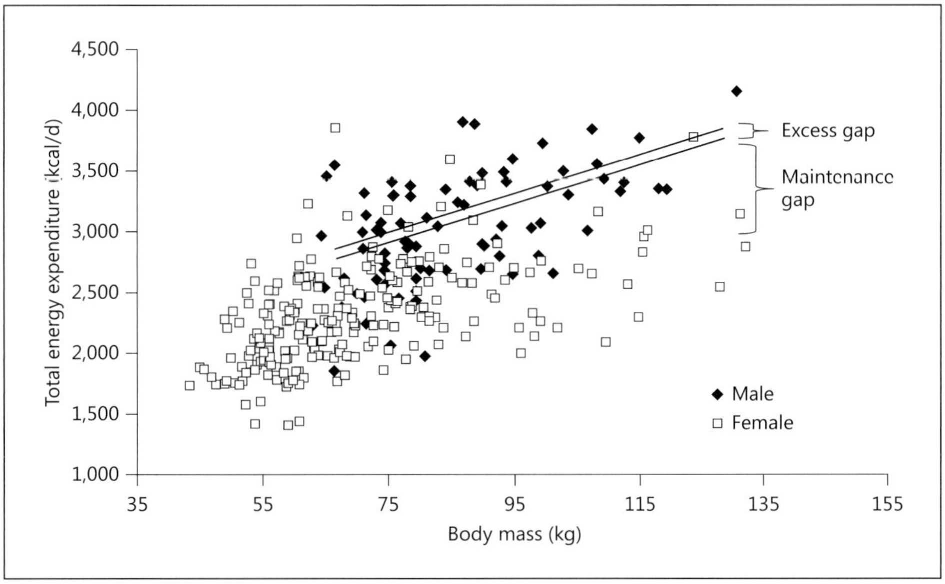

Fig. 2. TEE increases with weight in both men and women. This reflects increases in RMR due to increased fat-free mass and increased costs of physical activity due to the larger mass to be moved [5]. The energetic of a weight during adulthood can be described in terms of two energy gaps. The larger gap is the increase in weight maintenance energy requirement and a smaller positive energy balance over time that leads to energy storage and weight gain [8].

at healthy weight and one who is overweight (fig. 2). The first is the positive energy balance gap that results in energy deposition and weight, and the second is the difference in energy requirement between the two different body weights.

Energy Imbalance and Weight Change

Not surprisingly, individuals cannot measure energy intake or energy expenditure with adequate accuracy to predict weight change. Even personalized devices for tracking energy intake and expenditure are not sufficiently accurate for this task, and tracking changes in weight remains the best indicator of systematic energy imbalance. In doing so, however, it should be remembered that day-to-day changes in body mass (range ± 1 kg) usually reflect changes in intestinal contents and total body water, and detecting weight changes in response to systematic energy balance fluctuations requires long-term monitoring.

Online Weight Change Models

The use of weight change models can summarize the components of energy metabolism as they capture weight-dependent changes in energy balance. These models [9, 10] are based on the first law of thermodynamics. These are dependent on baseline body composition, age, height, gender, and degree of caloric restriction, and result in a curvilinear self-limiting pattern of weight change over time. These complex models have been successfully simplified for the physician for clinical application through web-based software (http://pbrc.edu/research-and-faculty/calculators/, http://bwsimulator.niddk.nih.gov/).

Specifically, thermodynamically based models describe changes in energy balance resulting from altering energy intake and/or PAEE by developing specific terms for each component of the energy balance equation. These models divide the rate of energy stored into two compartments, namely changes in energy resulting from changes in fat mass and fat-free mass to account for energy storage and resulting changes in energy expenditure. For example, a patient placed on a 500 kcal/day energy deficit diet for weight loss who loses 3–4 kg in 6 weeks is probably in compliance with the diet prescription, while one who loses less than 1–2 kg is probably not. Such models can be valuable tools for assessing dietary compliance during physician-assisted weight loss.

Conclusions

- Energy balance and body composition are intricately tied to energy intake and expenditure. Accurate measurements of body composition, energy expenditure components, and intake require expensive equipment and contribute to patient burden.
- Body weight, which is a much more easily measured parameter, provides a summary of these individual components and can be translated to a measure of health status.
- While single weights provide some insight into past energy balance and current health status, a better measure of health should also include serial weights tracked over time.
- Time trends in an individual's weight can indicate potential energy imbalance, for example indicating a trend toward obesity and increased risk for related illnesses.

References

1 Gallagher D, Heymsfield SB, Heo M, et al: Healthy percentage body fat ranges: an approach for developing guidelines based on body mass index. Am J Clin Nutr 2000;72:694–701.

2 Després JP, Lemieux I, Prud'homme D: Treatment of obesity: need to focus on high risk abdominally obese patients. BMJ 2001;322:716–720.

3 Ellis KJ: Human body composition: in vivo methods. Physiol Rev 2000;80:649–680.

4 Dugas LR, Harders R, Merrill S, et al: Energy expenditure in adults living in developing compared with industrialized countries: a meta-analysis of doubly labeled water studies. Am J Clin Nutr 2011;93:427–441.

5 Institute of Medicine: Dietary Reference Intakes for Energy, Carbohydrate, Fiber, Fat, Fatty Acids, Cholesterol, Protein and Amino Acids. Washington, National Academic Press, 2002, pp 154–185.

6 Yanovski JA, Yanovski SZ, Sovik KN, et al: A prospective study of holiday weight gain. N Engl J Med 2000;342:861–867.

7 Casazza K, Fontaine KR, Astrup A, et al: Myths, presumptions, and facts about obesity. N Engl J Med 2013;368:446–454.

8 Swinburn BA, Sacks G, Lo SK, et al: Estimating the changes in energy flux that characterize the rise in obesity prevalence. Am J Clin Nutr 2009;89:1723–1728.

9 Hall KD, Sacks G, Chandramohan D, et al: Quantification of the effect of energy imbalance on bodyweight. Lancet 2011;378:826–837.

10 Thomas DM, Schoeller DA, Redman LA, et al: A computational model to determine energy intake during weight loss. Am J Clin Nutr 2010;92:1326–1331.

Nutrition for Health

Bier D, et al. (eds): Nutrition for the Primary Care Provider. World Rev Nutr Diet. Basel, Karger, 2015, vol 111, pp 19–23
DOI: 10.1159/000362292

Appetite: Measurement and Management

Richard D. Mattes

Department of Nutrition Science, Purdue University, West Lafayette, Ind., USA

Key Words

Hunger · Satiation · Satiety · Food intake · Eating pattern

Key Messages

- Appetitive sensations and food intake stem from a complex interplay of factors that ultimately influence body weight and body composition.
- Appetite is a central focus in the management of several disorders, including undernutrition, eating disorders (anorexia, bulimia) and obesity. However, appetitive sensations are not a reliable marker of food intake.
- Appetite is multidimensional and, in research and clinical practice, is often divided into selected components, including hunger, desire to eat, and fullness. There are no reliable biological markers for quantifying appetite.
- Satiety hormones can modulate appetite and/or food intake, but their functional roles are not clear because their release and activity are influenced by cognitive, physiological, and lifestyle factors.
- Clinicians who wish to modulate appetite in patients may apply diet or lifestyle interventions, but only subtle effects should be expected. Pharmacological agents have varying efficacies and are best used in combination with nonpharmacological approaches.

Introduction

Much has been and continues to be debated about the controls or regulation of appetite, food intake, body weight and body composition. Of course, not all these factors can be regulated as some must be free to vary to account for the regulation of the other factors. Arguably, the weakest evidence for active regulation applies to appetitive sensations, which are widely viewed as fluctuating in concert with energy needs to promote energy balance. Whether this is, in fact, their role and the degree to which they can drive behavior are controversial. Some evidence indicates the appetitive system is biased towards excess energy intake as insurance against future energy deficits. If so, advice to better attune ingestive behavior with appetite could be counterproductive for weight management. Alternatively, under customary dietary conditions, the signals from the appetitive system may be trumped by other systems guiding ingestive behavior such as neural reward centers. In this case, appetitive signals would not be sufficiently powerful to achieve energy balance in environments where food is abundant, accessible and palatable. A better understanding of this biological system should inform clinical practice.

Role of Appetite and Definitions

The high prevalence of dysfunctional eating resulting in outcomes ranging from undernutrition to eating disorders (anorexia, bulimia, etc.) and obesity has prompted considerable interest in the role of appetite in ingestive behavior. Appetite is multidimensional and, in research and clinical practice, is often divided into selected components. Hunger comprises those sensations that motivate food seeking and ingestion and is commonly viewed as stemming from a biological need for energy. The latter differentiates hunger from sensations labeled 'desire to eat', which also prompt ingestive behaviors but do so based more on the rewarding properties of foods. Thus, it is possible to have low hunger and a strong desire to eat, such as when a highly palatable dessert is provided after a large meal. Fullness represents the sensations that diminish interest in eating, and while it appears to be on the opposite pole on a continuum with hunger, they are controlled by different mechanisms. Fullness may play out over different time frames. Within an eating event, these sensations terminate intake and are referred to as satiation. Fullness may also delay the onset of the next eating event and is then termed satiety. Thirst is another appetitive sensation and is most closely linked with hydration status, though beverages now contribute about 20% of daily energy in the US diet. While these biological systems are available to guide ingestive behavior, much eating and drinking occurs in the absence of hunger or thirst and in the presence of reasonably strong fullness sensations [1]. Furthermore, eating and drinking frequently do not occur despite high levels of hunger and thirst or low levels of fullness, often due to practical issues of daily living. The purposeful overriding of these signals may occur for various reasons such as anticipated future food limitations or maximization of present pleasure. Thus, appetitive sensations are important but not reliable markers of food intake.

Specific appetites are special cases where there is a strong motivation to ingest a particular nutrient (e.g. salt, iron, protein). Animals express these appetites (e.g. herbivores' attraction to salt licks), but humans have demonstrated them only under extreme conditions. Pica, the ingestion of non-food items, is often attributed to a nutrient deficiency, but rarely is this substantiated [2]. There appears to be a stronger sociocultural basis to the practice.

Appetitive sensations are of clinical interest in several regards. First, when the sensations are strong, most view them as unpleasant, and they can compromise the quality of life. This has prompted considerable research on the development of products and eating patterns to ameliorate or emphasize sensations without exacerbating possible energy balance problems (e.g. weight loss or gain). Second, therapeutic dietary regimens are only effective if followed, and strong appetitive sensation may lead to poor compliance. Third, by guiding food choice, appetitive sensations directly influence nutrient intake and nutritional status.

Measurement Options

There is no universally accepted method to quantify appetite. The most common approach is to assess the sensations via questionnaires. Participants are asked to rate their hunger, desire to eat (generally or for selected qualities such as sweet or savory foods), fullness, prospective consumption (how much could you eat right now) and thirst according to category or visual analog scales with end anchors of 'not at all' to 'extremely'. Primary limitations of this approach are that, generally, there is no control over individual differences in understanding of the descriptive terms, lack of training in quantifying them, assumptions that sensations change linearly over time and the act of completing the questionnaires may alter the underlying sensations themselves (expectation

Table 1. Selected peptides associated with appetitive sensations

Hormone	Appetitive effect	Primary site of release	Primary nutrient stimuli
Ghrelin	hunger (initiates an eating event)	fundus of stomach	total energy, possibly carbohydrate suppress strongest
Cholecystokinin	satiation	I cells of duodenum	protein, fat > carbohydrate
Glucagon-like peptide-1	satiation	L cells of ilium and colon	protein > carbohydrate > fat
Glucose-dependent insulino-tropic polypeptide	satiation	K cells of duodenum	carbohydrate, fat
Peptide YY	satiation	L cells of ilium and colon	protein > fat > carbohydrate
Pancreatic polypeptide	satiation	F cells in endocrine pancreas	neural, individual nutrients weak
Apolipoprotein A-IV	satiation	enterocytes during lipid packaging	fat
Gastric leptin	satiety	P cells of fundus and pepsinogen-secreting chief cells	total energy
Insulin	satiety	pancreatic β-cell	carbohydrate
Amylin	satiation and satiety	pancreatic β-cell	carbohydrate
Oxyntomodulin	satiation	L cells of ilium and colon	total energy
Enterostatin	inhibits fat intake (satiation)	pancreas	fat, protein

effects). Open-ended questionnaires have also been used, but the lack of standardized response options limits their interpretation.

Due to concerns about subjective reports, there has been considerable interest in identifying objective biomarkers of appetitive sensations. Many have been identified, but none substantiated. Glucose and/or insulin concentrations have been proposed and form the basis of the glycemic index or load theory of appetite regulation. It is proposed that foods prompting rapid glucose absorption elicit a strong insulin response that leads to a rebound hypoglycemic state and augmented hunger. However, euglycemic clamp studies indicate independent manipulation of either glucose or insulin does not lead to a change of appetite (noted changes are associative rather than causal) [3]. Many peptides secreted from enteroendocrine cells throughout the GI tract, the pancreas and adipocytes have been labeled satiety hormones (see table 1 for common candidates) [4]. Under nonphysiological conditions, each can be shown to modulate appetite and/or intake, but their role under customary dietary conditions is less clear because they have both neural (including cognitive) and nutrient bases for secretion, their release is influenced by lifestyle, they are highly interactive, and humans can willfully ignore the sensations they reportedly elicit.

Time is another proxy measure as it is assumed that hunger grows and fullness diminishes directly with time since the last eating event. However, for most people, the overnight fast is the longest interval between eating events and few are most hungry upon awakening. Also, sensations adapt to lifestyles and expected meal times. The association between meal size and intermeal interval is stronger than the effect of time since the last eating event on energy intake at the next eating event [5].

Table 2. Selected dietary and behavioral approaches to modulate appetite for therapeutic purposes

Food/ingredient/practice	Purported satiation/satiety value	Dominant suggested mechanism	Strength of evidence
Clear beverages	weak	weak compensatory dietary response	strong
Sweet foods/beverages	weak	activation of reward system	weak
Highly palatable foods	weak	activation of reward system	weak
High-fat items	weak	passive overconsumption	moderate
High sensory variety	weak	activation of reward system	moderate
Timing of eating events	weak when occurring at night	weak compensation potential	weak
Nuts	high	unknown	strong
Fiber	high	gastric stretch	weak-moderate
Protein	high	gut peptide secretion	moderate
Soup	moderate-high	cognitive	moderate
Fruits/vegetables/high volume	moderate-high	gastric stretch	weak
High eating frequency	high	modulation of appetitive swings	weak
Low-glycemic-index foods	high	moderation of glycemia	weak
Chewing gum	moderate	neural activation of satiety centers	weak
Physical activity	moderate	uncertain	moderate

Items or practices that have weak satiety effects may be useful adjuncts to diets intended to increase energy intake.

Gastric load (volume, composition) has been proposed as an important determinant of appetitive sensations. However, the volume of a meal or snack outside the body has little correlation with its volume in the stomach due to masticatory degradation of foods and differential rates of gastric emptying. Plus, a given load will have different effects based on gastric volume and tone [6]. It should also be noted that gastrectomized patients experience largely normal appetitive sensations [7].

Motivational or behavioral indices may also be used to quantify appetite, such as how hard an individual would be willing to work to obtain food. Marked interindividual variability in appetitive sensations has been documented; whether or not they predict ingestive behavior remains to be established [8].

Modulation of Appetite through Food Properties and Eating Patterns

A number of options are available to the clinician wishing to modulate appetitive sensations in a given patient. The goal may be to increase hunger, desire to eat and intake in individuals with early satiety (e.g. the elderly, patients with selected cancers), or the opposite in individuals where energy restriction is desired (e.g. overweight/obese individuals). Table 2 contains a list of popularized food attributes or eating practices that reportedly lend themselves to manipulation of appetite and feeding. In all cases, the entries are generalizations as subtle differences can alter responses. For example, protein has strong satiety value in solid foods, but less so in beverages. Generally, each manipulation of diet or lifestyle may be used to move in an intended direction, but in all cases, only subtle effects should be expected.

Pharmacological management of appetite has proven especially problematic [9]. Appetite reflects the contributions of multiple redundant biological systems that subserve core survival functions. As a consequence, pharmacological interventions tend to evoke undesired consequences resulting in their failure to reach the market or remain on it. The FDA has recently approved two new agents for managing hunger and desire to eat: Belviq (a serotonin 2C receptor agonist that promotes satiety) and Qsymia (a combination of phentermine, a stimulant, and topiramate, an anti-seizure agent). Currently approved agents may be expected to promote about a 5–10% reduction of body weight, comparable to dietary interventions. A number of orexigenic agents are available, also with varying efficacy and often uncertain mechanisms that are most effective when combined with nonpharmacological interventions [10].

Conclusions

- Appetite encompasses sensations that may motivate or inhibit feeding behavior, but their influence on energy balance has yet to be clearly characterized.
- Appetitive sensations are clinically important as they influence food choice, and this influences nutrient intake, quality of life and adherence to and benefit from therapeutic dietary regimens.
- There is no single accepted approach to quantify appetitive sensations.
- The properties of foods and lifestyle practices of individuals may be exploited to selectively enhance or inhibit appetite for directed purposes, but the magnitude of effects is generally limited.
- Pharmacological approaches to appetite management are frequently associated with unacceptable side effects, but have a role in weight management, especially when combined with nonpharmacological approaches.

References

1 McKiernan F, Hollis JH, McGabe G, Mattes RD: Thirst-drinking, hunger-eating; tight coupling? J Am Diet Assoc 2009;109:486–490.
2 MacClancy J, Henry J, Macbeth H (eds): Consuming the Inedible: Neglected Dimensions of Food Choice. New York, Berghahn Books, 2007.
3 Chapman IM, Goble EA, Wittert GA, et al: Effect of intravenous glucose and euglycemic insulin infusions on short-term appetite and food intake. Am J Physiol 1998;274:R596–R603.
4 Karhunen LJ, Juvonen KR, Purhonen AK, Herzig KH: Effect of protein, fat, carbohydrate and fibre on gastrointestinal peptide release in humans. Regul Pept 2008;149:70–78.
5 Bernstein IL, Zimmerman JC, Czeisler CA, Weitzman ED: Meal patterns in 'free-running' humans. Physiol Behav 1981;27:621–623.
6 Delgado-Aros S, Cremonini F, Castillo JE, et al: Independent influences of body mass and gastric volumes on satiation in humans. Gastroenterology 2004;126:432–440.
7 Kamiji MM, Troncon LEA, Suen VMM, de Oliveira RB: Gastrointestinal transit, appetite, and energy balance in gastrectomized patients. Am J Clin Nutr 2009;89:231–239.
8 McKiernan F, Houchins JA, Mattes RD: Relationships between human thirst, hunger, drinking, and feeding. Physiol Behav 2008;94:700–708.
9 Kabra DG, Karba UD, Tschop MH, Hoffman S: Pharmacological treatment of obesity; in Shiromani PJ, Horvath T, Redline S, van Cauter E (eds): Sleep Loss and Obesity: Intersecting Epidemics. New York, Springer, 2012, pp 203–225.
10 Nasr SZ, Drury D: Appetite stimulants use in cystic fibrosis. Pediatr Pulmonol 2008;43:209–219.

Nutrition for Health

Bier D, et al. (eds): Nutrition for the Primary Care Provider. World Rev Nutr Diet. Basel, Karger, 2015, vol 111, pp 24–29
DOI: 10.1159/000362293

Macronutrients: Requirements and Distribution

Jim Mann

Department of Human Nutrition, University of Otago, Dunedin, New Zealand

Key Words

Macronutrients · Protein · Fat · Carbohydrate · Dietary fiber

Key Messages

- A wide range of macronutrients is compatible with satisfactory growth and development, maintenance of good health and longevity.
- Intakes within the recommended range are readily achievable regardless of preferred dietary pattern.
- Other than in situations of food insecurity, advice to avoid excessive intakes of fat and free sugars, which contribute to an increased risk of overweight and obesity, is of particular importance.
- Consumption of even small amounts of meat protein or a wide variety of plant protein sources generally enables adequate intakes of total protein and indispensable amino acids.
- Advice regarding fat intake relates principally to a reduction of saturated fatty acids and elimination as far as possible of trans-fatty acids from manufactured foods. Linoleic acid and α-linolenic acid are essential fatty acids. A wide range of intakes of cis-monounsaturated fatty acids is acceptable.
- Carbohydrates should be derived principally from vegetables, fruits and minimally processed wholegrain cereals. This ensures an adequate intake of dietary fiber which protects against colon cancer, type 2 diabetes and coronary heart disease.

Introduction

Macronutrient requirements and the proportion of total energy which should be provided by carbohydrate, fat and protein are perennial topics for debate. An underlying principle, often forgotten, is that a wide range of dietary patterns, and hence macronutrient intakes, is compatible with satisfactory growth and development, maintenance of good health and longevity. For example, in most traditional Asian dietary patterns, a high proportion of total energy is provided by carbohydrate, and fat intake is relatively low, whereas in most 'Western' diets fat intake is appreciably higher. Yet, both approaches have the potential to achieve the expectations of optimal nutrition, suggesting that total energy intake and nature (quality) of macronutrients must be of greater importance than the precise distribution of intake. Table 1 shows the range of acceptable intakes recommended by the World Health Organization (WHO) considered appropriate for all populations.

Protein

Proteins are essential to the structure and function of all cells and are involved in many essential metabolic functions which are linked to the me-

Table 1. Macronutrient intake goals as recommended by the WHO [1, 2]

Fat	
Total	15–30
SFA	<10
PUFA	6–10
n-6 PUFA	5–8
n-3 PUFA	1–2
MUFA	by difference[1]
TFA	<1
Dietary cholesterol, mg/day	300
Carbohydrate	
Total	50–75
Free sugars	<10
Dietary fiber, g/day	>25
Protein	10–15

Unless otherwise stated, the goals are expressed as percentage total energy. SFA = Saturated fatty acids; PUFA = cis-polyunsaturated fatty acids; MUFA = cis-monounsaturated fatty acids; TFA = trans-fatty acids. The 2012 Nordic Nutrition Recommendations permit up to 40% total energy from fat but a restriction on the intake of SFA remains.

[1] Total fat = SFA + PUFA + TFA.

Table 2. Dispensable and indispensable amino acids

Indispensable amino acids	Partially indispensable	Dispensable amino acids
Histidine	Arginine	Alanine
Isoleucine	Asparagine	Aspartate
Leucine	Glutamine	Glutamate
Lysine	Glycine	
Methionine	Proline	
Phenylalanine	Serine	
Threonine		
Tryptophan	Cysteine[1]	
Valine	Tyrosine[1]	

[1] Requires essential amino acid precursors methionine and phenylalanine.

Table 3. Amino acid requirements (mg/kg/day) as recommended by WHO/FAO UNU Expert Consultation (based on stable isotope studies)

Histidine	10
Isoleucine	20
Leucine	39
Lysine	30
Methionine and cysteine	15
Phenylalanine and tyrosine	25
Threonine	15
Tryptophan	4
Valine	26
Total	184

tabolism of other nutrients. Protein is the second most abundant chemical compound in the body (after water) contributing about 16% (i.e. 11 kg) of the weight of a 70-kg man. Dietary proteins are absorbed, following digestion, as amino acids which then contribute to the total amino acid pool, from which the body's proteins are synthesized. All 20 amino acids are essential for protein synthesis but some can be synthesized from other metabolic precursors and are described as 'dispensable' amino acids. Nine of the 20 amino acids required for protein synthesis cannot be found in the body and therefore must be obtained from the diet. These are termed as 'indispensable' amino acids with the remainder being 'partially dispensable', i.e. they have the potential to be synthesized but not to the extent that fulfils the body's requirements (table 2).

Requirements for protein are expressed in terms of total protein and individual amino acids. The estimated average requirement for total protein in order for an individual to remain in nitrogen balance is estimated to be about 0.65 g protein/kg/day, with two standard deviations added to define the recommended daily intake, i.e. 0.83 g/kg/day, with specified amounts of essential amino acids (table 3). Protein requirements may also be considered in terms of nutrient density [protein (P):energy (E) ratios] when giving advice about types of diet and foods. Because infants and children have very high energy requirements, their protein needs, at least in most societies, are met by diets with a relatively low P:E ratio. As energy requirements reduce with age, the P:E ratio needs to increase and protein dense foods are more important. This applies especially for the elderly.

With even relatively small amounts of meat protein or a wide variety of plant protein sources, most populations achieve adequate intakes of total protein and indispensable amino acids. However, when only a limited range of vegetable sources of protein are available, lysine and tryptophan deficiencies may occur. Protein deficiency is commonly seen in association with famine, resulting from natural disasters or conflict and in conditions of extreme poverty. In any society and in association with any dietary pattern, deficiency may occur in situations of increased demand (e.g. infections or stress), increased losses (e.g. hemorrhage or burns) or when individuals are living in adverse social and physical conditions.

Protein intake from nonmeat sources is remarkably similar throughout the world, around 50 g/day. However, protein from meat sources varies enormously from very small amounts in countries such as Nigeria, Zimbabwe and India to average intakes of around 50 g/day or more in affluent countries. This equates to intakes of between 10 and 15% total energy. This has traditionally been considered to be an appropriate range of intake.

Somewhat more controversial has been the recent discussion as to whether diets containing larger amounts of protein might facilitate weight reduction and maintenance in overweight and obese individuals and populations, management of diabetes and enhanced bone health in the elderly. Relatively high-protein, low-carbohydrate diets such as the 'South Beach' and 'Zone' diets provide up to 30% total energy as protein and have been shown in relatively short-term studies to be more effective than high-carbohydrate diets in these respects. However, there is no convincing evidence of long-term benefit, and issues of cost, sustainability and long-term safety also require further consideration before such a recommendation can be endorsed.

Fats

Some people in high-income countries regard fats and most oils as foods to be avoided as far as possible because of their roles in obesity and coronary heart disease. However, lipids form an essential component of adequate nutrition as sources of energy and some, which cannot be synthesized by the body, are essential nutrients. They are important structural components of all membranes and have roles in cell signaling. They are the only form in which the body can store energy for prolonged periods of time and are essential for the provision and absorption of fat-soluble vitamins.

Most fatty acids can be made in the body, except for two essential fatty acids, linoleic and α-linolenic acids. Specific deficiencies are very rare even when intakes are very low, as is the case in some African and Asian countries. However, to ensure adequate intakes, some organizations have suggested minimum desirable intakes. For example, the WHO recommends that at least 2% total daily energy be derived from ω6 (n-6) polyunsaturated fatty acids, which includes linoleic acid, and 0.5% total energy from ω3 (n-3) polyunsaturated fatty acids, which includes α-linolenic acid. There are also recommendations for eicosapentaenoic (EPA) and docosahexaenoic (DHA) acids (the WHO recommends 0.25–2.00 g/day of EPA plus DHA), especially during pregnancy and lactation, to ensure adequate levels for the fetus and young infant. Infant formulae, especially those intended for premature infants, should contain EPA and DHA in similar proportions to those found in breast milk.

While much of the discussion around fat intake centers on acceptable upper limits, it is important to appreciate that dietary fat is essential for ensuring that energy needs are met in addition to providing the source of fat-soluble vitamins and essential fatty acids. It is generally assumed that for most adults, fat should provide at least 15% of the total energy requirements and 20% for women of reproductive age. A much higher proportion is generally assumed to be required by infants and young children in order to meet energy requirements for growth. Fifty to 60% of the energy content of breast milk is derived from fat, and during weaning it is necessary to ensure that fat intake is reduced gradually. At least until the age of 2 years, fat should provide about 40% total energy.

The dietary patterns of many Asian countries and the traditional diets of some other populations include fat intakes at these lower limits. Given the low rates of ischemic heart disease, low levels of LDL cholesterol and relatively long life expectancy, for example amongst the Japanese, it has been widely assumed that, regardless of dietary pattern, optimal fat intake should be much lower than those which characterize the diets of most Western populations. Diets low in saturated fat and with moderate amounts of cis-unsaturated fatty acids have been shown in dietary intervention trials to reduce indicators of cardiometabolic risk and in a limited number of longer term trials to reduce clinical ischemic heart disease. Guidelines have varied from country to country and according to whether individuals or populations are at particularly high risk of ischemic heart disease, but have generally suggested upper limits of total fat intakes ranging between 30 and 35% total energy with intakes even below 30% in those at high risk of ischemic heart disease or where a low-fat dietary pattern is preferred. The recommendations have particularly focused on reductions of saturated fatty acids to around 10% total energy (or less for those at risk of ischemic heart disease), well below that currently consumed in many countries with typical 'Western' dietary patterns.

More recently, the concern that a high intake of carbohydrate and sugars in particular may be a cause of obesity and some of its comorbidities, the observation that saturated fatty acids may only adversely affect the nonatherogenic forms of LDL and the demonstration in relatively short-term studies that high-fat diets may facilitate weight loss and improve some cardiometabolic risk indicators, have led to the suggestion that a high fat intake (up to 40% or even more) may be acceptable or even desirable, especially when consumed in conjunction with a high protein intake. It is argued that epidemiological data, most notably the potential health benefits of various Mediterranean dietary patterns, relatively high in mono- and polyunsaturated fat, support such an approach. A strong counter-argument to liberalizing total fat intake in populations prone to overweight and obesity is the association between higher total fat intakes and excess body weight. The only official endorsement, at least in part of this approach is to be found in the 2012 Nordic nutrition recommendations which permit a total fat intake as high as 40% total energy, though the restriction on saturated fat intake to 10% total energy remains.

A total polyunsaturated fatty acid intake of between 6 and 10% has been recommended, the greater proportion (5–8% total energy) being n-6 cis-polyunsaturated fatty acids and intake of cis-monounsaturated fatty acids being determined by difference, assuming a saturated fat intake of no greater than 10% total energy. These ranges permit a wide variety of food choices, compatible with most dietary patterns. Trans-fatty acids from manufactured foods, which increase the risk of ischemic heart disease and some cancers, should be eliminated as far as possible from the diet.

Carbohydrate

Carbohydrates are the most important source of food energy in the world. A wide range of cereals including rice, wheat, maize, barley, rye, oats, millet and sorghum are staple foods in many different dietary patterns. Starchy roots, pulses, other vegetables, fruit and sugar all contribute to a varying extent to the energy derived from carbohydrate, which generally ranges between 40 and 80% of total food energy, depending upon personal preference, culture and economic status. Carbohydrate-containing foods are also important sources of antioxidants, protein, vitamins, minerals, phytochemicals and sterols.

Glucose is essential as an energy source for the brain, red blood cells and the renal medulla. The body can generate approximately 130 g of the 180 g glucose required from noncarbohydrate sources via gluconeogenesis. Thus, the recommended minimum intake is considered to be about 50 g/day. However, utilizing gluconeogenesis is not a particularly efficient means of generating glucose and could necessitate a protein intake above usual requirements or, where protein intakes are marginal, an increase in muscle protein breakdown. A carbohydrate intake greater than the recommended minimum intake is preferable. If sufficient glucose is not available from the diet or via gluconeogenesis, these organs adapt by using ketones derived from fatty acid oxidation as an energy source. Ketosis may impair cognitive function, and other possible long-term effects are unknown. Requirements for glucose are increased during pregnancy and lactation, and the fetus may be adversely affected by ketosis, so the minimum recommended intake of carbohydrate during these phases of the life cycle should be around 100 g/day.

Most dietary patterns provide an appreciably higher intake than these minimum requirements. Average intakes range from around 200–250 g in countries where a 'Western' dietary pattern is the norm (e.g. USA, UK, Australia, The Netherlands) to over 400 g in some Asian countries and elsewhere where indigenous populations consume traditional diets (e.g. Papua New Guinea and many African countries). Epidemiologic observations and dietary intervention studies, mostly involving intermediate end points (biomarkers or risk indicators) have led many national and international organizations to recommend a range of intakes higher than those typically consumed in Western countries. From a health perspective, the major justification for recommending a relatively high intake of carbohydrate is the expectation of a reduced risk of ischemic heart disease by facilitating a reduction in intake of fat. The FAO/WHO Scientific Update on Carbohydrates recommended a range of 50–75% total energy. The European Food Safety Authority suggests that for adults and children intakes should range between 45 and 60% total energy, a range more compatible with current European and North American practices. The nature of carbohydrate is arguably more important than the quantity. Avoidance of excess intakes of sugars is recommended, either in the form of food-based guidelines (e.g. in South Africa) or in quantitative terms (e.g. WHO recommends that free sugars should provide less than 10% total energy) to reduce the risk of overweight and obesity and rates of dental caries, now acknowledged worldwide as an important chronic disease. Of course, both obesity and dental caries have many causes other than intake of sugar. Recommendations regarding dietary fiber have been complicated by lack of agreement regarding definitions, but CODEX has now agreed on a definition which distinguishes between the naturally occurring fiber in plant-based foods from synthetic and extracted fiber. The WHO has recommended that at least 25 g of dietary fiber (20 g nonstarch polysaccharides) from plant foods should be consumed daily. This advice taken in conjunction with the recommendation to reduce sugars represents an attempt to ensure that the bulk of the carbohydrate intake is derived from minimally processed wholegrain cereals, vegetables, pulses and fruit. Foods rich in dietary fiber are associated with reduced risk of colon cancer, coronary heart disease and type 2 diabetes.

The recent argument that high-carbohydrate diets promote insulin resistance and increase the risk of obesity and associated diseases, especially type 2 diabetes, and conversely that a low carbohydrate intake is beneficial in these regards has led to the recommendation by some researchers and practitioners that reduction of carbohydrate (sometimes to levels as low as will cause ketosis) should be followed by all at-risk individuals and even populations with high rates of obesity. While there has been fairly widespread adoption of such practices, they have not been recommended by official bodies. Indeed, there is no evidence against the advice that a wide range of carbohydrate intake is acceptable, provided appropriate carbohydrate-containing foods predominate. A low glycemic response after eating carbohydrate-containing foods has been suggested as a useful means of identifying such foods. While many 'low-glycemic-index' foods do represent appropriate food choices, the approach is not generally accepted as being universally applicable. There is considerable inter- and intraindividual variation in glycemic responses to the same foods, the composition of many foods is not consistent, and many low-glycemic-index foods are high in fat or sugars.

Table 4. Dietary guidelines for which there is almost complete agreement

Eat a nutritionally adequate diet composed of a variety of foods
Eat less fat, particularly saturated fat
Adjust energy balance for body weight control – less energy intake, more exercise
Eat more wholegrain cereals, vegetables and fruits
Reduce intake of salt and foods rich in salt
Drink alcohol in moderation, if you do drink

Conclusions

- When adequate food supplies are available, macronutrient requirements are generally readily met regardless of the preferred dietary pattern.
- A wide range of intakes is compatible with satisfactory growth and development, maintenance of good health and longevity.
- Other than in situations of food insecurity, an excessive intake of energy-dense foods high in total fat and free sugars, which contribute to the global epidemic of obesity and its comorbidities, is arguably the issue relating to macronutrients which is of greatest importance to human health.
- Globally applicable dietary guidelines (table 4) can readily translate recommended ranges of macronutrient intakes into appropriate food choices.

References

1 Joint WHO/FAO Expert Consultation: Diet, nutrition and the prevention of chronic diseases. World Health Organ Tech Rep Ser 2003;916:i-viii, 1–149.
2 Joint FAO/WHO scientific update on carbohydrates in human nutrition. Eur J Clin Nutr 2007;61(suppl 1):S1–S137.
3 Joint FAO/WHO/UNU Expert Consultation: Protein and amino acid requirements in human nutrition. World Health Organ Tech Rep Ser 2007;935: 1–265.
4 Malhotra A: Saturated fat is not the major issue. BMJ 2013;347:f6340.
5 Hooper L, Abdelhamid A, Moore HJ, et al: Effect of reducing total fat intake on body weight: systematic review and meta-analysis of randomised controlled trials and cohort studies. BMJ 2012;345:e7666.
6 Te Morenga L, Mallard S, Mann J: Dietary sugars and body weight: systematic review and meta-analyses of randomised controlled trials and cohort studies. BMJ 2013;346:e7492.
7 Moynihan PJ, Kelly SA: Effect on caries of restricting sugars intake: systematic review to inform WHO guidelines. J Dent Res 2014;93:8–18.
8 Cummings JH, Mann JI, Nishida C, Vorster HH: Dietary fibre: an agreed definition. Lancet 2009;373:365–366.
9 Mensink RP, Zock PL, Kester AD, Katan MB: Effects of dietary fatty acids and carbohydrates on the ratio of serum total to HDL cholesterol and on serum lipids and apolipoproteins: a meta-analysis of 60 controlled trials. Am J Clin Nutr 2003;77: 1146–1155.

Bier D, et al. (eds): Nutrition for the Primary Care Provider. World Rev Nutr Diet. Basel, Karger, 2015, vol 111, pp 30–37
DOI: 10.1159/000362294

Water-Soluble Vitamins

Hamid M. Said

University of California – School of Medicine, Irvine, Calif., and VA Medical Center, Long Beach, Calif., USA

Key Words

Ascorbate · Biotin · Cobalamin · Folate · Niacin · Pantothenic acid · Pyridoxine · Riboflavin · Thiamin

Key Messages

- The two main sources of the water-soluble vitamins are dietary intake and the intestinal microflora.
- Although structurally unrelated, each of these vitamins plays key roles in a multitude of cellular and physiological processes.
- Deficiencies can result in various clinical abnormalities that range from anemia to growth retardation and neurological disorders.
- Deficiency of a vitamin could be localized (tissue specific) as in the case of vitamin B_1 deficiency in the autosomal recessive disorder thiamin-responsive megaloblastic anemia.
- This review outlines the main functions of vitamins B_1, B_2, B_3, B_5, B_6, B_9, C, and H, as well as the consequences of deficiencies and overdosage, the main sources, and recommended daily allowances for each of these essential micronutrients.

Introduction

The water-soluble vitamins are a group of structurally and functionally unrelated compounds that share the characteristics of being essential for normal cellular functions, growth and development. Deficiency of these micronutrients leads to a variety of clinical abnormalities that range from anemia to growth retardation and neurological disorders; on the other hand, optimizing their body levels brings about positive health outcomes. Humans cannot synthesize water-soluble vitamins (with the exception of some synthesis of niacin); thus, they must obtain them from exogenous sources via intestinal absorption. While diet has been considered as the main source of these micronutrients in humans, there has been a growing appreciation in recent years for the contribution of the normal microflora of the large intestine towards overall homeostasis of a number of these micronutrients [e.g. thiamin, biotin, folate, riboflavin (RF), pyridoxine, pantothenic acid], and especially towards the cellular nutrition and health of the local colonocytes [1, 2]. The aim of this review is to provide a summarized description of the metabolic roles of these micronutrients, conditions associated with their deficiency and the clinical consequences of these deficiencies, their physiology, occurrence, and the Recommended Daily Allowance (RDA) as well as description of any adverse effect(s) that may develop as a result of their overdosing.

Vitamin B_1 (Thiamin)

Thiamin was the first member of the water-soluble family of vitamins to be described. Reference to beriberi (a thiamin deficiency disease) in the Chinese medical literature dates back to as early as 2700 B.C. Thiamin plays an essential role in normal cellular functions via its involvement in a variety of critical metabolic reactions related to energy metabolism. It also plays a role in reducing cellular oxidative stress. Thus, cellular deficiency of thiamin leads to an impairment in energy metabolism and to a propensity for oxidative stress; cellular deficiency also leads to apoptosis. Recently, additional roles for thiamin (e.g. effect on the function of membrane chloride channels in nerve cells) have been reported [for review, see 3]. Clinically, systemic thiamin deficiency in humans leads to a variety of abnormalities including neurological (neuropathy and/or Wernicke-Korsakoff syndrome) and cardiovascular (peripheral vasodilatation, biventricular myocardial failure, edema and potentially acute fulminant cardiovascular collapse) disorders. Tissue-specific (i.e. localized) deficiency of thiamin also occurs, as can be seen in patients with thiamin-responsive megaloblastic anemia (TRMA), and in patients with thiamin-responsive Wernicke's-like encephalopathy [4, 5]. TRMA is an autosomal recessive disorder that is associated with megaloblastic anemia, sensorineural deafness, and non-type 1 diabetes mellitus, and is caused by mutations in the human thiamin transporter-1, hTHTR-1 (product of the human *SLC19A2* gene), which is highly expressed in the affected tissues [4]. Thiamin-responsive Wernicke's-like encephalopathy is a genetic disorder that is associated with seizure, ophthalmoplegia, nystagmus, and ataxia and is caused by mutations in hTHTR-2 (product of the human *SLC19A3* gene) [5]. Both of these genetic disorders respond favorably to high doses of thiamin.

Thiamin deficiency represents a significant nutritional problem in both developing and developed countries. In developing countries, the main cause of thiamin deficiency is poor dietary intake of the vitamin (i.e. consumption of thiamin-deficient or depleted diets). In developed countries, chronic alcoholism is the main cause of thiamin deficiency, although the condition can also be seen in patients with diabetes mellitus, inflammatory bowel disease, celiac disease, renal diseases, AIDS, cancer, and in those with congestive heart failure, as well as in subjects on chronic diuretic therapy [for review, see 3]. Thiamin deficiency and suboptimal levels have also been reported in the elderly despite an average daily intake of the vitamin that exceeds the recommended requirement.

Chronic thiamin deficiency leads to two distinct types of conditions: beriberi and Wernicke's encephalopathy. Beriberi is recognized in three different forms: (a) dry beriberi, which is a symmetrical ascending peripheral neuritis that usually affects older individuals and is associated with wasting; it may also be associated with cardiac involvement; (b) wet (or edematous) beriberi, which involves the heart and leads to edema of the lower extremities resulting from the ensuing heart failure, and (c) acute 'fulminating' beriberi (which is also called shoshin beriberi), which occurs more frequently in infants and is associated with heart failure and metabolic abnormalities (with little evidence of peripheral neuritis).

Thiamin deficiency in the human central nervous system may lead to Wernicke's encephalopathy and Korsakoff's psychosis, conditions that are associated with chronic alcoholism and manifest as the Wernicke-Korsakoff syndrome. Some evidence, however, exists to suggest that thiamin deficiency alone is not sufficient to cause Wernicke-Korsakoff syndrome but that alcohol is a necessary factor for the induction of this abnormality. Korsakoff's psychosis is associated with confusion and loss of recent memory, although long-term memory may continue to be intact. Wernicke's encephalopathy develops later and is associated with clear neurological abnormalities (nystagmus, extraocular palsy, ataxia, confabulation, coma) and anatomic lesions (including hemorrhagic lesions in the thalamus pontine tegmentum, and mammillary body with severe damage to astrocytes, neuronal dendrites and myelin sheaths).

Two sources of thiamin are available to humans, one being the diet (absorbed in the small intestine), and the other is the normal microflora of the large intestine (absorbed in the colon). While the relative contribution of the bacterial source to total body nutrition of thiamin is not clear, the existence of an efficient carrier-mediated mechanism for thiamin uptake by human colonocytes, combined with the considerably longer transit time in the colon, suggests that this source of thiamin contributes to host nutrition, especially towards the cellular nutrition of the local colonocytes. Intestinal absorption of thiamin and its transport into other cell types is via a specific, carrier-mediated process that involves both hTHTR-1 and -2 [for review, see 1].

Good dietary sources of thiamin include rice bran, dried baker's yeast, wholegrain cereal, nuts, and dried legumes. Attention should be paid, however, to diets that contain thiamin antagonists or thiaminases. Sulfites (a food preservative) and a number of heat-stable polyhydroxyphenolic compounds (which exist in certain types of food like ferns, tea leaves, blueberry, red chicory, red beetroot, black currant, red beetroot, Brussels sprouts, and red cabbage) can cleave the thiamin molecule. Certain foods (e.g. fern, crab the African silkworm *Anaphe* spp. which is a protein source in certain part of Africa) contain thiaminase I and II, thiaminolytic enzymes that degrade thiamin leading to the generation of thiamin antagonists.

The RDA for thiamin is 1.4, 1.1, 1.5, and 1.6 mg/day for adult men, adult women, and during pregnancy and lactation, respectively. Since the requirement for thiamin is dependent on total caloric intake (especially that from carbohydrate), consumption of a calorie-rich diet may affect these RDA levels.

No toxic effects have been reported in humans as a result of ingestion of high doses of thiamin (up to 500 mg), or as a result of parenteral administration of the vitamin (single or repeat injections), although in very rare cases symptoms resembling anaphylactic shock and minor allergy have been described when the vitamin was given via the parenteral route.

Vitamin B_2 (Riboflavin)

RF in its coenzyme forms, riboflavin-5-phosphate and flavin adenosine dinucleotide, plays key roles in a variety of reactions involving carbohydrate, amino acid, and lipid metabolism, and in the conversion of folic acid and vitamin B_6 into their active coenzyme forms [for review, see 6]. Deficiency and suboptimal levels of RF occur in patients with inflammatory bowel disease and in subjects with chronic alcohol use; it also occurs in Brown-Vialetto-Van Laere syndrome (BVVL), a rare neurodegenerative disorder characterized by pontobulbar palsy, sensorineural hearing loss, and respiratory problems. BVVL is caused by mutations in the RF transporter-2 (see below) and responds to RF supplementation [7]. Systemic RF deficiency leads to a variety of clinical abnormalities that include degenerative changes in the nervous system, endocrine dysfunction, skin disorders, and anemia. In contrast, optimization of RF status reduces the risk of esophageal squamous cell carcinoma.

Two sources of RF are available to humans: a dietary source, which is absorbed in the small intestine, and a bacterial (normal microflora of the large intestine) source, which is absorbed in the colon. Transport of RF into human cells occurs via a carrier-mediated process that involves RF transporters-1, -2 and/or -3 (RFT-1, -2 and -3, respectively). The intestine utilizes RFT-1 and -2 for absorption of the vitamin [for review, see 1].

RF is widely available in many foods, with vegetables, meats, and milk products being particularly rich in the vitamin. The RDA for RF is 1.3, 1.1, 1.4, and 1.6 mg for adult males, adult females, and during pregnancy and lactation, respectively. No adverse effects are known for RF overdosing even at high levels.

Vitamin B_3 (Niacin, Nicotinic Acid)

Niacin is a precursor of the coenzymes nicotinamide adenine dinucleotide and nicotinamide adenine dinucleotide phosphate, both of which are involved in metabolic reactions (including glycolysis and the pentose phosphate shunt) that maintain the redox state of the cell. At high doses, the vitamin also has a lipid-lowering effect, and thus, has been used in the treatment of hypercholesterolemia and the prevention of atherosclerosis. Niacin deficiency leads to pellagra, a disease that is characterized by inflammation of the mucous membranes, skin lesions, diarrhea and neurological disorders. Deficiency and suboptimal levels occur in alcoholics and in patients with Hartnup's disease. Patients with the latter disease have mutations in the membrane transporter of the amino acid tryptophan (which is the precursor of endogenous niacin synthesis). Humans obtain their requirements of niacin from endogenous and exogenous sources. The former source is provided via the metabolic conversion of tryptophan to niacin, while the latter source is the diet.

Transport of niacin into human cells (including its absorption in the intestine) is via a specific, carrier-mediated process [for review, see 1]. Good dietary sources for niacin include meat products, cereals and brewers' yeast. The RDA for niacin (i.e. niacin equivalents) is 16, 14, 18, and 17 mg/day for adult males, adult females, and during pregnancy and lactation, respectively. No adverse effects have been reported with low doses of niacin. Chronic use of large doses of niacin (3–9 g/day), however, is associated with skin flushing, itching, and gastrointestinal and liver disorders.

Vitamin B_5 (Pantothenic Acid)

Pantothenic acid is needed for the synthesis of coenzyme A and acyl carrier protein, which are involved in carbohydrate, fat, and protein metabolism. Due to the ubiquitous distribution of pantothenic acid in foods, no known cases of spontaneous deficiency of the vitamin have been reported in humans. However, an inherited disorder, pantothenate kinase-associated neurodegenerative disorder (an autosomal recessive neurodegenerative disease with iron accumulation in the basal ganglia of the brain; previously called Hallervorden-Spatz syndrome), has been described in humans and is believed to be due to mutations in the gene encoding pantothenate kinase 2 PANK2.

Humans obtain pantothenate from dietary sources and from the colonic microflora. Absorption of pantothenate from both sources occurs via a carrier-mediated process that is shared with biotin and lipoate and involves the sodium-dependent multivitamin transporter [for review, see 1].

Rich sources of pantothenic acids include meats (liver and heart in particular), vegetables, and yeast. The RDA for pantothenic acid is not well defined; however, adequate intake has been estimated to be between 5 and 7 mg for adults (including during pregnancy and lactation). No adverse effects have been reported as a result of consumption of large doses of pantothenic acid of up to 10 g/day.

Vitamin B_6 (Pyridoxine and Derivatives)

Vitamin B_6 refers to three naturally occurring compounds: pyridoxal, pyridoxine, and pyridoxamine. The vitamin acts as a cofactor in a number of metabolic reactions involving carbohydrate, protein and lipid metabolism. Pyridoxal 5′-phosphate is the most biologically active form of the vitamin. Deficiency of vitamin B_6 (which leads to a variety of clinical abnormalities including neurological disorders and anemia) occurs in chronic alcoholism, in patients with diabetes mellitus and in those with celiac disease; it also occurs in subjects on long-term therapy with the agents isoniazid and penicillamine. Suboptimal levels of vitamin B_6 have also been reported in patients with vitamin B_6-dependent seizure, an autosomal-recessive disorder believed to be due to impairment in pyridoxine transport into cells [8].

Humans obtain vitamin B_6 from dietary and colonic bacterial sources. Absorption of these sources of vitamin B_6 occurs via a carrier-mediated uptake process [for review, see 1]. No information is currently available about the molecular identity of the transport system(s) involved.

Good sources of dietary vitamin B_6 include meats, wholegrain products, vegetables, and nuts. The RDA for vitamin B_6 is 2.0, 1.6, 2.1, and 2.1 mg/day for adult males, adult females, and during pregnancy and lactation, respectively. Incidences of adverse effects of overdosing of vitamin B_6 are relatively low, although a few cases of sensory neuronopathy, which is associated with gait and peripheral sensation, have been reported.

Vitamin B_9 (Folate)

Folate is a generic term for folic acid and its derivatives, compounds that act as coenzymes for cellular one-carbon metabolism and consequently for the synthesis of thymidine and purine as well as for the interconversion of amino acids. Folate deficiency is a highly prevalent vitamin deficiency and is associated with megaloblastic anemia, neural tube defects, growth retardation, cardiovascular disease and increased risk of certain types of cancer. On the other hand, optimizing folate body homeostasis leads to a significant reduction in the incidence of neural tube defects. A variety of conditions and factors interfere with the normal physiology and metabolism of folate, especially with its intestinal absorption process. This includes congenital defects in the absorptive system, i.e. mutations in the folate transport proton-coupled folate transporter (PCFT) system, which occurs in patients with hereditary folate malabsorption syndrome (HFMS) [9], intestinal diseases (e.g. celiac disease and tropical sprue), as a result of prolonged use of certain medications (e.g. sulfasalazine, trimethoprim, pyrimethamine, diphenylhydantoin), and in subjects with chronic alcoholism.

Two sources of folate are available to humans, a dietary source (absorbed in the small intestine) and a large intestinal bacterial source (absorbed in the colon). A positive relationship has been demonstrated in humans between fiber intake (which translates to flourishing intestinal microflora) and serum folate levels.

Transport of folate into human cells is via a specific and saturable process that involves three systems: the reduced folate carrier, PCFT and the folate receptor systems. In the intestine, the PCFT and reduced folate carrier systems are involved, with evidence supporting a predominant role for the former system coming from findings in patients with HFMS, where loss-of-function mutations in PCFT have been identified [for review, see 1]. HFMS is a rare autosomal recessive disorder that is characterized by anemia, hypoimmunoglobulinemia (with recurrent infections), diarrhea, and neurological abnormalities. When diagnosed early, the condition can be effectively treated with parenteral administration of folate or with oral administration of high pharmacological doses of the vitamin. If treatment of the disease is delayed, the neurological disorders could become permanent; if untreated, the condition is fatal.

Good dietary sources of folate include fruits, fortified cereals, vegetables, dairy products and liver. The RDA for folate for adults (both males and females) is 400 μg/day; during pregnancy and lactation it is 600 and 500 μg/day, respectively. No adverse effects have been reported as a result of large oral doses of folate, although allergic reaction has been observed in a few cases.

Vitamin B_{12} (Cobalamin)

Cobalamin (Cbl), in its coenzyme forms methyl-Cbl and adenosyl-Cbl, plays critical roles in the metabolism of propionate, amino acids, and in single-carbon exchange reactions. Cbl deficiency in humans occurs in a variety of conditions including intrinsic factor-deficient subjects (due to gastric atrophy, inborn lack of the factor, total gastrectomy), subjects with inflammatory bowel disease, vegans, in diabetic patients treated with metformin, and in subjects with genetic defects in the receptors and proteins responsible for the intestinal and cellular uptake of vitamin B_{12}. This deficiency leads to megaloblastic anemia, neurological disorders, and growth retardation. The deficiency can be corrected by parenteral administration of the vitamin, or by oral administration of high pharmacological doses of the vitamin.

Cbl is obtained from foods of animal origin. The vitamin is first liberated from its dietary binding proteins and then binds to haptocorrin (a protein that is synthesized by the salivary glands) to protect it against the effect of low gastric pH [for review, see 8]. In the jejunum, haptocorrin is degraded by pancreatic proteases, and the released Cbl then binds to the intrinsic factor (which is produced by parietal cells in the stomach). The intrinsic factor-bound Cbl is then recognized by a specific receptor complex, cubam, present on the apical brush border membrane of the intestinal cells in the distal part of ileum [for review, see 10].

Meat and microbes are the main source of Cbl, and the vitamin is virtually absent from a vegetarian or vegan diet; therefore, such individuals are at risk of developing Cbl deficiency. In addition, an impaired absorption of Cbl is frequently observed in elderly people, in whom a poor Cbl status is believed to have a prevalence of around 20%. The RDA for Cbl is 2.0, 2.0, 2.6 and 2.8 μg/day for adult males, adult females, and during pregnancy and lactation, respectively. No major toxicity has been reported in humans even with high doses of vitamin B_{12}.

Vitamin C (Ascorbate, Dehydroascorbate)

Dietary ascorbate (vitamin C) exists in the reduced (i.e. ascorbic acid, AA) and oxidized (dehydro-L-ascorbic acid, DHAA) forms. The vitamin acts as a cofactor in a variety of critical metabolic reactions that include the synthesis of collagen, carnitine, and catecholamine as well as in peptide amidation and tyrosine metabolism; it is also involved in maintaining metal ions (like iron and copper) in their reduced forms, and serves as a scavenger for free radicals. A role for AA in the regulation of cystic fibrosis transmembrane conductance regulator-mediated chloride secretion in epithelial cells has also been suggested. DHAA is structurally different from AA; rather, it is structurally similar to glucose. DHAA is converted to AA intracellularly via the action of DHAA reductase. Converting DHAA to AA helps maintain low (nontoxic) levels of the compound. Deficiency of this vitamin leads to a variety of clinical abnormalities that include scurvy, poor wound healing, vasomotor instability and connective tissue disorders.

Humans cannot synthesize vitamin C endogenously as they lack the enzyme L-gulonolactone oxidase; rather, they obtain the vitamin from dietary sources via intestinal absorption. Unlike a number of other water-soluble vitamins (e.g. thiamin, biotin, folate), which are also produced by the normal microflora of the large intestine, there appears to be no net production of ascorbate by these bacteria. Cellular uptake of AA, including its absorption in the intestine, involves the sodium-dependent vitamin C transporter-1 (SVCT-1; product of the *SLC23A1* gene), and SVCT-2 (product of the *SLC23A2* gene) [for review, see 1]. Transport of DHAA into cells, including its intestinal absorption, also occurs via a carrier-mediated process and involves the glucose transporters GLUT1, GLUT3 and GLUT4 [for review, see 1].

Vitamin C is widely distributed in fruits (e.g. orange, strawberry, cantaloupe, grapefruit, mango) and vegetables (e.g. broccoli, Brussels sprouts, cabbage, pepper, cauliflower) occurring mostly (up to 90%) as AA and the remaining portion as DHAA; this ratio could change with prolonged storage, exposure to air, and in aqueous solution. Because the body can reduce DHAA to AA, this form also has biological activity. The RDA for vitamin C is 90, 75, 85, and 120 mg/day for adult males, adult females, and during pregnancy and lactation, respectively.

Toxic effects of vitamin C are few and are dependent on the level of intake. Oral ingestion of large doses of vitamin C (3–5 g) can cause gastrointestinal problems (diarrhea and bloating); it may also cause transient hyperuricosuria and an increase in oxalate production and excretion. The latter may increase the risk of urinary calculi formation.

Vitamin H (Biotin)

In mammals, biotin serves as a cofactor for a number of carboxylases that are involved in a variety of metabolic reactions including fatty acid biosynthesis, gluconeogenesis, and catabolism of certain amino acids and fatty acids. The vitamin also plays a role in regulating the expression of oncogenes [for review, see 11]. Deficiency of biotin leads to dermatitis around body orifices, alopecia, conjunctivitis, and neurological disorders. Animal studies have shown that during pregnancy, biotin deficiency may lead to congenital malformation and death. Biotin deficiency and suboptimal levels occur in subjects with biotinidase deficiency (an autosomal-recessive inherited metabolic disorder in which the enzyme biotinidase is defective and biotin is not recycled; the condition can be treated with biotin supplementation) [12], those on long-term therapy with anticonvulsant drugs, those on long-term parenteral nutrition, after prolonged consumption of raw eggs, in chronic alcoholics, during pregnancy, and in subjects with inflammatory bowel disease.

Humans obtain biotin from dietary and colonic bacterial sources. Absorption of biotin in the small and large intestine as well as transport into cells occurs via a carrier-mediated uptake process that is shared with the vitamin pantothenic acid and with the metabolically important substrate lipoate (a potent intracellular and extracellular antioxidant) and involves the sodium-dependent multivitamin transporter [for review, see 1].

Biotin is widely distributed in foodstuff with dairy products, meat (liver), egg yolk, and vegetables representing good sources for the vitamin. The RDA for biotin is not well defined; however, adequate intake has been estimated at 30 μg/day for adult males and females (including pregnant women) and at 35 μg/day during lactation. No adverse effects have been reported as a result of large daily oral (up to 200 mg) or intravenous (20 mg) biotin doses.

Conclusion

Significant progress has been made in recent years with regard to physiology and pathophysiology of water-soluble vitamins and their involvement in different and previously unrecognized physiological events. With proper identifications, incidences of mutations in the involved transport systems for a number of these micronutrients have also been recognized allowing for proper treatment of the resulting clinical conditions in a timely manner. Also recognized now is the contribution of the intestinal microbiota toward overall vitamin body homeostasis and nutrition, and especially toward the cellular nutrition and health of the local colonocytes.

Acknowledgements

This study was supported by grants from the National Institutes of Health (DK56061 and DK58057) and the Department of Veterans Affairs.

References

1 Said HM: Intestinal absorption of water-soluble vitamins in health and disease. Biochem J 2011;437:357–372.
2 Arumugam M, Raes J, Pelletier E, et al: Enterotypes of the human gut microbiome. Nature 2011;473:174–180.
3 Said HM: Thiamin; in Coats PM, Betz JM, Blackman MR, et al (eds): Encyclopedia of Dietary Supplements. New York, Informa Healthcare, 2010, pp 752–757.
4 Neufeld EJ, Fleming JC, Tyartaglini E, Steinkamp MP: Thiamin-responsive megaloblastic anemia syndrome: a disorder of high-affinity thiamin transport. Blood Cells Mol Dis 2001;27:135–138.
5 Kono S, Miyajima H, Yoshida K, et al: Mutations in a thiamine-transporter gene and Wernicke's-like encephalopathy. N Engl J Med 2009;360:1792–1794.
6 Said HM, Ross C: Riboflavin; in Ross C, Caballero B, Cousins RJ, et al (eds): Modern Nutrition in Health and Disease, ed 11. New York, Lippincott Williams and Wilkins, 2012.
7 Bosch AM, Abeling NG, Ijlst L, et al: Brown-Vialetto-Van Laere and Fazio Londe syndrome is associated with a riboflavin transporter defect mimicking mild MADD: a new inborn error of metabolism with potential treatment. J Inherit Metab Dis 2011;34:159–164.
8 Gospe SM: Pyridoxine-dependent seizures: finding from recent studies pose new questions. Pediatr Neurol 2002;26:181–185.
9 Qiu A, Jansen M, Sakaris A, et al: Identification of an intestinal folate transporter and the molecular basis for hereditary folate malabsorption. Cell 2006;127:917–928.
10 Quadros EV: Advances in the understanding of cobalamin assimilation and metabolism. Br J Haematol 2010;148:195–204.
11 Said HM: Biotin: Biochemical, Physiological and Clinical Aspects; in Stanger O (ed): Water Soluble Vitamins. New York, Springer, 2012, pp 2–20.
12 Wolf B, Heard GS, Secor-McVoy JR, Raetz HM: Biotinidase deficiency: the possible role of biotinidase in the processing of dietary protein-bound biotin. J Inherit Metab Dis 1984;7:121–122.

Bier D, et al. (eds): Nutrition for the Primary Care Provider. World Rev Nutr Diet. Basel, Karger, 2015, vol 111, pp 38–44
DOI: 10.1159/000362295

Fat-Soluble Vitamins

Elizabeth J. Johnson Emily S. Mohn

Jean Mayer USDA Human Nutrition Center on Aging, Tufts University, Boston, Mass., USA

Key Words

Fat-soluble vitamins · Absorption · Transport · Storage · Functions · Requirements

Key Messages

- The four fat-soluble vitamins are vitamins A, D, E, and K. Due to their fat-soluble properties, they have similar absorption, transport, and storage as dietary fat.
- Fat-soluble vitamins play essential roles in various bodily tissues, including (but not limited to) the retina, brain, nervous tissue, epithelial linings, immune cells, and bone.
- Inadequate intake or absorption of these vitamins can lead to a number of serious clinical complications at all stages of the human life cycle.

Introduction

The fat-soluble vitamins are vitamins A, D, E, and K (table 1). Fat-soluble vitamins follow the same absorption mechanism as fat [1]. For fat-soluble vitamins to be absorbed, they must be emulsified and incorporated into mixed micelles containing cholesterol, phospholipids, and fatty acids. This requires bile from the liver and gallbladder as well as pancreatic enzymes. Micelles are absorbed into intestinal enterocytes via passive diffusion or specific transporters. Fat-soluble vitamins are reorganized into chylomicrons and released into the lymphatic system. Chylomicrons are broken down by lipoprotein lipase, an enzyme on peripheral tissue surfaces, releasing fat-soluble vitamins into the tissue. Chylomicron remnants are taken up by the liver and broken down. Fat-soluble vitamins can either be stored in the liver or repackaged and released into the bloodstream for uptake into various tissues either for use or storage. Requirements for these vitamins are found in table 2. Tolerable upper limits have been set for these vitamins, except for vitamin K (table 3).

Vitamin A

Dietary Sources

Vitamin A is found in foods as either fatty acid esters of retinol (retinyl esters) or provitamin A carotenoids (β-carotene, α-carotene, β-cryptoxanthin) [2, 3]. These carotenoids are converted to retinol with varying degrees of efficiency. Di-

Table 1. Fat-soluble vitamins

Vitamin	Chemical name	Structure
A	retinol	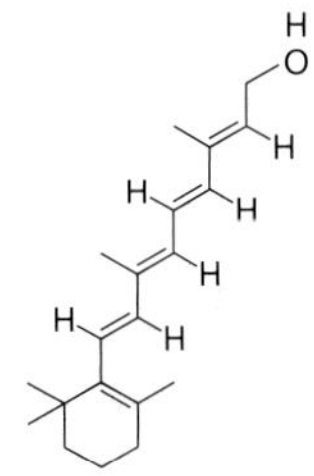
D	cholecalciferol (D_3)	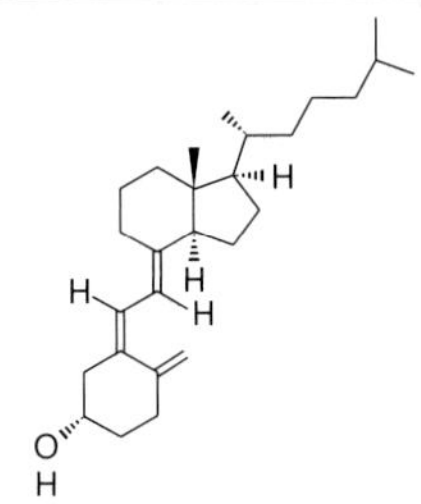
D	ergocalciferol (D_2)	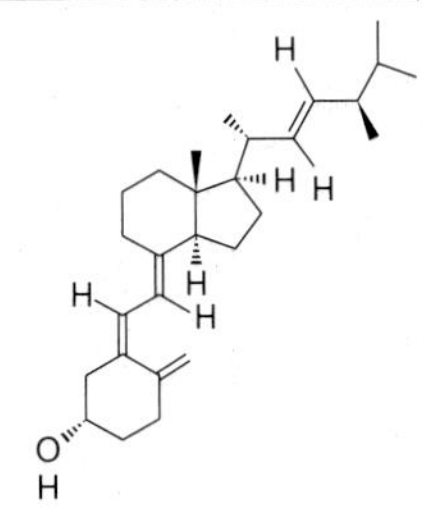
E	α-tocopherol	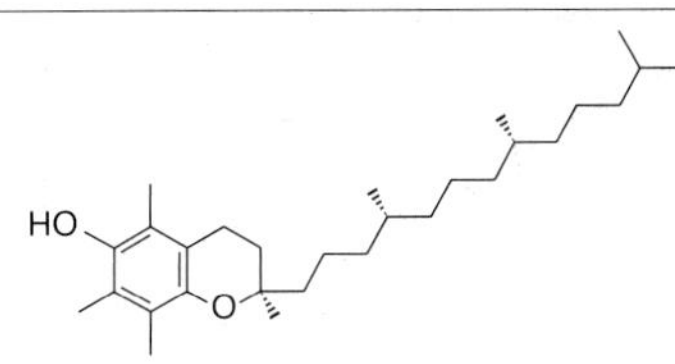
E	α-tocotrienol	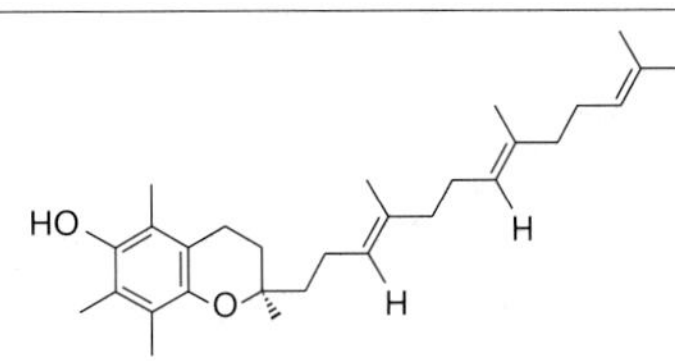
K	menaquinone (MK-7)	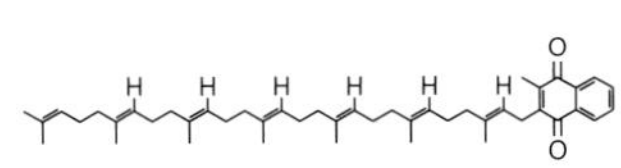
K	phylloquinone	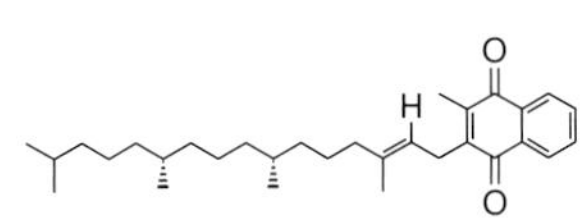

Table 2. RDA for fat-soluble vitamins

Age	Vitamin A, µg/day[1]	Vitamin D, µg/day	Vitamin E, mg/day	Vitamin K, µg/day[2]
Males				
Infants[2]				
0–6 months	400 (1,333)	10 (400)	4 (6)	2
7–12 months	500 (1,667)	10 (400)	5 (7.5)	2.5
Children				
1–3 years	300 (1,000	15 (600)	6 (9)	30
4–8 years	400 (1,333)	15 (600)	7 (10.5)	55
9–13 years	600 (2,000)	15 (600)	11 (16.5)	60
Adolescents (14–18 years)	900 (3,000)	15 (600)	15 (22.5)	75
Adults				
19–70 years	900 (3,000)	15 (600)	15 (22.5)	120
≥71 years	900 (3,000)	20 (800)	15 (22.5)	120
Females				
Infants[2]				
0–6 months	400 (1,333)	10 (400)	4 (6)	2
7–12 months	500 (1,667)	10 (400)	5 (7.5)	2.5
Children				
1–3 years	300 (1,000)	15 (600)	6 (9)	30
4–8 years	400 (1,333)	15 (600)	7 (10.5)	55
9–13 years	600 (2,000)	15 (600)	11 (16.5)	60
Adolescents (14–18 years)	700 (2,333)	15 (600)	15 (22.5)	75
Adults				
19–70 years	700 (2,333)	15 (600)	15 (22.5)	90
≥71 years	700 (2,333)	20 (800)	15 (22.5)	90
Breastfeeding				
≤18 years	1,200 (4,000)	15 (600)	19 (28.5)	75
>18 years	1,300 (4,333)	15 (600)	19 (28.5)	90
Pregnancy				
≤18 years	750 (2,500)	15 (600)	15 (22.5)	75
>18 years	770 (2,567)	15 (600)	15 (22.5)	90

Figures in parentheses indicate IU. [1] Retinol activity equivalents. [2] Adequate intake.

etary β-carotene is the most efficient (12 µg β-carotene = 1 µg of retinol, or 1 retinal activity equivalent). Dietary α-carotene and β-cryptoxanthin are approximately half as efficient. Vitamin A is obtained mostly from animal sources, including meats, cheeses, and fortified milk. Provitamin A carotenoids are found in fruits and vegetables.

Absorption and Transport

Retinyl esters and provitamin A carotenoids are often attached to food compounds and are hydrolyzed and freed for small intestine uptake. The small intestine releases pancreatic enzymes to release vitamin A from food to its free form. Brush border enzymes on the surface of intestinal cells also contribute to the release. A fraction of the

Table 3. Tolerable upper level for fat-soluble vitamins

Age	Vitamin A, µg/day	Vitamin D, µg/day	Vitamin E, mg/day
Infants			
0–6 months	600 (2,000)	25 (1,000)	not established
6–12 months	600 (2,000)	37.5 (1,500)	not established
Children			
1–3 years	600 (2,000)	62.5 (2,500)	200 (300)
4–8 years	900 (3,000)	75 (3,000)	300 (450)
9–13 years	1,700 (5,667)	100 (4,000)	600 (900)
Adolescents (14–18 years)	2,800 (9,333)	100 (4,000)	800 (1,200)
Adults (>18 years)	3,000 (10,000)	100 (4,000)	1,000 (1,500)

Figures in parentheses indicate IU.

provitamin A carotenoids are converted to vitamin A in the intestinal lumen prior to absorption or within intestinal cells. Vitamin A is then repackaged into chylomicrons and released into the lymphatic system, where it is taken up by peripheral tissues until it reaches the liver. The liver is the main storage site of vitamin A. Upon release from the liver, vitamin A is bound to retinol-binding protein (RBP) and travels through the bloodstream for uptake by tissues containing RBP receptors.

Functions

In the retina, vitamin A is converted to retinal and binds to the protein opsin forming rhodopsin. When light hits the retina cells, retinal changes conformation and detaches from opsin. Opsin also changes shape to generate an electrical impulse in the retina cells, which transfers the signal to nerve cells, and then to the brain. The brain interprets the signal as light. Some retinal is lost during every cycle. Therefore, vitamin A must be replenished through diet.

Vitamin A deficiency during pregnancy may lead to birth defects and high infant mortality rates. Retinoic acid, a form of vitamin A is vital for the differentiation of stem cells into epithelial tissues, red blood cells, and components of the eye. Vitamin A also plays an important role in immune function. It maintains the integrity of the epithelium inside and outside the body, which serves as a barrier against foreign pathogens.

Deficiency

Vitamin A deficiency symptoms develop once vitamin A liver stores are completely or nearly depleted. Night blindness occurs when there is not enough retinal to regenerate rhodopsin in the retina. This leads to the inability to immediately recover vision after light flashes, as well as vision loss in dark/dim light. Vitamin A deficiency also plays a role in permanent blindness where, due to inadequate mucus secretion in the front of the eye, the corneal cells become dry and hard, and keratin, a hard-water-insoluble protein accumulates.

Vitamin A deficiency can increase susceptibility to diseases and infection. Severe deficiencies can lead to death. A priority in international nutrition policy is vitamin A supplementation to developing nations, where vitamin A deficiencies are prevalent, to decrease infant morbidity/mortality. Keratinization can occur in prolonged vitamin A deficiency in external epithelial cells (or skin cells), leading to dry, red, bumpy skin.

Toxicity

Vitamin A toxicity occurs from either extremely high doses over a short period of time or chronic overexposure with high doses. This leads to the saturation of RBP, and free retinol can damage cells. Intakes above this limit may cause liver damage, changes in vision, headache, dry/itchy skin, and hair loss.

Vitamin D

Dietary Sources

A significant amount of the vitamin D is synthesized in the skin when exposed to UVB radiation from sunlight [4]. This form of vitamin D is biologically inactive and must undergo hydroxylation reactions in the liver and kidney before it can function within the body. The main form of vitamin D found in food is vitamin D_3. Many sources also contain D_2. D_3 is the form synthesized in the skin. The active form of vitamin D is calcitriol (1,25 dihydroxyvitamin D). Vitamin D naturally occurs in few foods, although it is naturally found in wild salmon and swordfish. Most dietary vitamin D is from fortified sources. Two main fortified sources of vitamin D are milk and ready-to-eat cereals [2].

Absorption, Transport and Activation

Vitamin D absorption follows the same path as dietary fat (see above). Adipose tissue is the main vitamin D storage site. Vitamin D synthesized in the skin enters the circulation and is taken up by the liver. Once there, vitamin D undergoes a hydroxylation reaction to form calcidiol (25-hydroxyvitamin D). This form binds to the vitamin D-binding protein and is released into the circulation. Calcidiol is the major form of vitamin D in serum and increases with increased vitamin D from the diet or sun.

Functions

When serum calcium and phosphorous levels drop too low, parathyroid glands secrete parathyroid hormone, which increases the activation of vitamin D via a hydroxylation reaction in the kidney, forming calcitriol (1,25-dihydroxyvitamin D). Calcitriol increases serum calcium and phosphorous concentrations by increasing intestinal absorption of calcium and phosphorous. Calcitriol increases the reabsorption of calcium filtered by kidneys and mobilizes calcium in bones. This allows for calcium and phosphorous levels to rise to the desired range.

Calcitriol has been shown to modulate a variety of processes through binding to its receptor and regulating gene expression, cell proliferation, and cell differentiation. Vitamin D status has been linked to the decreased risk for developing autoimmune diseases. Furthermore, vitamin D deficiency has been linked to increased inflammation.

Deficiency

In children, vitamin D deficiency causes rickets, a disease of inadequate bone mineralization. In rickets, weak bones bend under the body weight and sometimes there are deformed rib cages. For adults, lack of vitamin D can cause osteomalacia. Long-term vitamin D insufficiency is a factor for increased risk of osteoporosis. Osteoporosis is characterized by low bone density and bone tissue deterioration.

Toxicity

Vitamin D toxicity occurs due to oversupplementation, not from overexposure to sunlight. Excess vitamin D in the body causes high blood calcium levels above a healthy range leading to inappropriate deposition of calcium in soft tissues. Calcium deposition in the kidneys can lead to kidney stone formation. Blood vessels and arteries begin to harden with calcification in the heart. Increased vitamin D can also lead to increased bone resorption, leading to bone loss. Vitamin D tolerable upper intake levels have been determined for various age groups (table 3).

Vitamin E

Dietary Sources
Vitamin E exists in different forms, four of which are: α-tocopherol, γ-tocopherol, α-tocotrienol, and γ-tocotrienol [5]. α-Tocopherol is the main form stored and used by the body. The following information will be on this form. Vitamin E is naturally found in oils, such as sunflower and safflower oil, and oily foods, such as nuts [2].

Absorption, Transport and Storage
Dietary vitamin E is absorbed in the intestine through the same mechanisms as other fat-soluble vitamins. In the liver, the vitamin E forms (except α-tocopherol) are metabolized or excreted. α-Tocopherol is maintained in the liver through its binding to α-tocopherol transfer protein and is the only form that the liver releases. Liver release of α-tocopherol in lipoproteins is taken up by various tissues for use.

Functions
The main function of vitamin E is as an antioxidant. Oxidative stress is caused by environmental factors, such as smoke or alcohol. Oxidants are also formed endogenously through normal processes of energy metabolism. Vitamin E intercepts free radicals in lipid membranes to prevent the propagation of lipid peroxidation. In this way, vitamin E prevents the oxidation of tissue membranes and circulating lipoproteins. Vitamin E must be recycled by other antioxidants to continue to function. Vitamin C is one of the main antioxidants responsible for vitamin E regeneration.

Deficiency
Vitamin E deficiency leads to the breakdown of cell membranes and tissue damage due to oxidative stress. Hemolysis can occur. Common manifestations of vitamin E deficiency are peripheral neuropathy and degeneration of axons.

Toxicity
Oversupplementation is the main cause of vitamin E toxicity. Too much vitamin E can lead to blood coagulation problems and hemorrhaging.

Vitamin K

Dietary Sources
Vitamin K refers to several different molecules that all possess similar structural characteristics [3]. Phylloquinone is the main form of vitamin K found in foods. Some menaquinones can be found in food sources. Additionally, menaquinone-4 can be synthesized from phylloquinone in the body. Main sources of phylloquinone in the diet include green, leafy vegetables and broccoli [2]. Menaquinones with long side chains can be synthesized by microbiota in the human colon, although its contribution to overall vitamin K status is unknown.

Absorption and Transport
Vitamin K absorption in the intestine follows the same mechanism as dietary fat. In the liver, vitamin K is used or repackaged and released in triglyceride-rich lipoproteins. The major site of vitamin K storage is the adipose tissue. Unlike the other fat-soluble vitamins, a significant portion of vitamin K is excreted in the bile and urine.

Functions
The main role of vitamin K is the activation of vitamin K-dependent coagulation and bone formation proteins. Many observational studies have shown that vitamin K intake is associated with a decreased risk of hip fracture. However, other studies have shown no association between vitamin K intake and bone mineral density, and randomized controlled trials have failed to show an effect of vitamin K on bone health.

Deficiency
Vitamin K deficiency leads to increased risk for hemorrhaging. Vitamin K deficiency is a problem

for newborns due to poor vitamin K placental transfer. Injections of vitamin K are given to infants at birth to prevent any bleeding issues. Vitamin E may play a role in antagonizing vitamin K status; therefore, extremely high doses of vitamin E may increase the risk for vitamin K deficiency. Similarly, anticoagulants have been shown to antagonize the role of vitamin K. Those on such medication should monitor vitamin K intake.

Toxicity
To date, there is no clinical evidence that increased consumption of vitamin K is toxic in healthy individuals.

Conclusion

- Fat-soluble vitamins play an important role in human health.
- Main functions of these nutrients are known.
- Each fat-soluble vitamin has specific symptoms of deficiencies and toxicities.
- New roles for each fat-soluble vitamin are constantly being discovered.

References

1 Reboul E, Borel P: Proteins involved in uptake, intracellular transport and basolateral secretion of fat-soluble vitamins and carotenoids by mammalian enterocytes. Prog Lipid Res 2011;50:388–402.

2 USDA Agricultural Research Service, National Agricultrual Library: USDA National Nutrient Database for Standard Reference. ndb.nal.usda.gov/.

3 Food and Nutrition Board, Institute of Medicine: Dietary Reference Intakes for Vitamin A, Vitamin K, Arsenic, Boron, Chromium, Copper, Iodine, Iron, Manganese, Molybdenum, Nickel, Silicon, Vanadium, and Zinc. Washington, National Academy Press, 2014.

4 Food and Nutrition Board, Institute of Medicine: Dietary Reference Intakes for Calcium, Phosphorus, Magnesium, Vitamin D, and Fluoride. Washington, National Academy Press, 2010.

5 Food and Nutrition Board, Institute of Medicine: Dietary Reference Intakes for Vitamin C, Vitamin E, Selenium and Carotenoids. Washington, National Academy Press, 2000.

Bier D, et al. (eds): Nutrition for the Primary Care Provider. World Rev Nutr Diet. Basel, Karger, 2015, vol 111, pp 45–52
DOI: 10.1159/000362296

Minerals and Trace Elements

Susan J. Fairweather-Tait[a] Kevin Cashman[b, c]

[a]Norwich Medical School, University of East Anglia, Norwich, UK; [b]School of Food and Nutritional Sciences, and [c]Department of Medicine, University College Cork, Cork, Ireland

Key Words

Minerals · Trace elements · Deficiency · Toxicity

Key Messages

- Inappropriate intakes and/or elevated requirements resulting from a range of conditions, including disease, malabsorption, medications, and excessive losses, eventually lead to a state of deficiency or toxicity.
- Disorders that affect the organs can manifest as deficiencies in minerals or trace elements. For example, iron deficiency is common in inflammatory bowel disease.
- Excess levels of certain minerals or elements result in damage to the related organs, as demonstrated in the kidney where high phosphorus levels are associated with the parenchymal deposition of calcium phosphate precipitates.
- Vulnerable groups or conditions with increased risk of mineral deficiency include those with anorexia nervosa, pregnant women, infants and children, and patients on parenteral nutrition.
- The use of certain drugs and medications can also affect the body's mineral and trace element status. This can also be influenced by hereditary disorders such as hereditary hemochromatosis, Wilson's disease and Menkes' syndrome.

Introduction

Essential minerals and trace elements have well-characterized physiological functions within the body (table 1) and must be supplied by the diet [for more details, see 1]. Dietary Reference Intakes for the various minerals and by life stage groups have been derived by the North American Institute of Medicine [2]. Inappropriate intakes and/or elevated requirements resulting from a range of conditions, including disease, malabsorption, some medicines, and excessive losses, will eventually lead to a state of deficiency or toxicity with associated pathophysiology. For many minerals, there are no simple, sensitive and specific biomarkers of status (table 2), so deficiency or toxicity may not be diagnosed until fairly well advanced, at which point the patient may present with clinical signs or symptoms (table 3). With a poor diet, it is likely that multiple micronutrient deficiencies will occur, but there are also rare genetic mutations that affect the metabolism of single minerals or trace elements; these are usually unrelated to diet.

Table 1. Major functions of minerals and trace elements

Minerals	
Calcium	Structural (bones, teeth), extracellular cation (neural transmission, muscle contraction, vascular tone)
Magnesium	>300 enzymatic processes, bone health, maintenance of intracellular levels of K and Ca
Phosphorus	Structural (bones, teeth, phospholipids), acid-base balance, protein activation via phosphorylation
Potassium	Intracellular cation (neural transmission, muscle contraction, vascular tone)
Sodium	Extracellular cation, membrane potential, membrane transport
Chloride	Extracellular anion, fluid and electrolyte balance, gastric juice
Trace elements	
Copper	Metalloenzymes, red blood cell formation, connective tissues
Fluoride	Not an essential nutrient but present as fluorohydroxyapatite in tooth enamel
Iodine	Thyroid hormones
Iron	Heme proteins, flavoproteins, other enzymes
Manganese	Metalloenzymes, bone formation
Selenium	Selenoproteins, thyroid hormone, redox status
Zinc	>100 enzymes, growth, development, gene expression

The Role of Minerals and Trace Elements in the Etiology and Management of Various Diseases or Disorders

The following section will highlight conditions where the risk of deficiency can be increased and may warrant detailed investigations of mineral nutritional status (table 2).

GI Tract

Iron deficiency is frequent in inflammatory bowel disease (IBD) due to blood loss. Zinc deficiency is also a problem, and low serum zinc concentrations have also been reported in Crohn's disease and in ulcerative colitis. Serum selenium is low in IBD, and the activity of glutathione peroxidase, a selenium-dependent enzyme, is decreased in some patients with Crohn's disease and ulcerative colitis. Celiac disease patients have global malabsorption problems, and gluten-free diets may not contain an adequate level of some micronutrients such as magnesium; microcytic anemia (iron deficiency) is very common, and these patients are also at risk of developing low bone mineral density (BMD), where calcium and vitamin D play a key role.

Liver

Deficiencies of minerals occur in patients with liver disease due to steatorrhea (calcium), alcohol abuse and increased levels of aldosterone (potassium) and the use of diuretics (potassium, calcium, magnesium, zinc). Dietary treatment of ascites requires sodium restriction, depending on the severity, but very low sodium diets are impractical and unpalatable.

Pancreas

Patients with chronic pancreatitis are generally undernourished; selenium appears to be the mineral most frequently noted as being deficient, but this is thought to be due to malabsorption or increased oxidative stress rather than an inadequate intake.

Kidney

High phosphorus intakes are associated with the parenchymal deposition of calcium phosphate precipitates, which causes kidney damage; therefore, phosphorus intake should be reduced according to the glomerular filtration rate (GFR):

- GFR 25–70 ml/min, phosphorus 8–10 g/kg/day
- GFR <25 ml/min, phosphorus 5–10 g/kg/day.

Table 2. Biomarkers for assessing trace element/mineral exposure and status

Biomarkers of exposure or status (body levels)	Adult 'normal range'[1]	Comment on usefulness of biomarker
Calcium		
(1) Serum calcium (2) Serum ionized calcium (3) Mineral content of skeletal bone (DXA, CT) (4) Urinary and/or serum bone remodeling biomarkers (5) Serum PTH (6) 24-hour urinary calcium	(1) 2.15–2.55 mmol/l (86–102 mg/l) [10] (2) 1.16–1.32 mmol/l (46.4–52.8 mg/l) [10] (3) BMD as T scores; normal bone: T score better than –1; osteopenia: T score between –1 and –2.5; osteoporosis: T score less than –2.5 (5) 15–65 pg/ml [15] (6) 15–20 mmol (100–250 mg)/24 h (normal diet); 7.5–22.5 mmol (50–150 mg)/24 h (on low-calcium diet) [16]	(1, 2) Maintained within a narrow range (3) T score is the number of standard deviations below the average for a young adult at peak bone density (4) Large assay-dependent differences in values and thus in normal ranges (6) No clear relationship between dietary intake and 24-hour urinary excretion
Copper		
(1) Serum copper (2) Serum/plasma ceruloplasmin	(1) M 11.0–22.0 μmol/l (0.7–1.4 mg/l); F 12.6–24.4 μmol/l (0.8–1.9 mg/l) [10] (2) M 250–550 mg/l; F 200–450 mg/l	(1) Changes occur in response to pathological conditions (2) Decreases in Wilson's disease, increases in inflammatory conditions
Iodine [17, 18]		
(1) Urinary iodine (children and adults) (2) Serum thyroglobulin (children and adolescents) (3) Serum T_4 and T_3 (4) Serum thyroid-stimulating hormone (including women during pregnancy and lactation) (5) Goiter	(1) 100–300 μg/l (2) 4–40 μl (3) T_4 (free form) 11–18 pmol/l, T_3 (free form) 3.5–5.0 pmol/l (4) 0.1–5 mIU/l (5) Grade (0, 1, 2) scored by palpation	(1) Accurately reflects intake (24-hour samples best) (2) Useful biomarker of adequacy in children and adults (3) Less sensitive biomarker, not useful in pregnancy (4) Useful in newborn infants (5) Long-term measure of inadequate iodine intake
Iron		
(1) Hemoglobin (2) Ferritin (plasma or serum) (3) Soluble transferrin receptor (plasma or serum) (4) Erythrocyte zinc protoporphyrin (5) Serum iron (6) Bone marrow biopsy	(1) M 140–175 (mean 157) g/l [19] F 123–153 (mean 138) g/l [19] (2) M 16-328 μg/l (5th to 95th centile) [20] F 5–170 μg/l (5th to 95th centile) [20] (3) M 2.2–5.0 mg/l; F 1.9–4.4 mg/l [19] (4) >40 μmol/mol heme iron (washed erythrocytes), >80 μmol/mol heme iron (unwashed erythrocytes) indicates iron deficiency (5) M 11.6–31.3 μmol/l (0.65–1.65 mg/l); F 9.0–30.4 μmol/l (0.5–1.7 mg/l) [10]	(1) Detects IDA, low specificity and sensitivity (2) Accurate measure of stores but elevated with infection and inflammation (3) Good early indicator of iron deficiency (4) Sensitive measure of erythropoiesis (5) Fasting essential as changes after meals (6) Gold standard but invasive

Table 2 (continued)

Biomarkers of exposure or status (body levels)	Adult 'normal range'[1]	Comment on usefulness of biomarker
Magnesium (1) Serum/plasma magnesium (2) Erythrocyte magnesium (3) 24-hour urinary magnesium	(1) 0.66–1.07 mmol/l (16–26 mg/l) [10] (2) M 1.95 (SD 0.19) mmol/l, 47.5 (SD 4.5) mg/l F 2.03 (SD 0.21) mol/l, 49.4 (SD 5.2) mg/l (3) 120–140 mg/24 h	(1) There are changes in serum magnesium concentration associated with various pathological conditions (2) Insensitive biomarker (3) Used as biomarker of magnesium status primarily in association with magnesium load test (for screening for magnesium deficiency)
Phosphorus (1) Serum/plasma phosphorus	0.81–1.45 mmol/l (25–45 mg/l) [10]	
Potassium (1) 24-hour urinary potassium (2) Total body K^{40}	(1) M 76.7 (2.5th to 97.5th percentile 24.3 to 152.1) mmol/24 h [21] F 65.2 (2.5th to 97.5th percentile 22.4–127.0) mmol/24 h [21]	(1) 24-hour urine reflects intake, and thus varies by population; example opposite from UK National Diet and Nutrition Survey data for 19- to 64-year-olds (2) Total body K is a research tool
Selenium (1) Serum/plasma selenium (2) Plasma selenoprotein P (3) Plasma GPx3 (4) Toenail selenium (5) Hair selenium	(1) 46–143 µg/l [10]	All useful measures; GPx mainly used to detect deficiency; hair samples are particularly prone to contamination (2–5) Large assay-dependent differences in values and thus in normal ranges
Sodium (1) Serum/plasma sodium (2) 24-hour urinary sodium	(1) 134–143 mmol/l (3.08–3.29 g/l, 95% range) (2) 127 (2.5th to 97.5th percentile 53–274) mmol/24 h [21]	(1) Lowest recorded value 90 mmol/l, highest recorded values 170–200 mmol/l (2) 24-hour urine reflects intake, and thus varies by population; example opposite from UK National Diet and Nutrition Survey data for 19- to 64-year-olds
Zinc [22] (1) Serum/plasma zinc (2) Hair zinc	(1) 10.7–22.9 µmol/l (0.7–1.5 mg/l) [10] (2) M 180 (SD 25; 138–231) µg/g F 195 (SD 23; 154–277) µg/g	Zinc deficiency/excess can be detected using serum/plasma and hair zinc concentrations, but these biomarkers are insensitive and cannot be used to assess zinc status

[1] Values to represent 'normal ranges' taken from Milne [10], Lentner [11], Ayling and Marshall [12], Gibney et al. [13], Gibson [14] and NDNS [23].

Table 3. Signs and symptoms of deficiency and toxicity of minerals and trace elements

	Deficiency	Causes	Excess	Causes
Calcium	osteoporosis, pre-eclampsia	low intake or impaired absorption over many years	kidney stones; hypercalcemia; renal insufficiency	excessive intake of calcium supplements; peptic ulcer treatment
Copper	anemia, neutropenia, bone fractures; Menkes syndrome; X-linked cutis laxa (sagging skin, impaired connective tissues)	premature birth; excessive intakes of zinc; Menkes caused by a mutation of the *ATP7A* gene that encodes for Cu transport protein; cutis laxa is a mild form of Menkes	acute toxicity causes vomiting, diarrhea, hemolytic anemia; chronic toxicity causes hepatitis, cirrhosis, jaundice; Wilson's disease	contaminated drinks and foods (copper pipes); Wilson's caused by a mutation of the *ATP7B* gene that encodes for protein that transports copper into bile
Iodine	iodine deficiency disorders (goiter, cretinism); Pendred's syndrome	low intakes in areas where soil is iodine deficient; excessive intakes of goitrogens (brassica vegetables); mutations in Pendrin gene resulting in defective iodination of thyroglobulin	rapid heart rate, trembling, excessive sweating, lack of sleep, weight loss	high intakes of seafood or seaweed contaminated with iodine
Iron	iron deficiency anemia (tiredness, impaired work performance, failure to thrive in infants)	low bioavailable diets, increased requirement (blood loss, growth)	acute toxicity causes GI problems (constipation, diarrhea, cramps); chronic toxicity increased risk for bacterial infections, arthropathy, cardiomyopathy, endocrine dysfunctions; HH	overuse of iron supplements; HH is caused by mutations of the *HFE* gene which result in inappropriately high iron absorption
Phos-phorus	anorexia, muscle weakness, bone pain, rickets, osteomalacia	near-total starvation	adverse effects on calcium economy	excessive intake of cola beverages and food phosphate additives
Potas-sium	severe: cardiac arrhythmias, muscle weakness, glucose intolerance; moderate: high BP, high risk of kidney stones, CVD (stroke), increased bone turnover	low intake, diuretics; Cushing's disease, chronic renal disease, diarrhea, vomiting, laxative abuse	cardiac arrest	excessive intake of potassium supplements, metabolic acidosis, chronic renal failure, ACE inhibitors, Addison's disease, angiotensin receptor blockers and potassium-sparing diuretics
Selenium	associated with Keshan disease (cardiomyopathy) and Kashin-Beck disease (osteoarthropathy); impaired immune function	low intakes in areas where soil is selenium deficient	brittle hair and nails, skin lesions, garlic breath	excessive intake of supplements and high selenium foods e.g. Brazil nuts
Sodium	headache, muscle weakness and spasms/cramps, nausea, vomiting, confusion, lethargy, appetite loss	acute diarrhea, excessive sweat loss, diuretic overuse, cachexia, congestive heart failure	hypertension	high intake
Zinc	growth retardation, hair loss, skin lesions, loss of appetite, loss of taste sensation, delayed sexual maturation; acrodermatitis enteropathica	low intake, high cereal fibre and legume (phytate) diet; acrodermatitis enteropathica caused by a mutation of the *SLC39A4* gene which encodes a zinc uptake protein	acute toxicity causes nausea and vomiting; chronic toxicity causes copper deficiency	contaminated water (galvanized containers)

A low phosphorus (and protein) diet will reduce calcium intake; therefore, calcium supplements may be required. Patients with renal failure cannot maintain mineral homeostasis by urinary excretion, and this increases the risk for development of clinically hazardous blood or tissue concentrations. Patients with chronic kidney disease (CKD) need to consume a diet low in sodium, potassium and phosphorus, but may need additional calcium, iron and magnesium. CKD-mineral and bone disorder is a new term for a common clinical entity observed in patients with CKD that involves abnormal mineral metabolism, bone disease and vascular calcification. CKD-mineral and bone disorder can manifest as one or more abnormalities of calcium, phosphorus, vitamin D metabolism, or parathyroid hormone; abnormalities in bone turnover, mineralization, volume, linear growth, or strength, and vascular or other soft-tissue calcification. Specific clinical practice guidelines for kidney transplant patients include monitoring serum calcium and phosphorus and hematological measurements (to diagnose anemia) [3].

Bone

The human skeleton contains 1–1.5 kg of calcium and 0.8–1 kg of phosphorus. Rickets and osteomalacia are caused by calcium, phosphorus, and/or vitamin D deficiency, whereas osteoporosis is characterized by a reduction in BMD due to a combination of genetic and environmental factors. Long-standing calcium deficiency plays a contributory role in the etiology of osteoporosis, partly as a result of the reduced absorption associated with low vitamin D status (limited sunlight exposure and low dietary intake of vitamin D), but also from increased calcium excretion with diuretics and renal failure. Vitamin D and calcium supplements may be recommended for postmenopausal women who are housebound. Corticosteroid treatment for IBD, rheumatoid arthritis and other conditions leads to bone mineral loss. In systemic lupus erythematosus, significant reductions in BMD have been observed in premenopausal patients, related and unrelated to corticosteroid use. In IBD, where a low BMI may be an additional factor, there is a high prevalence of osteopenia, with Crohn's disease patients being more severely affected than those with ulcerative colitis. Patients undergoing organ transplantation are also at high risk of osteoporosis; bone loss is rapid after organ transplantation, and occurs mainly in the first 6 months. High intakes of calcium (e.g. 1,000 mg/day) and vitamin D (e.g. 500 IU/day) may reduce the rate of bone loss in some patients.

Cardiovascular System

Potassium deficiency or excess may predispose to cardiac rhythm disturbances. Intakes are inversely related to the incidence of hypertension and stroke. Water hardness (and hence calcium intake) is inversely related to coronary heart disease, as is magnesium intake. Recent evidence has emerged showing that disease-specific mortality risks are elevated for cardiovascular disease and ischemic heart disease with calcium intakes >1,400 or <600 mg/day. Risk of stroke may be increased with low calcium intakes (<700 mg/day). Sodium intakes are weakly associated with blood pressure in epidemiological studies, and the effect of reducing sodium intake varies between individuals, being most pronounced in the elderly and in Afro-Caribbeans.

Cancer

Mineral deficiencies can occur in some cancer patients due to low intake (cachexia), excessive losses (e.g. blood loss) and cytokine-mediated inflammatory response which reduces iron absorption. Low serum zinc can be normalized in a few weeks with zinc supplements of 50 mg/day. Serum copper, present mainly in ceruloplasmin, may be elevated in patients with tumors due to changes in ceruloplasmin metabolism. It is homeostatically controlled by desialylation in the liver but may be resialylated at the tumor cell surface leading to an increase in blood copper concentration.

Other Vulnerable Groups or Conditions with Increased Risk of Mineral Deficiency
The Academy of Nutrition and Dietetics (formerly American Dietetic Association) has published Evidence-Based Nutrition Practice Guidelines for a number of diseases and vulnerable groups [4].

Patients with Anorexia Nervosa
Calcium deficiency is common due to low intakes of dairy products. Iron and zinc deficiencies are also common because of the avoidance of red meat, leading to iron deficiency anemia, lack of appetite and loss of taste sensation. Potassium and phosphate losses may be high from vomiting and use of laxatives and diuretics, and this may lead to cardiac abnormalities and heart failure. Refeeding places additional demands on the heart through the increased requirements for potassium and phosphate, so care must be taken when instituting nutritional therapy in order to avoid refeeding syndrome.

Pregnancy
Iron deficiency anemia is one of the most common pregnancy complications. Screening should be carried out at the first prenatal visit and regularly throughout the pregnancy. The recent recommendations for antenatal care from the WHO are a daily supplement of 30–60 mg iron, together with 400 μg folic acid, to reduce the risk of low birthweight, maternal anemia and iron deficiency [5].

Studies have shown that high hemoglobin values are associated with adverse pregnancy outcomes; however, iron supplementation cannot, in itself, raise hemoglobin to these levels; thus, adverse outcomes are more likely secondary to underlying conditions that are responsible for the high hemoglobin values.

Infants and Children
Deficiencies of trace elements, particularly iron and zinc, are common due to low body stores, improper feeding, and/or increased losses e.g. recurrent infections. Iodine and selenium deficiencies are endemic in particular geographical areas where the mineral is lacking in the earth's crust. In infants and young children, deficiency impairs thyroid function and may have a negative impact on brain development, causing cretinism.

Parenteral Nutrition
This mode of nutrition should provide essential minerals and trace elements appropriate for the life stage [6], although not all essential nutrients can be mixed in a parenteral solution, e.g. iron. Mineral and trace element status should be monitored and nutrients supplied via other routes if necessary. Requirements of young children are different from those of adults (table 2) and specialist pediatric preparations must be used. Deficiencies in zinc and selenium occur most commonly because selenium is often not added to the solution and levels of added zinc may be too low. There are nutrition guidelines for critical care patients [7]. There are also comprehensive guidelines on pediatric parenteral nutrition [8].

Drugs/Medications
Some drugs may induce mineral deficiencies, for example:

- Aminoglycoside – magnesium and zinc
- Antacids – phosphorus
- Proton pump inhibitors – iron
- Diuretics – sodium, potassium, magnesium, zinc
- Laxatives – sodium, potassium, magnesium
- Platinum – magnesium, zinc.

Examples of Genetic Disorders of Minerals/Trace Elements

Hereditary hemochromatosis (HH) is an iron-loading disorder associated with *HFE* gene mutations. Wilson's disease, which leads to copper overload, is caused by a mutation in the *ATP7B* gene. Menkes' syndrome, a neurodegenerative disorder of infancy associated with copper deficiency, is caused by a mutation in the *ATP7A* gene. Acrodermatitis enteropathica, severe zinc deficiency observed in infants, is associated with mutations in the *SLC39A4* gene. The impact of these genetic disorders on mineral and trace element status has been reviewed elsewhere [9].

Conclusions

- Inappropriate intakes and/or elevated requirements resulting from a range of conditions, including disease, malabsorption, medications, and excessive losses, eventually lead to a state of deficiency or toxicity.
- For many minerals, there are no simple, sensitive and specific biomarkers of status, so deficiency or toxicity may not be diagnosed until fairly well advanced, at which point the patient may present with clinical signs and symptoms. For some minerals, there are relatively good biomarkers of status.
- Vulnerable groups or conditions with increased risk of mineral deficiency include those with anorexia nervosa, pregnant women, infants and children, and patients on parenteral nutrition.
- The use of certain drugs and medications can also affect the body's mineral and trace element status. This can also be influenced by hereditary disorders such as HH, Wilson's disease and Menkes' syndrome.

References

1 http://www.nlm.nih.gov/medlineplus/minerals.html.
2 http://www.iom.edu/Activities/Nutrition/SummaryDRIs/~/media/Files/Activity%20Files/Nutrition/DRIs/5_Summary%20Table%20Tables%201-4.pdf.
3 http://www.kdigo.org/clinical_practice_guidelines/kdigo_guideline_for_care_ktr.php.
4 http://andevidencelibrary.com/category.cfm?cid=14&cat=0.
5 http://www.who.int/nutrition/publications/micronutrients/guidelines/daily_ifa_supp_pregnanen/index.html.
6 https://www.nutritioncare.org/.
7 http://www.criticalcarenutrition.com/.
8 Koletzko B, Goulet O, Hunt J, et al: Guidelines on Paediatric Parenteral Nutrition of the European Society of Paediatric Gastroenterology, Hepatology and Nutrition (ESPGHAN) and the European Society for Clinical Nutrition and Metabolism (ESPEN), Supported by the European Society of Paediatric Research (ESPR). J Pediatr Gastroenterol Nutr 2005;41(suppl 2):81–84.
9 Strain JJ, Cashman KD: Minerals and trace elements; in Gibney MJ, Lanham-New S, Cassidy A, Vorster HH (eds): Introduction to Human Nutrition (The Nutrition Society Textbook), ed 2. Chichester, Wiley Blackwell, pp 188–237.
10 Milne DB: Laboratory assessment of trace element and mineral status; in Bogden JD, Klevay LM (eds): Clinical Nutrition of the Essential Trace Elements and Minerals: The Guide for Health Professionals. Totowa, Humana Press, 2000.
11 Lentner C: Geigy Scientific Tables. Basel, Ciba-Geigy, vol 3, 1984.
12 Ayling R, Marshall W: Nutrition and Laboratory Medicine. London, Association for Clinical Biochemistry, 2007.
13 Gibney MJ, Elia M, Ljungqvist O, Dowsett J: Clinical Nutrition. Oxford, Blackwell Science, 2006.
14 Gibson RS: Principles of Nutritional Assessment, ed 2. Oxford, Oxford University Press, 2005.
15 http://www.mayomedicallaboratories.com/test-catalog/Clinical+and+Interpretive/28379.
16 http://www.nlm.nih.gov/medlineplus/ency/article/003690.htm.
17 EFSA Panel on Dietic Products, Nutrition and Allergies: Scientific opinion on dietary reference values for iodine. EFSA J 2014;12:3660.
18 Zimmermann MB: Methods to assess iron and iodine status. Br J Nutr 2008;99(suppl 3):S2–S9.
19 http://emedicine.medscape.com/article/2086300-overview.
20 WHO: Serum ferritin concentrations for the assessment of iron status and iron deficiency in populations. WHO/NMH/NHD/MNM/11.2. Geneva, WHO, 2011.
21 http://webarchive.nationalarchives.gov.uk/20130402145952/http://transparency.dh.gov.uk/2012/06/21/sodium-levels-among-adults/.
22 McKenzie JM: Content of zinc in serum, urine, hair, and toenails of New Zealand adults. Am J Clin Nutr 1979;32:570–579.
23 http://multimedia.food.gov.uk/multimedia/pdfs/ndnsv3.pdf.

Bier D, et al. (eds): Nutrition for the Primary Care Provider. World Rev Nutr Diet. Basel, Karger, 2015, vol 111, pp 53–57
DOI: 10.1159/000362297

Vegetarian Diets

Susan I. Barr

Food, Nutrition and Health, The University of British Columbia, Vancouver, BC, Canada

Key Words

Vegetarian diets · Iron · Zinc · Calcium · Vitamin B_{12} · Omega-3 fatty acids

Key Messages

- Dietary patterns of vegetarians fall on a continuum, ranging from minimal to complete avoidance of animal foods. The specific nutritional implications of vegetarian diets therefore depend upon the foods included and excluded.
- The nutrients of concern for vegetarians are protein, iron, zinc, calcium, vitamin D, vitamin B_{12} and omega-3 fatty acids.
- Iron and zinc are less bioavailable in vegetarian diets. Accordingly, the recommended intakes of these minerals for vegetarians are higher than those for omnivores.
- Although dairy products and eggs contain vitamin B_{12}, deficiency of this nutrient is relatively common among lacto-ovo vegetarians and vegans. Fortified foods or supplements are recommended.
- Vegetarians should also include good dietary sources of the omega-3 fatty acid, α-linolenic acid.
- Though vegetarian diets vary widely in composition, good dietary planning can meet the nutritional needs of individuals across the entire spectrum of vegetarianism.

Introduction

Vegetarianism is said to be increasing in many Western countries, and is associated with significantly lower ischemic heart disease mortality and cancer incidence [1]. Vegetarian diets are often defined as those excluding all meat, poultry, fish and seafood, and may be adopted for a variety of reasons including perceived health benefits, religious or cultural practices, and concerns about animal welfare or environmental sustainability [2]. Among US adults, the prevalence of vegetarianism (defined as 'never' eating meat, fish or poultry) appears to be about 4%, including 1% who are vegan [3]. Prevalence is slightly higher in women than men and in younger than older adults (in both cases, approx. 5 vs. approx. 3%), but varies little according to income and educational attainment [3]. Although well-planned vegetarian diets can meet all nutrient requirements and recommendations for health [2], the nutritional implications vary depending on the type of vegetarian diet followed. Accordingly, the purpose of this article is to describe different types of vegetarian diets, highlight particular nutrients or situations of potential concern, and identify vegetarian food sources of key nutrients.

Table 1. Foods included in and excluded from vegetarian diets

Type of diet	Animal foods excluded	Animal foods included
Semi-vegetarian	may avoid red meat but include poultry and/or fish and seafood	dairy products, eggs
Lacto-ovo-vegetarian	all meat, poultry, fish and seafood	dairy products, eggs
Lacto-vegetarian	meat, poultry, fish, seafood and eggs	dairy products
Vegan	all	none

Types of Vegetarian Diets

Vegetarian diets are typically classified based on the exclusion of meat, fish, poultry, dairy products and eggs (table 1). However, this simple classification does not convey the variability of the dietary practices of those who consider themselves to be vegetarian. In practice, there is a continuum from those who may avoid red meat but consume fish or poultry, through to vegans who avoid all animal-derived foods or ingredients (e.g. gelatin, honey, and vitamin D_3) and may also avoid the use of any animal products (e.g. leather, wool, silk, down).

The nutritional implications of vegetarian diets depend upon the foods included and excluded. Thus, upon hearing that a patient or client is vegetarian, the healthcare practitioner should always ask 'Can you tell me which types of foods you eat and which ones you avoid?' It is also useful to ascertain how often various categories of foods are consumed. For example, questioning might reveal that someone who says she is a lacto-ovo vegetarian consumes dairy products less than once a day, and only eats eggs when they are included as ingredients in other foods (e.g. baked goods). Further to this, it is important to ask these questions at regular intervals, as many individuals transition their diets over time, in some cases reverting to an omnivorous diet and in others progressing farther along the vegetarian continuum.

Nutrients of Potential Concern

Nutrients that may be of concern in vegetarian diets are discussed briefly below, and vegetarian food sources are listed in table 2.

Protein

Although many consumers are concerned about the adequacy of protein in vegetarian diets, these concerns are generally unfounded [2]. Even vegan diets typically provide over 10% of energy as protein, and if energy needs are met, this intake level almost always exceeds the Recommended Dietary Allowance (RDA) for protein. Both dairy products and eggs are high-quality proteins, as is soy protein. And while other plant-based proteins are limiting in one or more indispensable amino acids, provided a variety of plant protein sources is consumed throughout the day (e.g. soy products, legumes, nuts and seeds, grains), there is no need to consume complementary proteins (with different limiting amino acids) at the same meal [2].

Iron

The RDAs for iron are based on consumption of an omnivorous diet including both heme and nonheme iron, in which iron absorption averages about 18% [4]. In contrast, iron absorption averages about 10% on vegetarian diets, which provide only the less well-absorbed nonheme form of iron. Accordingly, recommended iron intakes for vegetarians are 1.8 times higher than those for

Table 2. Nutrients of concern in vegetarian diets and selected food sources

Nutrient	Vegetarian food sources
Iron	dark leafy greens, legumes, enriched grains, nuts, fortified[1] breakfast cereals; include a vitamin C source (e.g. citrus fruits, leafy greens, bell peppers, potatoes, cauliflower) to increase absorption
Calcium	milk and dairy products[2], calcium-fortified[1] beverages (e.g. soy milk, orange juice), calcium-set tofu, low-oxalate dark green vegetables (e.g. kale, broccoli, collards), almonds
Zinc	legumes (e.g. baked beans, chickpeas), soy products, dairy products[2], nuts, grains, fortified[1] breakfast cereals; leavened breads have lower phytic acid content and improved zinc absorption
Vitamin B_{12}	milk and dairy products[2], eggs[2]; vitamin B_{12} is not found naturally in plant-based foods, but fortified[1] products are available (e.g. meat analogues, fortified soy beverages, nutritional yeast)
Vitamin D	fortified cow's milk[2], fortified[1] plant-based beverages (e.g. soy, rice, etc.), fortified[1] orange juice; vitamin D_2 is considered a 'vegan' source
Omega-3 fatty acids	eggs[2], flaxseed, walnuts, canola oil, soybean oil, soybeans

[1] Note that fortification policies vary among countries; accordingly, the nutrient contribution of fortified foods will also vary. [2] Not a vegan source.

omnivores [3]: 32 mg/day (vs. 18 mg/day) for premenopausal adult women and 14 mg/day (vs. 8 mg/day) for adult men and postmenopausal women. It is relatively easy for vegetarian men and postmenopausal women to meet these recommendations. However, since typical diets do not provide iron in amounts recommended for premenopausal vegetarian women, occasional monitoring of iron status may be warranted in this group.

Zinc

Bioavailability of zinc is lower in vegetarian diets, largely due to its binding by phytic acid (found in nuts, grains and legumes). For this reason, it is suggested that the requirement for zinc may be as much as 50% higher on vegan vegetarian diets [4]. The implications of this for Western vegetarians are not clear: although there is no evidence of frank zinc deficiency, detection of marginal deficiency is challenging.

Calcium

Individuals who consume the recommended amounts of milk and dairy products (or fortified plant-based alternatives) as part of a healthy varied diet should meet RDAs for calcium (1,000 mg for women aged 19–50 and men aged 19–70; 1,200 mg for women >50 and men >70), whether they are omnivorous, vegetarian or vegan. However, many adults (regardless of their dietary pattern) do not meet these recommendations, and thus calcium is a nutrient of concern for much of the population. This is particularly true for vegan vegetarians who choose not to use fortified foods, among whom very low calcium intakes and increased fracture risk have been reported [5]. Because of unresolved concerns about potential adverse effects of high calcium intakes achieved through supplementation [6], the recommended approach for those with low calcium intakes is to first maximize calcium intake from food, and to recommend supplements only if necessary to meet the RDA.

Vitamin D

Vitamin D plays an established role in bone health [4], and is also being examined for other possible health outcomes. It is obtained through dietary intake and sunlight exposure (with the amounts synthesized influenced by latitude, season, time of day, skin pigmentation, sunscreen use and age). The RDAs for vitamin D reflect the intake needed to support adequate serum 25(OH)D levels in the absence of sunlight exposure. Both vitamin D_2 and vitamin D_3 are used to fortify foods and are available as supplements. Vitamin D_2 is derived from ultraviolet (UV) irradiation of the plant sterol, ergosterol, and is considered acceptable by vegetarians, while vitamin D_3 is considered an animal source as it is derived from UV irradiation of 7-dehydrocholesterol. When consumed on a daily basis, vitamin D_2 appears to be as effective as vitamin D_3 in supporting serum 25(OH)D levels [7].

Vitamin B_{12}
Although dairy products and eggs contain vitamin B_{12}, deficiency is relatively common among both lacto-ovo vegetarians and vegans [8]. Unfortified plant foods do not contain vitamin B_{12}, so fortified foods or supplements must be used by vegans. It is important to emphasize the need for adequate intakes of this nutrient as high folate intakes typical of vegetarian diets will prevent the megaloblastic anemia typically seen with vitamin B_{12} deficiency. This means that neurological damage may progress without being detected.

Omega-3 Fatty Acids
The nutritionally essential fatty acids include linoleic acid (LA; C18:2n-6) and α-linolenic acid (ALA; C18:3n-3). Both are formed in plants and undergo elongation and desaturation in animal tissues to form arachidonic acid (AA; C20:4n-6, an eicosanoid precursor) and docosahexaenoic acid (DHA; C22:6n-3, a constituent of membrane lipids in the brain and retina). These longer-chain polyunsaturates are found in small amounts in animal foods, but do not occur in vegan diets. And although AA and DHA can be synthesized from LA and ALA, respectively, the amount of DHA formed from ALA is limited. Moreover, n-3 and n-6 fatty acids compete for elongation and desaturation, and vegetarian diets typically contain a high ratio of LA (n-6):ALA (n-3), further limiting DHA synthesis. This, in addition to minimal or zero intake of preformed DHA, leads to tissue DHA levels that are lower in vegetarians, and to an even greater extent in vegans, than in omnivores [9]. DHA is associated with protection against cardiovascular disease and with eye and brain development; accordingly, questions have been raised about the health consequences of lower DHA status among vegetarians. At this point, there is no good evidence of any adverse health effects [9]. Nevertheless, it seems prudent for vegetarians to include good dietary sources of ALA (see table 2).

Vegetarian Diets and Eating Disorders

A very high prevalence of vegetarianism (approx. 50%) has been reported in studies of patients with anorexia nervosa [e.g. 10], leading some to speculate that vegetarianism may contribute to the onset of eating disorders. However, subsequent work has demonstrated that eating attitudes and behaviors of otherwise healthy individuals do not vary meaningfully between vegetarians and non-vegetarians, suggesting that the eating disorder may lead to the vegetarianism, rather than the converse. While further research is needed, unexpected weight loss in individuals who have recently transitioned to a vegetarian diet may serve as a warning sign of a developing eating disorder, and should be evaluated.

Conclusions

- Well-planned vegetarian diets can satisfy all nutrient requirements and recommendations for healthful eating.
- Dietary patterns of those who consider themselves to be vegetarian fall along a continuum, ranging from minimal to complete avoidance of animal foods. Clarifying where an individual falls along this continuum is essential for providing appropriate dietary guidance.
- Potential 'nutrients of concern' for vegetarians include iron, calcium, zinc, vitamin B_{12}, vitamin D, and omega-3 fatty acids. In many cases,

good vegetarian sources of these nutrients are available. For some nutrients (e.g. vitamin B_{12}, calcium, vitamin D, iron in younger women), use of supplements or sufficient quantities of fortified foods may be required, particularly for those following vegan diets.

- Referral to a dietitian with expertise in vegetarian diets may be warranted for individuals who choose to follow vegan diets. A number of websites also provide additional information and dietary guidance (table 3).

Table 3. Websites on vegetarianism and vegetarian diets

www.nlm.nih.gov/medlineplus/vegetariandiet.html. Website on vegetarian diets from Medline Plus, US National Institutes of Health
www.vegetariannutrition.net. Website of the Vegetarian Nutrition Practice Group of the Academy of Nutrition and Dietetics
www.vegsoc.org. Website of the Vegetarian Society of the United Kingdom
www.vrg.org. Website of the Vegetarian Resource Group

References

1 Huang T, Yang B, Zheng J, et al: Cardiovascular disease mortality and cancer incidence in vegetarians: a meta-analysis and systematic review. Ann Nutr Metab 2012;60:233–240.

2 American Dietetic Association: Position of the American Dietetic Association: vegetarian diets. J Am Diet Assoc 2009; 109:1266–1282.

3 Stahler C: How often do Americans eat vegetarian meals? And how many adults in the US are vegetarian? http://www.vrg.org/blog/2012/05/18/how-often-do-americans-eat-vegetarian-meals-and-how-many-adults-in-the-u-s-are-vegetarian/ (accessed April 25, 2013).

4 Otten JJ, Hellwig JP, Meyers LD (eds): Dietary Reference Intakes. The Essential Guide to Nutrient Requirements. Washington, The National Academies Press, 2006.

5 Appleby P, Roddam A, Allen N, Key T: Comparative fracture risk in vegetarians and nonvegetarians in EPIC-Oxford. Eur J Clin Nutr 2007;61:1400–1406.

6 Spence LA, Weaver CM: Calcium intake, vascular calcification, and vascular disease. Nutr Rev 2013;71:15–22.

7 Tripkovic L, Lambert H, Hart K, et al: Comparison of vitamin D_2 and vitamin D_3 supplementation in raising serum 25-hydroxyvitamin D status: a systematic review and meta-analysis. Am J Clin Nutr 2012;95:1357–1364.

8 Pawlak R, Parrott SJ, Raj S, et al: How prevalent is vitamin B_{12} deficiency among vegetarians? Nutr Rev 2013;71:110–117.

9 Sanders TAB: DHA status of vegetarians. Prostaglandins Leukot Essent Fatty Acids 2009;81:137–141.

10 O'Connor MA, Touyz SW, Dunn SM, Beumont PJV: Vegetarianism in anorexia nervosa? A review of 116 consecutive cases. Med J Aust 1987;147:540–542.

Bier D, et al. (eds): Nutrition for the Primary Care Provider. World Rev Nutr Diet. Basel, Karger, 2015, vol 111, pp 58–63
DOI: 10.1159/000362298

Dietary Supplements

Paul M. Coates Paul R. Thomas

Office of Dietary Supplements, National Institutes of Health, Bethesda, Md., USA

Key Words

Dietary supplements · Multivitamin-multimineral supplements · Efficacy · Safety · Food and Drug Administration

Key Messages

- Dietary supplements are widely available and are commonly used by the general public.
- The two main categories of dietary supplements are products composed of vitamins and minerals, and products used for specific health purposes.
- Some dietary supplements, such as calcium, vitamin D and folic acid, may benefit certain groups.
- For the many dietary supplements whose marketing implies specific health benefits, one should refer to recommendations made on their usage by relevant professional societies or other expert bodies.
- Primary-care practitioners should carefully balance the efficacy and safety of a particular supplement to maximize its potential benefits and minimize any risks to the patient.

Introduction

Dietary supplements contain one or any combination of nutrients, herbs and botanicals, amino acids, enzymes, and other ingredients. These constituents are either extracted from their natural sources or chemically synthesized into finished products. Widely available for purchase without a prescription, they are found in many forms, including pills, powders, drinks, and energy bars. Dietary supplements are often promoted as providing health benefits beyond basic nutrition. They are used by people of all ages as a health measure to ensure adequate intake of nutrients, maintain health, prevent illnesses, and to treat or manage various health problems and diseases, both minor (such as indigestion) and those requiring medical attention (such as cancer).

The number and diversity of dietary supplement products in the US marketplace continue to grow. More than 85,000 are estimated to be avail-

Table 1. Recommended Dietary Allowances (RDAs) and tolerable upper intake levels (ULs) for selected nutrients for adults in the United States and Canada

Nutrient	RDA	Tolerable UL
Vitamin B12	2.4 μg (men and women ≥19 years)	data insufficient to set
Vitamin C	90 mg (men ≥19 years) 75 mg (women ≥19 years)	2,000 mg
Vitamin D	600 IU (men and women 19–70 years) 800 IU (men and women >70 years)	4,000 IU
Calcium	1,000 mg (men 19–70 years) 1,200 mg (men >70 years) 1,000 mg (women 19–50 years) 1,200 mg (women >50 years)	2,500 mg (men and women 19–50 years) 2,000 mg (men and women >50 years)
Iron	8 mg (men ≥19 years) 18 mg (women 19–50 years) 8 mg (women >50 years)	45 mg

For simplicity, this table provides the RDAs and ULs for only a few nutrients for adults. The NIH Office of Dietary Supplements website provides the full set of nutrient recommendations as established by the Food and Nutrition Board of the Institute of Medicine, National Academy of Sciences (at http://ods.od.nih.gov/Health_Information/Dietary_Reference_Intakes.aspx).

able, with total sales exceeding USD 32 billion per year in 2012 – an average of almost USD 100 spent by each individual in the United States [1]. Primary-care practitioners (PCPs) should query patients about their supplement use and interests in these products to provide them with the best health care.

Use of Dietary Supplements

There are two broad categories of dietary supplements: products composed of vitamins and minerals, for which recommended and tolerable upper levels of intake exist (table 1), and products used for specific purposes, such as for managing bodily discomforts and illnesses or more generally in the hope of enhancing health or resistance to disease.

Approximately one-half of all Americans use dietary supplements, most commonly basic multivitamin-multimineral (MVMM) supplements whose nutrients are in amounts that approximate a good-quality diet [2]. For people who do not eat as well as they should, supplements may help them to receive adequate amounts of nutrients, even though these products cannot replace the variety of foods that are important to a healthy diet.

Individual nutrients may also be used for nutritional purposes; for example, calcium and vitamin D for bone health and iron for anemia. One reason consumers give for taking dietary supplements is 'to supplement the diet,' but the two most common reasons are 'to improve overall health' and 'to maintain health (stay healthy)' [3].

Dietary supplements taken for nonnutritional purposes include coenzyme Q10 to lower blood pressure and reduce side effects from treatment with a statin medication, the herb echinacea to boost immunity and prevent or treat colds and the flu, and probiotics to treat antibiotic-associated diarrhea or constipation. Available scientific research may or may not support these uses, and in many cases the evidence is insufficient to make a definitive judgment.

To address the appropriate use of dietary supplements with individual patients, the PCP should consider the efficacy and safety of the ingredients and the quality of available product options.

Efficacy

Manufacturers of dietary supplements are not required to prove effectiveness prior to marketing these products. The PCP and patients must use various resources to learn which supplements may promote or improve health, and in whom and under what conditions they may do so.

No US government health agency, private health group, or health professional organization promotes regular use of an MVMM or individual nutrients without considering first the quality of a person's diet. Food, enriched and fortified food products, and even water contribute to one's total nutrient intake. However, individuals with poor nutrient intakes from diet alone, who consume low-calorie diets, or who avoid certain foods (such as strict vegetarians and vegans) might benefit from taking MVMMs. PCPs may prescribe MVMMs for people with medical conditions and diseases that impair digestion, absorption, or use of nutrients. They may also recommend prenatal MVMMs to pregnant patients.

Some nutrients might benefit certain population groups [4]. For example:

- Supplementation with calcium and vitamin D might increase bone mineral density and decrease fracture rates in postmenopausal women.
- Women of childbearing age who might become pregnant should obtain 400 μg/day of synthetic folic acid from fortified foods or dietary supplements. Taking sufficient amounts of folic acid in the first month of pregnancy (a time when many women do not yet know that they are pregnant) reduces the risk of neural tube defects in newborns.
- People over the age of 50 should obtain the recommended intakes of vitamin B_{12} mainly from fortified foods or dietary supplements, because they may be less able than younger people to absorb the protein-bound, naturally occurring vitamin B_{12} in food. In addition, vegans should ensure that their intakes of vitamin B_{12} from fortified foods or supplements are adequate.
- Pregnant women should take an iron supplement as recommended by an obstetrician or other healthcare provider.
- The American Academy of Pediatrics recommends that exclusively and partially breastfed infants receive supplements of 400 IU/day of vitamin D shortly after birth and continue to receive these supplements until they are weaned and consume at least 1,000 ml/day of vitamin D-fortified formula or whole milk [5]. Similarly, all nonbreastfed infants ingesting less than 1,000 ml/day of vitamin D-fortified formula or milk should receive a vitamin D supplement of 400 IU/day.
- The American Academy of Pediatrics advises that children at nutritional risk who might benefit from supplementation include those who have anorexia or an inadequate appetite, follow fad diets, have chronic disease, come from deprived families or suffer parental neglect or abuse, participate in dietary programs for managing obesity, consume a vegetarian diet without adequate dairy products, and have failure to thrive [6].

For the many dietary supplements whose marketing implies or suggests more specific health benefits and improvements, recommendations about their use are in some cases made by relevant professional societies or other expert bodies. For example, the American Heart Association recommends consumption of approximately 1 g/day of the fatty acids EPA and DHA for patients with documented heart disease, from oily fish or supplements [7]. The American Association of Orthopedic Surgeons advises that glu-

Table 2. Information sources on dietary supplements

Source	Access	Notes
Office of Dietary Supplements (NIH)	http://ods.od.nih.gov/ free	comprehensive source of information on supplements, including fact sheets for health professionals and consumers on many supplement ingredients
National Center for Complementary and Alternative Medicine (NIH)	http://nccam.nih.gov free	news, information, and fact sheets on dietary supplements, especially nonnutrient ingredients (e.g. botanicals)
PubMed, National Library of Medicine (NIH)	www.ncbi.nlm.nih.gov/pubmed free	search the biomedical literature on a supplement topic of interest by applying the subject filter of 'dietary supplements'
MedlinePlus, National Library of Medicine (NIH)	http://www.nlm.nih.gov/medlineplus/ free	consumer-friendly reviews of supplement ingredients addressing effectiveness, usual dosage, and drug interactions
US Food and Drug Administration	http://www.fda.gov/Food/DietarySupplements/ free	information on dietary supplement regulations and policies, alerts, and product warnings
Natural Medicines Comprehensive Database	http://naturaldatabase.com subscription based	comprehensive monographs on supplement ingredients; search by ingredient, product name, or medical condition
Natural Standard	http://www.naturalstandard.com subscription based	comprehensive monographs on supplement ingredients; search by ingredient, product name, or medical condition
ConsumerLab.com	http://www.consumerlab.com subscription based	monographs on dietary supplement ingredients with independent evaluations of product quality

NIH = National Institutes of Health.

cosamine and chondroitin not be prescribed for symptomatic osteoarthritis of the knee [8].

Other resources to discover evidence-based information on dietary supplements are described in table 2.

Safety

Most biologically active constituents in dietary supplements are toxic at some dose. Too much vitamin A can cause headaches, liver damage and birth defects, for example, and excess iron causes nausea and vomiting and may damage the liver and other organs. Good information sources on supplement efficacy will address dosing as well as symptoms associated with toxicity.

Nutrients are usually safe when consumed below the tolerable upper intake levels. Most patients who take a basic MVMM or recommended doses of individual nutrients do not exceed these amounts. In some cases, under the care of a healthcare provider, nutrients may be used in high doses for specific medical reasons, and the potential for adverse effects must be monitored. Large doses of the B vitamin niacin, for example, may be used in the medical management of dyslipidemia.

The PCP should consider that some dietary supplements may interact with certain medications and lead to adverse events. For example, vitamin K supplements can reduce warfarin's ability to reduce blood clotting. St. John's wort can speed the breakdown of many drugs from the body (including antidepressants and birth control pills), thereby reducing their effectiveness. Antioxidant supplements such as those with large amounts of vitamins C and E may reduce the effectiveness of some types of cancer chemotherapy.

The PCP and patient should be alert to the possibility of an unexpected side effect from taking a dietary supplement, especially from a product with ingredients other than nutrients at nutritional levels. PCPs in the United States who believe a patient suffered an adverse event from taking a supplement should report it to the US Food and Drug Administration (FDA), call 800-FDA-1088 or complete a form at http://www.fda.gov/Safety/MedWatch/HowToReport. (Other countries may have their own reporting systems.) The FDA relies on these voluntary reports as signals that a product may present safety risks to consumers. Also, report the event to the supplement's manufacturer using contact information on the label. A company is required to report to the FDA any serious adverse event report it receives (e.g. resulting in hospitalization, being life threatening, or causing disability).

PCPs may well be wary about supplement use (beyond basic nutrients at nutritional levels) by children or by pregnant or lactating women. The safety aspects of most supplements have not been well tested in these groups.

Quality

Dietary supplements are often complex products containing multiple ingredients sourced from across the globe. Ensuring consistent high quality in products is a critical task. In the United States, the FDA has established quality standards to help ensure product identity, purity, strength, and composition by preventing the inclusion of the wrong ingredient, too much or too little of an ingredient, the possibility of contamination, and improper packaging and labeling. The FDA periodically inspects manufacturing facilities.

Some supplements in the marketplace are of substandard quality, but the extent of the problem is not known. ConsumerLab.com, a private company that has independently tested the contents of >2,400 supplement products over more than 12 years, identifies approximately 1 in 4 with a quality problem, primarily because of an ingredient present below the labeled amounts or of substandard quality, followed by contamination with heavy metals [9]. FDA has identified hundreds of dietary supplements marketed for sexual enhancement, weight loss, and bodybuilding that have been adulterated with prescription medications [10].

The PCP should recommend supplement products from well-known and established brands and those that have a reputation for rigorous quality control. Several independent organizations offer quality testing and allow the products that pass these tests to display their seals of approval. Organizations that offer this quality testing include the US Pharmacopeia, ConsumerLab.com, and NSF International. Such seals are no guarantee of product safety and effectiveness, however.

Regulation and Oversight

In the United States, dietary supplements, like medications, are overseen by the FDA but are regulated quite differently. Supplements do not require premarket review or approval. They are allowed to make certain health-related, though not disease-related, claims.

The FDA has the authority to remove supplements from the market shown to be unsafe or improperly manufactured. The agency may also take legal action when companies make false or deceptive statements about their products or promote them as disease treatments or cures. The Federal Trade Commission monitors and regulates advertising, marketing, and promotion of supplements in the various media.

Many countries have their own regulatory structure for products known as dietary supplements in the United States. In Canada, for example, they are called Natural Health Products and must be authorized for sale.

Resources

Helpful information sources on dietary supplements are listed in table 2.

Conclusions

- As PCPs pay attention to the health and lifestyle practices of their patients to provide the best medical care, discussions about the dietary supplements they take, or those that might be recommended, are of value.
- The PCP may need to initiate the conversation, as many patients are reluctant to do so. Use of dietary supplements is largely self-determined. Less than a quarter of supplements used by adults are recommended by a physician or other healthcare provider [2].
- The PCP and patient should discuss what supplements may be helpful in particular situations and which may pose any risks. Ideally, they should come to agreement on the best approaches to maximize potential benefits and minimize any risk of harm from using these products.
- Among the questions to discuss are: What are the potential health benefits of each supplement? Might it provide specific benefits to the patient? Does it pose any safety risks? What is a proper dose to take? How, when, and for how long should it be taken?

References

1 NBJ's Supplement Business Report 2013. Nutr Bus J 2013.
2 Bailey RL, Gahche JJ, Lentino CV, et al: Dietary supplement use in the United States, 2003–2006. J Nutr 2011;141:261–266.
3 Bailey RL, Gahche JJ, Miller PE, et al: Why US adults use dietary supplements. JAMA Intern Med 2013;173:355–361.
4 Office of Dietary Supplements, National Institutes of Health: Dietary supplement fact sheet for the health professional: multivitamin/mineral supplements. January 2013. http://ods.od.nih.gov/factsheets/MVMS-HealthProfessional/.
5 Wagner CL, Greer FR; American Academy of Pediatrics Section on Breastfeeding; American Academy of Pediatrics Committee on Nutrition: Prevention of rickets and vitamin D deficiency in infants, children, and adolescents. Pediatrics 2008;122:1142–1152.
6 Kleinman RE (ed): Feeding the child; in Pediatric Nutrition Handbook, ed 5. Washington, American Academy of Pediatrics, chapter 7, 2004.
7 Kris-Etherton PM, Harris WS, Appel LJ: AHA scientific statement: fish consumption, fish oil, omega-3 fatty acids, and cardiovascular disease. Circulation 2002; 106:2747–2757.
8 American Academy of Orthopaedic Surgeons: Treatment of osteoarthritis of the knee (non-arthroplasty). December 6, 2008. www.aaos.org/Research/guidelines/GuidelineOAKnee.asp.
9 Cooperman T: Third party dietary supplement testing: ConsumerLab.com; in Bonakdar RA (ed): The H.E.R.B.A.L. Guide: Dietary Supplement Resources for the Clinician. Philadelphia, Lippincott Williams & Wilkins, 2010, pp 126–130.
10 US Food and Drug Administration: Beware of fraudulent 'dietary supplements'. FDA Consumer Health Information, March 2011. http://www.fda.gov/downloads/ForConsumers/ConsumerUpdates/UCM247107.pdf.

Bier D, et al. (eds): Nutrition for the Primary Care Provider. World Rev Nutr Diet. Basel, Karger, 2015, vol 111, pp 64–70
DOI: 10.1159/000362299

Nutrition in Pregnancy and Lactation

H. Salome Kruger[a] Nancy F. Butte[b]

[a]Centre of Excellence for Nutrition, North-West University, Potchefstroom, South Africa; [b]USDA/ARS Children's Nutrition Research Center, Department of Pediatrics, Baylor College of Medicine, Houston, Tex., USA

Key Words

Pregnancy · Lactation · Weight gain · Iron deficiency · Supplements · Hypertension · Gestational diabetes

Key Messages

- Target women to prevent both insufficient and excessive weight gain.
- Provide prenatal dietary supplementation for nutritionally at-risk mothers to reduce perinatal morbidity.
- Implement weight monitoring and supplementation through primary healthcare.
- Implement periconceptional folic acid supplementation for the prevention of neural tube defects in populations with low folate intakes.
- Promote intermittent rather than daily iron or iron + folic acid supplementation to reduce risk of maternal anemia and iron deficiency at term.
- Counsel pregnant and lactating women to omit alcohol and to drink caffeine-containing drinks in moderation (equivalent of two cups of coffee).

Introduction

Optimal maternal health during pregnancy reduces the risk of suboptimal fetal development [1]. Obesity prevalence is increasing among women of childbearing age in both developed and developing countries. Although teenage pregnancies remain common in some countries, generally women are getting pregnant at an older age, resulting in increased prevalence of hypertension and gestational diabetes [1]. Weight gain within the Institute of Medicine's recommendations is associated with favorable fetal and maternal outcomes, whereas insufficient weight gain is associated with low birthweight (LBW), and excessive gain is associated with infant macrosomia [1]. The key components of nutritional management during pregnancy include consumption of a variety of foods, appropriate weight gain, appropriate micronutrient supplementation, physical activity and avoidance of alcohol, tobacco, and other harmful substances [2].

Table 1. New recommendations for total and rate of weight gain during pregnancy, by prepregnancy BMI

Prepregnancy BMI	Total weight gain range		Rates of weight gain[1]	
	kg	lb	kg/week	lb/week
Underweight (<18.5)	12.5–18	28–40	0.51 (0.44–0.58)	1 (1–1.3)
Normal weight (18.5–24.9)	11.5–16	25–35	0.42 (0.35–0.50)	1 (0.8–1)
Overweight (25.0–29.9)	7–11.5	15–25	0.28 (0.23–0.33)	0.6 (0.5–0.7)
Obese (≥30.0)	5–9	11–20	0.22 (0.17–0.27)	0.5 (0.4–0.6)

Data from Institute of Medicine and National Research Council [1]. Reproduced with permission.
[1] Second and third trimester. Calculations assume a 0.5–2 kg (1.1–4.4 lb) weight gain in the first trimester. Values are expressed as mean (range).

Nutritional Assessment during Pregnancy

Weight monitoring in pregnancy helps clinicians to target women at risk of poor pregnancy outcome. Body mass index (BMI) remains a useful index for evaluating prepregnancy nutritional status in clinical settings; thus, measuring height at the first visit is recommended [1]. Chronically energy-deficient women with short stature (<145 cm), and/or low prepregnancy weight (<45 kg), and/or mid-upper arm circumference <22 cm are considered to be vulnerable to poor pregnancy outcomes such as obstructed labor due to cephalopelvic disproportion [3]. Adolescent pregnancy, high caffeine consumption, smoking and psychosocial stress of the mother were associated with LBW in underweight mothers [1]. Obese women were more likely to deliver infants with macrosomia and require admittance to intensive care than their normal-weight counterparts. Obese women were also more likely to develop hypertension, diabetes mellitus, or urinary tract infections during pregnancy than normal-weight women [3].

Most pregnant women in developing countries seek antenatal care late during pregnancy, so that prepregnancy weight is not available and therefore antenatal care can be based only on rate of gestational weight gain [4]. The recommended mean weekly weight gains range from 0.22 kg/week for obese women to 0.51 kg/week for underweight women from the second trimester of pregnancy onwards (table 1) [1]. Women with established weight gain deviations, less than 1 kg per month or more than 3 kg per month, should receive individualized dietary counseling. Erratically high weight gain is likely to represent edema. A sharp increase in weight gain, edema and hypertension indicate preeclampsia, a serious pregnancy complication [1].

A review of studies supports prenatal programming of childhood obesity. The Dutch famine study found that exposure to maternal malnutrition in early, but not late, gestation was associated with increased odds of childhood obesity [5]. Furthermore, prenatal exposure to maternal smoking showed significantly increased odds of childhood obesity [6]. The use of anthropometric indicators becomes more complex in developing countries, where a large proportion of women are short, but overweight and the prevalence of HIV infection is high among pregnant women [4].

Energy and Nutrient Requirements and Supplementation during Pregnancy

The energy requirement of pregnant women increases throughout pregnancy [7]. For most vitamins and minerals, adequate intakes can be achieved by increasing dietary intake of a variety of foods according to increased energy requirements, but for others, such as folate and iron, supplementation is necessary [2]. There is an association between periconceptional folate intake and the prevention of neural tube defects. Few women use supplements regularly during the periconceptional period, but national fortification programs usually ensure sufficient folate intakes in women of childbearing age to prevent neural tube defects [8, 9].

Anemia in pregnancy remains a public health problem associated with increased risk of LBW in developing countries. A study in Indian pregnant women showed that iron supplementation was associated with significantly increased mean birthweight [10]. Oral iron supplements improve maternal health and pregnancy outcomes, but may cause side effects, such as constipation and nausea. A systematic review to assess the effectiveness and safety of daily versus intermittent iron supplementation in pregnant women showed reduced risk of maternal iron deficiency at term, with no significant difference between the two groups. Side effects were reported more often only in daily supplement users than in placebo groups [11]. Another review showed that fortified beverages and foods generally decreased maternal anemia and iron deficiency and increased birthweight, and also increased birth length and reduced preterm delivery in some studies in developing countries [12]. A systematic review comparing the effect of supplementation with multiple micronutrients versus iron and folic acid on pregnancy outcomes in developing countries showed that multiple micronutrient supplementation was more effective than iron and folic acid supplementation at reducing the risk of LBW [13]. Findings summarized in a recent review of evidence-based interventions for improvement of maternal and child nutrition support the replacement of iron-folate supplements with multiple micronutrient supplements for pregnant women in populations at risk. Multiple micronutrient supplements reduced the risk of LBW and small-for-gestational-age births in vulnerable populations [14].

Evidence suggests that adequate intakes of omega-3 fatty acids, docosahexaenoic acid (DHA) and eicosapentaenoic acid, reduce the incidence of preterm birth and improve infant cognitive and visual performance. Research results on prenatal omega-3 intake and outcomes are, however, inconclusive [15]. Still, studies in low-income countries showed that omega-3 fatty acid intakes were below the recommended minimum for pregnant women [14].

International agencies recommend similar intakes of calcium for pregnant and nonpregnant women [2, 9]. A review of studies in developed countries on the relationship between supplemental calcium and hypertension concluded that a relationship between calcium and risk of pregnancy-induced hypertension and preeclampsia is unlikely [16]. A more recent systematic review of studies including populations with low calcium intakes indicates that risk of high blood pressure, preeclampsia and preterm birth was reduced with calcium supplementation [14, 17]. Iodine deficiency during pregnancy is the main cause of preventable mental retardation in childhood [18]. The results of a systematic review suggest that iodized salt is an effective means of improving iodine status [19]. The WHO recommendation for iodine intake during pregnancy and lactation has recently increased from 200 to 250 μg/day in countries where less than 90% of households use iodized salt. The use of iodized salt in households might not be sufficient to cope with the increased iodine demand during pregnancy. Therefore, iodine supplementation of 150 μg/day in pregnant women is recommended [8]. There is currently insufficient evidence to draw conclusions on the usefulness and safety of isolated zinc supplementation or vitamin D supplementation during pregnancy [14].

Table 2. The management of nutrition-related complications of pregnancy [16, 17, 20]

Complication	Nutritional management
Insufficient weight gain	dietary counseling, food supplementation
Excessive weight gain	dietary counseling, physical activity under supervision
Nausea, hyperemesis	small frequent meals, limit intakes of fats and fried foods; fluid and electrolyte replacement, hospitalization if necessary for intravenous fluids and electrolytes
Poor dietary habits	dietary counseling
Constipation with/without hemorrhoids	dietary counseling to increase fiber and fluid intakes, fiber supplements, dried prunes and figs
Heartburn	smaller, more frequent meals, sit upright after meals
Edema	lie down to rest during the day
Diabetes mellitus/gestational diabetes	individually adapted meal plan in consultation with a dietitian
Pregnancy-induced hypertension	hospitalization, individually adapted meal plan in consultation with a dietitian, calcium supplementation may be useful in persons with low calcium intakes

Nutrition-Related Complications of Pregnancy

Pregnant women with inappropriate weight gain, hyperemesis, poor dietary habits, gestational diabetes or hypertension should be referred to a qualified nutrition professional [2]. Pregnancy during adolescence is a time of nutritional risk due to competition for nutrients between the growing pregnant adolescent and her fetus. The management of nutrition-related complications of pregnancy is summarized in table 2 [20].

Nutritional Assessment and Supplementation during Lactation

Energy requirements of lactating women are increased up to 6 months postpartum [7]. For most vitamins and minerals, adequate intakes can be achieved by increasing dietary intake from a variety of foods according to increased energy requirements [12]. Breastfed infants whose mothers received DHA versus placebo during lactation performed significantly better on the Sustained Attention Subscale of the Leiter International Performance Scale, but there were no statistically significant differences between groups on other neuropsychological domains. At the age of 5 years, the children performed better on a test of sustained attention. This suggests that DHA intake during early infancy confers long-term benefits on specific aspects of neurodevelopment [21].

Problems Experienced by Lactating Women

There is a negative association between maternal obesity and the initiation as well as the continuation of breastfeeding, suggesting that excessive body fat may inhibit lactation performance [22]. Excessive gestational weight gain, insufficient physical activity, excessive food intake and short period or no breastfeeding were each significantly related to postpartum weight retention [23].

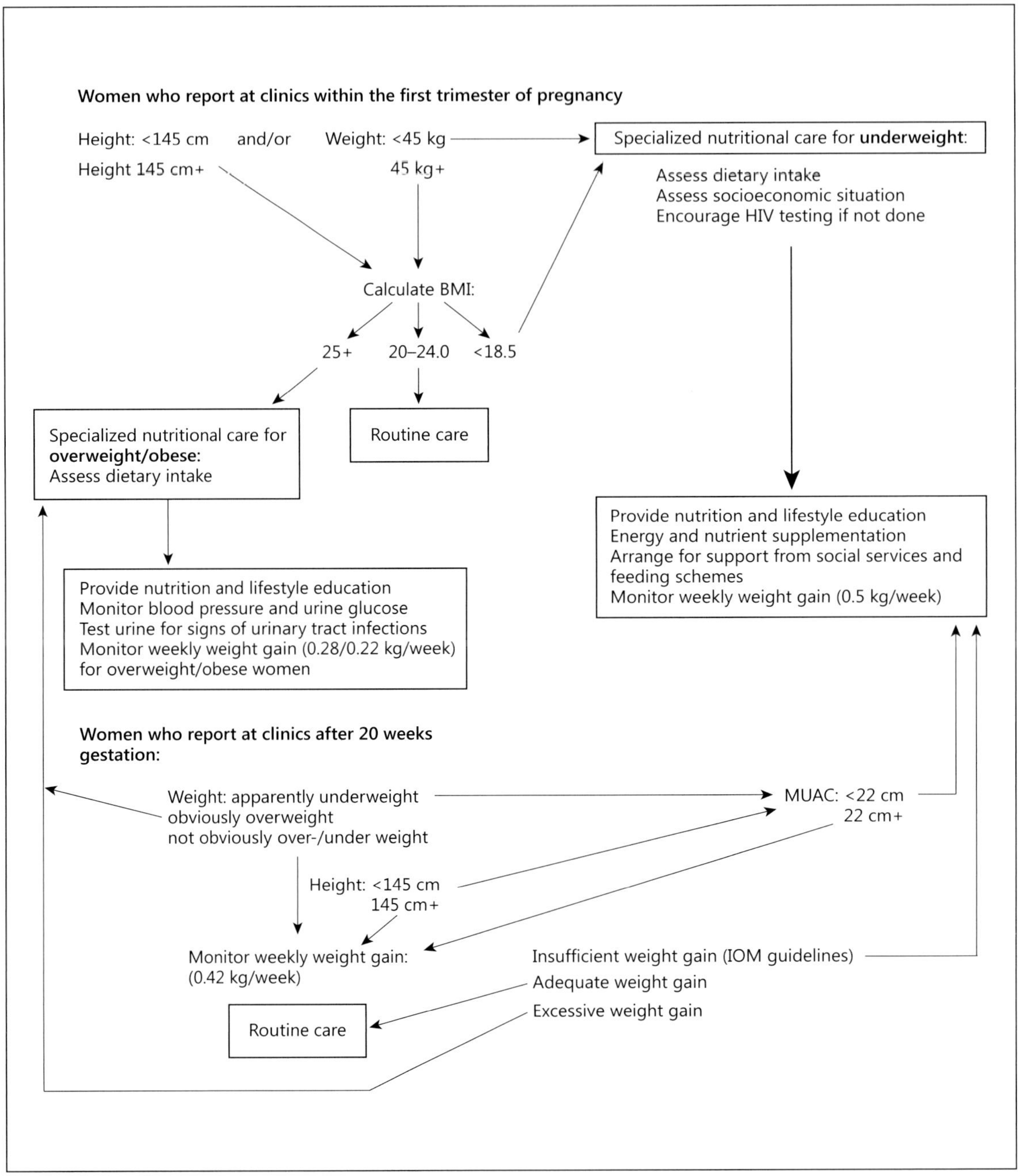

Fig. 1. A framework for the management of pregnancy weight gain [24]. Reproduced with permission from Curationis, AOSIS Open Journals under the Creative Commons Attribution License; http://dx.doi.org/10.4102/curationis.v28i4.1012. MUAC = Mid-upper arm circumference; IOM = Institute of Medicine.

Integrated Intervention

Figure 1 shows a proposed framework for the management of pregnancy weight gain [24]. Health care providers should explain to underweight women why weight gain is important, and they should be counseled to promote a balanced diet consistent with cultural and financial considerations. Undernourished women should receive micronutrient-rich food supplements for at least the last trimester of pregnancy [12]. Special attention to foods rich in or supplements of iron, calcium, and folate may help to decrease perinatal morbidity [2]. Overweight women should receive advice about a balanced diet and be monitored to prevent excessive weight gain [1].

Conclusions

- Women with a weight below 45 kg and/or a height below 145 cm and/or a mid-upper arm circumference smaller than 22 cm during any stage of pregnancy should be referred for specialized nutritional care during pregnancy.
- Women who gain less than 1 kg per month or more than 3 kg per month should be referred to a dietician.
- Overweight women should also receive nutritional care, and their weekly weight gain, blood pressure, urinary glucose and indicators of urinary tract infections should be monitored closely.
- More overweight but micronutrient-deficient women enter pregnancy and produce malnourished infants.
- Strategies to ensure the optimal nutritional status of pregnant and lactating women and their infants include nutrition education, micronutrient fortification and supplementation programs [2, 8, 11, 19].

References

1 Institute of Medicine and National Research Council: Weight Gain During Pregnancy: Reexamining the Guidelines. Washington, The National Academies Press, 2009.

2 Kaiser LL, Allen LH: Position of the American Dietetic Association: nutrition and lifestyle for a healthy pregnancy outcome. J Am Dietet Assoc 2008; 108:553–561.

3 Perlow JH, Morgan MA, Montgomery D, et al: Perinatal outcome in pregnancy complicated by massive obesity. Am J Obstet Gynecol 1992;167(suppl 4):958–962.

4 Villamor E, Msamanga G, Spiegelman D, et al: HIV status and sociodemographic correlates of maternal body size and wasting during pregnancy. Eur J Clin Nutr 2002;56:415–424.

5 Roseboom TJ, Painter RC, van Abeelen AFM, et al: Hungry in the womb: what are the consequences? Lessons from the Dutch famine. Maturitas 2011;70:141–145.

6 Huang JS, Lee TA, Lu MC: Prenatal programming of childhood overweight and obesity. Matern Child Health J 2007; 11(suppl 5):461–473.

7 Butte NF, King JC: Energy requirements during pregnancy and lactation. Public Health Nutr 2005;8:1010–1027.

8 Berti C, Biesalski HK, Gärtner R, et al: Micronutrients in pregnancy: current knowledge and unresolved questions. Clin Nutr 2011;30:689–701.

9 WHO: Vitamin and mineral requirements in human nutrition. Geneva, WHO, 2004.

10 Sharma A, Patnaik R, Garg S, et al: Detection and management of anaemia in pregnancy in an urban primary health care institution. Indian J Med Res 2008; 128:45–51.

11 Peña-Rosas JP, Viteri FE: Effects and safety of preventive oral iron or iron+folic acid supplementation for women during pregnancy. Cochrane Database Syst Rev 2009;CD004736.

12 Yang Z, Huffman SL: Review of fortified food and beverage products for pregnant and lactating women and their impact on nutritional status. Matern Child Nutr 2011;7(suppl 3):19–43.

13 Kawai K, Spiegelman D, Shankarb AH, et al: Maternal multiple micronutrient supplementation and pregnancy outcomes in developing countries: meta-analysis and meta-regression. Bull WHO 2011;89:402–411.

14 Bhutta ZA, Das JK, Rizvi A, et al: Maternal and child nutrition 2. Evidence-based interventions for improvement of maternal and child nutrition: what can be done and at what cost? Lancet 2013; 382:452–477.

15 Guesnet P, Alessandri JM: Docosahexaenoic acid (DHA) and the developing central nervous system (CNS). Implications for dietary recommendations. Biochimie 2011;93:7–12.
16 Trumbo PR, Ellwood KC: Supplemental calcium and risk reduction of hypertension, pregnancy-induced hypertension, and preeclampsia: an evidence-based review by the US Food and Drug Administration. Nutr Rev 2007;65:78–87.
17 Hofmeyr GJ, Lawrie TA, Atallah AN, et al: Calcium supplementation during pregnancy for preventing hypertensive disorders and related problems. Cochrane Database Syst Rev 2010;CD001059.
18 Walker SP, Wachs TD, Gardner JM, et al: Child development: risk factors for adverse outcomes in developing countries. Lancet 2007;369:145–157.
19 Wu T, Liu GJ, Li P, et al: Iodised salt for preventing iodine deficiency disorders. Cochrane Database Syst Rev 2002; CD003204.
20 Erick M: Nutrition in pregnancy and lactation; in Mahan LK, Escott-Stump S, Raymond JL (eds): Krause's Food and the Nutrition Care Process. St Louis, Elsevier Saunders, 2011, pp 340–374.
21 Jensen CL, Voigt RG, Llorente AM, et al: Effects of early maternal docosahexaenoic acid intake on neuropsychological status and visual acuity at five years of age of breast-fed term infants. J Pediatr 2010;157:900–905.
22 Rasmussen KM: Association of maternal obesity before conception with poor lactation performance. Annu Rev Nutr 2007;27:103–121.
23 Olson CM, Strawderman MS, Hinton PS, et al: Gestational weight gain and postpartum behaviors associated with weight change from early pregnancy to 1 y postpartum. Int J Obes Relat Metab Disord 2003;27:117–127.
24 Kruger HS: Maternal anthropometry and pregnancy outcomes: a proposal for the monitoring of pregnancy weight gain in outpatient clinics in South Africa. Curationis 2005;28:40–49.

Bier D, et al. (eds): Nutrition for the Primary Care Provider. World Rev Nutr Diet. Basel, Karger, 2015, vol 111, pp 71–75
DOI: 10.1159/000362301

Exercise and Sports

Ronald J. Maughan[a] Susan M. Shirreffs[b]

[a]School of Sport, Exercise and Health Sciences, Loughborough University, Loughborough, and
[b]New Product Research, GlaxoSmithKline, Brentford, UK

Key Words

Exercise · Athlete · Diet · Energy requirements · Nutrient requirements · Hydration

Key Messages

- Diet and food choices can have a significant impact on athletic performance, with profound implications for health and performance.
- The metabolic and nutritional demands vary between different sports, as well as across the annual cycle of training versus competition.
- Both fat and carbohydrate contribute to energy supply during exercise, with protein contributing a relatively low amount. At low intensities, fat oxidation predominates with a progressive increase in the relative contribution of carbohydrate with increasing intensity.
- Hydration status is important for health and performance as exercise increases water requirements due to additional loss in sweat.
- Athletes should be aware of their needs for specific nutrients, especially calcium, iron and vitamin D. Although supplements do not compensate for an inadequate diet, supplements may be a short-term option when food intake or food choices are restricted.
- Athletes should adopt specific nutrition strategies tailored to their exercise and training needs in order to optimize performance and support good health.

Introduction

With the growing recognition that lifestyle choices have a profound effect on health outcomes, the population has become increasingly polarized. At a time when rates of obesity, diabetes and other noncommunicable diseases continue to rise rapidly, so too is regular recreational exercise becoming more common in at least some parts of the general population. Diet and exercise go hand in hand as key parts of a healthy lifestyle. Neither is completely effective on its own, and attention to both will pay many rewards over a lifetime. Along with recreational exercise, many are tempted to engage in competitive sports: the tens of thousands who successfully complete the big city marathon races are testimony to what can be achieved with regular training, though many others have more modest goals. The elite athlete is often seen as a role model for healthy active lifestyles, but these athletes face a number of nutritional challenges. It is clear that diet can significantly influence athletic performance and the food choices that an athlete makes will have profound implications for both health and performance.

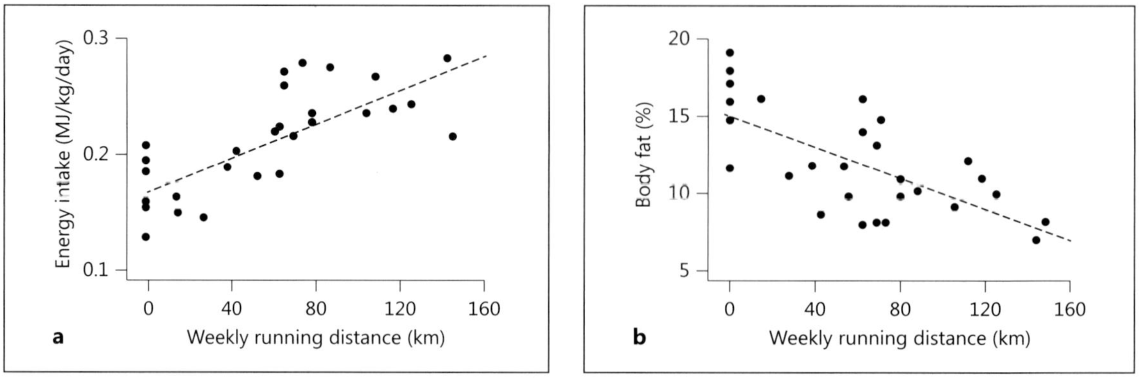

Fig. 1. a Cross-sectional data showing the relationship between energy intake and exercise load (expressed as average weekly running distance for the preceding 10 weeks). All subjects were weight stable and had been active (or sedentary) for at least 2 years. Based on data from Maughan et al. [11]. **b** Cross-sectional data showing the relationship between body fat content and exercise load (expressed as average weekly running distance for the preceding 10 weeks). All subjects were weight stable and had been active (or sedentary) for at least 2 years. In spite of the higher energy intake, those with the highest training loads had the lowest body fat content. Based on data from Maughan et al. [11].

Energy and Nutrient Needs for the Physically Active

The most obvious effect of exercise is to increase the rate of energy expenditure. Resting metabolic rate is about 1–1.5 kcal/min, but the energy cost of walking, jogging or running is about 1 kcal per kg of body mass per km covered, independent of speed. Completing a distance of 5 km therefore requires about 350 kcal for a 70-kg person. At walking speed, this takes an hour, at jogging speed about 30 min and for the serious athlete about 13–16 min. Exercise, if sufficiently intense and prolonged, can therefore impose a high energy demand, and this energy demand must be met from food that is consumed or from the body's endogenous stores, including especially the fat stores. Many of the health benefits of exercise are independent of its effects on body mass and fat levels [1], but if energy intake stays constant, a regular program of exercise should reduce body fat content. Most exercise programs will also increase muscle mass. The available evidence suggests that exercise does stimulate appetite, and an increased food intake will attenuate any reduction in body fat content, but the compensation is not complete and a fall in fat mass should ensue if the exercise program is adhered to (fig. 1). This may require more exercise than is currently recommended to improve cardiovascular and metabolic health: about 200 min or more of moderately vigorous exercise may be required to achieve long-term weight loss and prevent weight regain [2]. Recent studies have suggested that many of the cardiovascular benefits of exercise can be achieved with only a few high-intensity efforts on a few days of the week [3], even though this has little impact on energy balance. Studies with modest exercise programs and diets that are high in protein content have confirmed that it is possible to lose fat mass and gain muscle mass at the same time [4].

Both fat and carbohydrate contribute to energy supply during exercise: there is little change in the rate of net protein catabolism. At low intensities, fat oxidation predominates with a progressive increase in the relative contribution of carbohydrate as intensity increases. At low intensities, however, the rate of energy expenditure is also low, and moderate exercise intensity is likely to have the greatest impact on fat oxidation and potentially also on energy balance [5]. Exercise intensities that are too high are uncomfortable, and only the most motivated will persist.

Although the body has ample fat stores, the carbohydrate store is small – about 80–100 g as glycogen in the liver and about 300–500 g in skeletal muscle. Obligatory glucose use amounts to about 100 g per day, and glycogen use in endurance exercise can reach 2–4 g/min, so an adequate intake of carbohydrate is essential, especially for those who are active. A carbohydrate intake of 4–6 g/kg/day may be recommended on exercise days [6]. Exercise with low carbohydrate availability increases fat use, but the exercise is harder and feels harder. For those likely to be discouraged by effort, this may lead to lack of adherence, especially in the early stages of an exercise program.

Hard physical exercise may lead to a slight increase in the requirement for protein due to a greater protein oxidation during exercise, especially during the early stages of a training program. Protein catabolism is also increased during exercise if glycogen stores are inadequate or if carbohydrate is not consumed during exercise. The extra protein required can, however, be met from the diet: if the training load is sufficient to increase protein requirement, it will usually also increase total energy intake and therefore protein intake. The exception might be when energy intake is restricted to achieve weight loss, when a higher protein intake is advised. A similar consideration is applied to vitamin and mineral requirements. High energy intake will generally result in all needs being met, provided that a varied diet is consumed.

Hydration status is important for health and performance, and regular exercise will increase water requirements because of additional losses in sweat. It is seldom necessary to drink during exercise that lasts less than about 30–40 min, but occasional sips of water may help reduce the perception of effort and thus encourage adherence to the exercise program. In longer exercise sessions, particularly in warm and humid weather, sweat losses may be substantial and consumption of water or a carbohydrate-electrolyte sports drink may be encouraged [7]. One of the primary benefits of maintaining hydration may be a reduction in the perception of effort during exercise: if the exercise feels easier, adherence is likely to be improved. There is now some evidence that simply rinsing the mouth with a carbohydrate-containing drink may enhance performance, perhaps by activation of carbohydrate receptors in the mouth [8].

Energy and Nutrient Needs for Competitive Sport

The elite athlete is characterized by a unique genetic endowment, to which is allied a high degree of motivation and the changes induced by consistent intensive training. The impact of nutrition is relatively small, but at the highest level of sport, the outcome is determined by such small differences.

The metabolic and nutritional demands of sport vary greatly between different sports, and the balance between training and competition also varies between sports and across the annual cycle of training and competition. It is well established that diet significantly influences athletic performance, and athletes are encouraged to adopt specific nutritional strategies before, during and after training and competition to maximize their mental and physical performance. Energy demands depend on the periodized training load and competition program, and will vary from day to day and across the season. A diet that provides adequate energy from a wide range of commonly available foods can meet the carbohydrate, protein, fat and micronutrient requirements of training and competition. Low energy availability should be avoided, as it can impair performance and adaptation to training and may be harmful to brain, reproductive, metabolic and immune function, and to bone health. An appropriate diet will help athletes reach an optimum physique to achieve success in their sport. Careful selection of nutrient-rich foods to reduce the risk of developing nutrient deficiencies that impair both health and performance is especially important when energy intake is restricted to reduce body and/or fat mass.

During high-intensity training, particularly of long duration, athletes should aim to achieve carbohydrate intakes that meet the needs of their training programs and also adequately replace carbohydrate stores during recovery between training sessions and competitions: this may require up to 10–12 g/kg/day of carbohydrate from various sources for some athletes in peak training periods, but athletes in technical events may need only 4–6 g/kg/day [6]. For events lasting an hour or more, the athlete should aim to begin competition with body carbohydrate stores sufficient to meet their needs by consuming carbohydrate-rich foods in the hours and days beforehand. Ingestion of even small amounts of carbohydrate during exercise can enhance cognitive and physical performance in competition lasting 1 h. As the duration of the event increases, so does the amount of carbohydrate needed to optimize performance. To achieve the high rates of intake (up to 90 g/h) needed to optimize performance in events lasting more than about 3 h, athletes should practice consuming carbohydrate during training to develop an individual strategy, and should make use of sports foods and drinks containing carbohydrate combinations that will maximize absorption from the gut and minimize gastrointestinal disturbances.

Dietary protein may be needed in amounts greater (1.2–1.8 g/kg/day) than those recommended for the general population (0.8 g/kg/day), but a varied diet that meets energy needs will generally provide protein in excess of requirements. Foods or snacks that contain high-quality proteins should be consumed regularly throughout the day as part of the day's total protein intake, and in particular soon after exercise, in quantities sufficient to maximize the synthesis of proteins, to aid in long-term maintenance or gain of muscle and bone and in the repair of damaged tissues. Ingestion of foods or drinks providing 15–25 g of such protein after each training session will maximize the synthesis of proteins that underpin these goals.

Dehydration, if sufficiently severe, can impair performance in most events, particularly in warm and high-altitude environments. Athletes should be well hydrated before exercise, and should generally drink sufficient fluid during exercise to limit dehydration to less than about 2% of body mass [7]. Chilled fluids may benefit performance in hot conditions. Athletes should not drink so much that they gain weight during exercise. There are large individual differences in the amount of salt lost in sweat, and some sodium should be included in drinks when sweat losses are high, especially when exercise lasts more than about 2 h. During recovery from exercise, rehydration should include replacement of both water and salts lost in sweat [9].

Athletes should be particularly aware of their needs for some specific nutrients, especially calcium, iron and vitamin D, but supplements are not generally necessary if a varied diet is chosen. The use of supplements does not compensate for poor food choices and an inadequate diet, but supplements that provide essential nutrients may be a short-term option when food intake or food choices are restricted due to travel or other factors [10]. Vitamin D may be needed in supplemental form when sun exposure is inadequate. Of the many different dietary ergogenic aids available to athletes, a very small number may enhance performance for some athletes when used appropriately: examples might include caffeine, creatine, buffering agents and nitrate. Athletes contemplating the use of supplements and sports foods should consider their efficacy, their cost, the risk to health and performance, and the potential for a positive doping test. Supplement use in young athletes should be discouraged, and the focus should be on consuming a nutrient-rich, well-chosen diet to allow for growth while maintaining a healthy body composition. Robust immunity and reduced risk of infection can be achieved by consuming a varied diet adequate in energy and micronutrients, ensuring adequate sleep and limiting other life stress.

Conclusions

- To enjoy all the benefits of sport, athletes and active individuals, whether they compete at the elite level or exercise on a recreational basis, should adopt specific nutrition strategies that can optimize mental and physical performance and support good health.
- An active lifestyle allows more food to be eaten without unwanted weight gain and, provided that a varied diet is eaten, this will provide increased amounts of all essential nutrients.
- A high carbohydrate diet supports a regular exercise program, as carbohydrate is the primary fuel for the exercising muscles.
- Protein requirements are increased by regular exercise, but a varied diet that meets energy needs will provide more than enough protein.
- Maintaining hydration status is important, and extra salt may be needed by some individuals when sweat losses are high.
- Dietary supplements are heavily promoted to athletes and active individuals: most are not beneficial, but a few may help if used appropriately.

References

1 Lee DC, Sui X, Blair SN: Does physical activity ameliorate the health hazards of obesity? Br J Sports Med 2009;43:49–51.

2 Jakicic JM, Davis KK: Obesity and physical activity. Psychiatr Clin North Am 2011;34:829–840.

3 Gibala MJ, McGee SL: Metabolic adaptations to short-term high-intensity interval training: a little pain for a lot of gain? Exerc Sport Sci Rev 2008;36:58–63.

4 Josse AR, Atkinson SA, Tarnopolsky MA, Phillips SM: Increased consumption of dairy foods and protein during diet- and exercise-induced weight loss promotes fat mass loss and lean mass gain in overweight and obese premenopausal women. J Nutr 2011;1419:1626–1634.

5 Achten J, Jeukendrup AE: Maximal fat oxidation during exercise in trained men. Int J Sports Med 2003;24:603–608.

6 Burke LM, Hawley JA, Wong SH, Jeukendrup AE: Carbohydrates for training and competition. J Sports Sci 2011;29 (suppl 1):S17–S27.

7 Shirreffs SM, Sawka MN: Fluid and electrolyte needs for training, competition and recovery. J Sports Sci 2011;29(suppl 1):S39–S46.

8 Carter JM, Jeukendrup AE, Jones DA: The effect of carbohydrate mouth rinse on 1-h cycle time trial performance. Med Sci Sports Exerc 2004;36:2107–2111.

9 Maughan RJ, Shirreffs SM: Dehydration and rehydration in competitive sport. Scand J Med Sci Sports 2010;20(suppl 3):40–47.

10 Maughan RJ, Greenhaff PL, Hespel P: Dietary supplements for athletes: emerging trends and recurring themes. J Sports Sci 2011;29(suppl 1):S57–S66.

11 Maughan RJ, Robertson JD, Bruce AC: Dietary energy and carbohydrate intakes of runners in relation to training load. Proc Nutr Soc 1989;48:170A.

Bier D, et al. (eds): Nutrition for the Primary Care Provider. World Rev Nutr Diet. Basel, Karger, 2015, vol 111, pp 76–81
DOI: 10.1159/000362302

Food Allergy and Food Intolerance

John Leung[a–d] Sheila E. Crowe[e]

[a]Food Allergy Center at Tufts Medical Center and Floating Hospital for Children, and Departments of [b]Gastroenterology, [c]Pediatric Gastroenterology, and [d]Allergy and Immunology, Tufts Medical Center, Boston, Mass., and [e]Division of Gastroenterology, Department of Medicine, University of California at San Diego, San Diego, Calif., USA

Key Words

Food allergy · Food intolerance · IgE · Dietary restriction · Nutritional deficiency

Key Messages

- Adverse reactions to food can be classified as either immune mediated (e.g. food allergy, FA) or non-immune mediated (e.g. food intolerance, FI). Non-immune-mediated reactions are the most prevalent.
- Eight foods (milk, eggs, peanuts, tree nuts, soy, wheat, fish and shellfish) account for 90% of all IgE-mediated food allergies.
- Celiac disease is a classical example of a non-IgE-mediated adverse food reaction that affects 1% of the population. Examples of other immune-mediated adverse food reactions are food protein-induced enterocolitis syndrome, eosinophilic esophagitis and eosinophilic gastrointestinal disorders.
- FI is much more common than FA. Examples of FI include food poisoning, lactose intolerance, as well as toxic, pharmacological, and functional adverse reactions to foods. Quite often, these reactions mimic reactions due to FA.
- Appropriate diagnosis is important in order to avoid the unnecessary elimination of a particular food item from the diet.
- When a restricted diet is clinically indicated for long-term management, it should be undertaken under close supervision from an experienced nutritionist and expert physician to reduce the risk of nutritional deficiencies.

Introduction

Food allergy (FA) is defined as an adverse health effect arising from a specific immune response that occurs reproducibly on exposure to a given food. FA is a growing public health concern and its prevalence seems to be on the rise. It is estimated that 9 million, or 4%, of adults have FA in the United States. Up to 20% of the population, however, frequently confuses food intolerance (FI) with FA, leading to unnecessary dietary restriction and potential nutritional deficiency. In

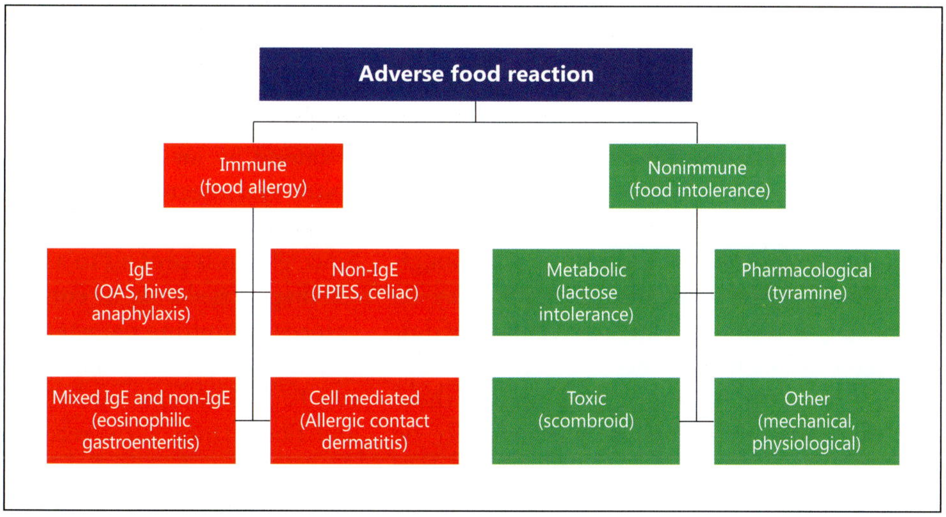

Fig. 1. Classification of adverse food reactions. FPIES = Food protein-induced enterocolitis syndrome; OAS = oral allergy syndrome. Adapted from Boyce et al. [1].

this chapter, we will discuss the key clinical features that distinguish FA from FI, with a special focus on the nutritional deficiency and its management.

Food Allergy versus Food Intolerance

In general, any adverse reaction to food can be classified into either immune mediated (e.g. FA) or nonimmune mediated (FI), with the latter being the most prevalent (fig. 1). The fundamental difference between FA and FI is that the former is immune mediated, while the latter is not [1]. In clinical practice, it is of paramount importance to distinguish the two, because their clinical implication and nutritional needs are distinctly different. For instance, while consumption of milk in a patient with lactose intolerance causes self-limited symptoms such as diarrhea, bloating and abdominal discomfort, ingestion of even a trace amount of milk by a patient with cow milk allergy (CMA) can trigger potentially life-threatening anaphylactic shock.

Food Allergy

To understand FA, we first need to understand the nomenclature. 'Allergy' has conventionally been associated with IgE-mediated processes. It is therefore not surprising that FA is often equated to IgE-mediated FA, though there are other food allergies that are not IgE mediated. For our discussion, we will use the term 'IgE-mediated food allergy' to specifically refer to FA that are mediated by IgE. Another term you may encounter in the literature is food hypersensitivity. It is often used to describe FA, although some have used this term more broadly to include FI. For this reason, we will avoid using the term food hypersensitivity in our discussion.

Eight foods account for 90% of all IgE-mediated food allergies: milk, eggs, peanuts, tree nuts, soy, wheat, fish and shellfish [1].The onset of symptoms is rapid and even minute amounts of the allergen can trigger severe reactions. The reactions can range from self-limited localized hives to life-threatening generalized anaphylaxis. Common symptoms include hives, pruritus, erythema, angioedema, nasal congestion, cough, chest tightness, vomiting, nausea, diarrhea, dizziness, wheezing and rhinoconjunctivitis. Patients with suspected IgE-mediated FA should be referred to an allergist for evaluation and management.

Shellfish, peanut, tree nuts and fish are responsible for most of the FA in adults. Although these foods contain valuable nutrients, they do not usually account for a large percentage of daily dietary intake in a Western diet. Many other foods can supply the nutrients found in these specific foods, and substitution can easily be made. Although significant nutritional deficiency secondary to a single FA is rare among adults in the US, CMA, wheat allergy and multiple food allergies (MFA) remain a significant challenge for nutritionists and clinicians. Adults with CMA are at risk of vitamin D and calcium deficiency because it is difficult to meet calcium needs through nondairy sources without careful substitution. Therefore, calcium supplements should always be considered in patients with CMA to reduce the risk of osteoporosis and fracture [2].

Wheat is present in many processed foods such as crackers, cookies, cakes, pasta, bread and cereal. Moreover, wheat is also a minor ingredient in condiments, marinades, cold cuts, soy sauce, hard candies, low-fat products, etc. The major product of wheat, wheat flour, is a great source of carbohydrates, iron, thiamine, riboflavin, niacin, folic acid, vitamin B_6, magnesium and fiber. Fortunately, there are a wide variety of wheat-free products made from alternative flours (rice, corn, oat, barley, buckwheat, rye, amaranth, millet and quinoa). The availability of gluten-free foods can also benefit those with wheat allergy. It is important to note that up to 20% of the individuals with an allergy to one grain will have allergies to other grains. Use of these alternative grain products should be individualized and based upon tolerance as determined by an allergy specialist.

Non-IgE-Mediated Adverse Reactions to Food

Celiac disease is a classical example of non-IgE-mediated adverse food reaction found in adults. It is caused by an abnormal immune reaction to gluten and affects 1% of the population [3]. Life-long elimination of gluten is the only treatment. Since gluten is present in a variety of food items, the diagnosis should be confirmed by a specialist before committing patients to a life-long gluten-free diet. Gluten-free diets are often low in vitamin B, calcium, vitamin D, iron, zinc, magnesium and fiber. Until fairly recently, few gluten-free products were enriched or fortified, adding to the risk of nutritional deficiency. Food protein-induced enteropathy is another non-IgE-mediated adverse reaction to food, and is most commonly seen in young infants.

Other Immune-Mediated Adverse Reactions to Food

Examples of other immune-mediated adverse food reactions are food-induced allergic contact dermatitis, eosinophilic gastrointestinal disorders and eosinophilic esophagitis (EoE). EoE deserves special attention because a subset of patients respond very well to elimination diets, which pose significant nutritional risks. EoE is a chronic immune-/antigen-mediated disorder characterized by eosinophilic infiltration of the esophagus [4]. Adults with EoE often present with refractory reflux, epigastric or chest pain, dysphagia and food impaction. The majority of affected adults are men in their 20s or 30s. Over the past few years, the treatment modality for adults has shifted from primarily medical (swallowed topical corticosteroids) to dietary approach (elimination diet) [5]. The three primary dietary treatment options are testing-directed elimination (foods are eliminated based on allergy testing results), empirical elimination (milk, soy, egg, wheat, peanut/tree nuts, and fish/shellfish are eliminated) and elemental diet (amino-acid based formula that eliminates all potential food allergens). If a dietary approach is employed, patients should be closely followed by a registered dietitian to avoid nutritional deficiency.

Food Intolerance

FI is much more common than FA. Examples of FI include food poisoning, lactose intolerance, as well as toxic, pharmacological, and functional adverse reactions to foods. Quite often, these reactions mimic reactions due to FA. It is therefore important to keep in mind the differential diagnosis when evaluating patients with suspected FA.

Food poisoning typically manifests as nausea, vomiting, fever, abdominal pain and diarrhea. A good history and physical examination is usually sufficient to distinguish such reactions from FA. GI infections can also result in transient lactose intolerance. Since most food poisoning episodes are self-limited, they do not pose a significant risk for malnutrition.

Lactose intolerance is the most common adverse reaction to a specific food, with most cases resulting from a genetically regulated reduction of intestinal lactase activity later in adult life [6]. The lactose intolerance breath test provides a simple, accurate and noninvasive way to confirm the diagnosis. It is important to confirm the diagnosis so patients will not unnecessarily avoid milk consumption, which is one of the most bioavailable sources of ingested calcium and vitamin D. Naturally low-lactose dairy products such as yogurt, hard cheeses and kefir are typically well tolerated in patients with lactose intolerance. Commercially available lactase enzymes can be added to lactose-containing food or ingested with meals containing lactose to reduce symptoms. Moreover, lactose-free milk products are readily available in grocery stores. Since patients with lactose intolerance often have significantly lower calcium intake, calcium supplementation should be considered to reduce the risk for osteoporosis and fracture [7].

Scombroid fish poisoning is the most common seafood-associated disease in the US. Shortly after ingesting contaminated fish, patients experience acute onset of flushing, a sensation of warmth, an erythematous rash, palpations and tachycardia [8]. The symptoms resemble an IgE-mediated allergic reaction and are often misdiagnosed as FA, leading to unnecessary diet restriction and nutritional compromise.

Pharmacological reactions to food or food additives represent a relatively common type of FI. Ingestion of foods with high histamine content such as well-ripened cheese, pickled cabbage, red wine and tuna fish can cause a wide range of allergic-like symptoms in susceptible individuals with a genetic defect in the metabolism of exogenous histamine [9]. In some instances, FI can result from drug-food interactions. A classic example is hypertensive crisis observed in individuals taking monoamine oxidase inhibitors and ingesting tyramine-rich food (e.g. wine and cheese). Adverse reactions to food additives such as artificial colors (FD&C yellow No. 5) and various preservatives (for example, sulfites) are other examples of FI. Avoidance is the only treatment. Management of the nutritional needs for these FI is similar to that of food allergies, but they are typically not a concern given a less restricted list of foods to be avoided in such disorders. Functional FI no doubt exists and appears to be more prevalent in patients with irritable bowel syndrome and other functional GI disorders with or without underlying psychiatric disorders [10]. Patients often report adverse reactions to multiple foods. They often self-eliminate multiple food classes from their diet and are at particular high risk for nutritional deficiency. Since some patients may be willing to reintroduce foods into their diet if diagnostic tests fail to confirm a food-related reaction, targeted skin testing, specific IgE serology and/or food challenges may be helpful in liberalizing

Table 1. Useful resources for patients suffering from FA

General information
http://www.foodallergy.org/
http://www.niaid.nih.gov/topics/foodallergy/Pages/default.aspx
http://www.aaaai.org/conditions-and-treatments/allergies/food-allergies.aspx
http://www.acaai.org/allergist/allergies/Types/food-allergies/Pages/default.aspx
http://community.kidswithfoodallergies.org/about
Food allergy recipes
http://www.realfoodallergyfree.com/allergy-free-recipe-index/
http://www.kidswithfoodallergies.org/recipes/allergy-friendly-recipes.php
http://www.foodallergykitchen.com/pages/recipes.php

their diet and minimizing nutritional risk. On the other hand, this same group of patients is also more likely to supplement their diet with supratherapeutic amounts of 'health food' preparations and nutritional supplements. The dangers of oversupplementation are well described.

Symptoms triggered by physiological reactions to food are frequently encountered in clinical practice. Fatty foods, chocolate, peppermint, colas, red wine, orange juice and excessive alcohol are known to reduce lower esophageal sphincter pressure and worsen symptoms of gastroesophageal reflux disease. Legumes, onions, cabbage, bran fiber, and grains serve as a substrate for gas production by colonic flora and can aggravate bloating symptoms. These physiological reactions to foods are typically noted by patients with functional GI disease, many of whom appear to exhibit heightened sensory responses to normal digestive events. As long as a balanced diet is maintained, avoidance of the specific food items described herein has virtually no impact on nutritional status.

Special Nutritional Issues of Multiple Food Allergies

In the previous sections, we discussed the nutritional management of patients with a particular FA. Patients with MFA present a unique diagnostic and nutritional challenge. They are at high risk for malnutrition. Although MFA is more commonly seen in pediatric patients, it is infrequently seen in adults. One example is adult patients undergoing multiple food elimination diet for the treatment of EoE. Close monitoring of nutritional status is warranted, and supplements should be considered in appropriate settings. The same applies to patients with specific immune-mediated food-induced conditions who are on a restricted diet for other reasons (e.g. a strict vegetarian with celiac disease). Clinicians should be sensitive to a patient's dietary preference and understand that changing one's diet might not be acceptable to the individual for cultural, religious or other reasons. Some useful resources for patients suffering from FA are listed in table 1.

Conclusions

- Dietary limitation due to adverse reactions to food can have a significant impact on nutritional intake.
- It is therefore important to identify individuals in whom restricted diets are truly justified.
- When a restricted diet is clinically indicated for long-term management, it should be undertaken under close supervision from an experienced nutritionist and expert physician to reduce the risk of nutritional deficiencies.

References

1 Boyce JA, Assa'ad A, Burks AW, et al: Guidelines for the diagnosis and management of food allergy in the United States: report of the NIAID-sponsored expert panel. J Allergy Clin Immunol 2010;126:S1–S58.

2 Jensen VB, Jørgensen IM, Rasmussen KB, et al: Bone mineral status in children with cow milk allergy. Pediatr Allergy Immunol 2004;15:562–565.

3 Rubio-Tapia A, Hill ID, Kelly CP, et al: ACG clinical guidelines: diagnosis and management of celiac disease. Am J Gastroenterol 2013;108:656–676.

4 Dellon ES, Gonsalves N, Hirano I, et al: ACG clinical guideline: evidenced based approach to the diagnosis and management of esophageal eosinophilia and eosinophilic esophagitis (EoE). Am J Gastroenterol 2013;108:679–692 .

5 Vashi R, Hirano I: Diet therapy for eosinophilic esophagitis: when, why and how. Curr Opin Gastroenterol 2013;29: 407–415.

6 Swagerty DL, Walling AD, Klein RM: Lactose intolerance. Am Fam Physician 2002;65:1845–1850.

7 Di Stefano M, Veneto G, Malservisi S, et al: Lactose malabsorption and intolerance and peak bone mass. Gastroenterology 2002;122:1793–1799.

8 Hungerford JM: Scombroid poisoning: a review. Toxicon 2010;56:231–243.

9 Maintz L, Novak N: Histamine and histamine intolerance. Am J Clin Nutr 2007;85:1185–1196.

10 Kelsay K: Psychological aspects of food allergy. Curr Allergy Asthma Rep 2003; 3:41–46.

Bier D, et al. (eds): Nutrition for the Primary Care Provider. World Rev Nutr Diet. Basel, Karger, 2015, vol 111, pp 82–86
DOI: 10.1159/000362303

Religion and Culture

H.H. Vorster

Centre of Excellence for Nutrition, North-West University, Potchefstroom Campus, Potchefstroom, South Africa

Key Words

Religion · Culture · Ethnicity · Traditional dietary practices · Medical and spiritual care

Key Messages

- Health professionals (HPs) should be aware, sensitive and respectfully support differences in religion, cultural values and dietary practices of clients and patients.
- HPs should develop cultural competency and follow ethical guidelines to interact with patients to ensure good communication and treatment compliance.
- HPs should not depart from evidence-based practices, nor use religious and cultural practices as part of treatment, but may discuss medical and dietary issues in context of a shared faith and culture.
- In the cultural process, HPs should not generalize, be condescending, biased or patronizing.
- A good caring relationship may overcome cultural missteps and mistakes.

Introduction

Modern medicine is evidence based. Nevertheless, all health professionals (HPs) will at some time in their career have to consult and treat clients and patients with religious beliefs and from cultures other than their own, who may regard evidence less important than their own convictions. HPs should therefore develop awareness and skills to become culturally competent.

A patient's religion and culture will determine what it means to be ill and how an individual will behave as a client or patient. Religion and culture will influence communication and rapport between HPs and patients, as well as treatment compliance and follow through. It could, therefore, determine a patient's response to treatment recommendations, including dietary prescriptions. Dietary practice is a learned behavior, and food has great symbolic meaning in many cultures and religions.

Development of Cultural Competency

To develop cultural competency for the best possible treatment and prevention outcomes, three main facets of culture, ethnicity, religion, spirituality and health should be understood by HPs: (1) the problematic area about the scientific evidence that religion and prayer influence health outcomes; (2) the need to acquire knowledge about the beliefs and practices of different religions and cultures that could impact on dietary practices and health care; (3) the necessity to develop awareness about ethical guidelines for interaction with patients with different religious and cultural persuasions and eating patterns, and skills to apply these guidelines in practice.

Religion

An individual's religion is the personal awareness, conviction, belief and commitment to and serving of God or a god (a supreme being of supernatural powers) with worshipful devotion and conduct in accordance with divine commands as found in sacred writings or declared by authoritative teachers [1].

Science and religion share a complex history and relationship. In the past, spiritual and medical care, including dietary prescriptions and advice, were often dispensed by the same person [2].

Although many believe that religion and prayers contribute to healing, and many can cope better with ill-health because of the comfort and strength of their religion, there is no convincing scientific evidence that prayers can heal [2]. The evidence is weak and inconsistent. Part of the problem to prove the relationship between religion and health is methodological. Examining this relationship would depend on how religion as exposure and health as outcome are defined and measured. Such a relationship would be confounded by a host of factors such as genetics, epigenetics, age, sex, education, socioeconomic status, health status, and health behaviors such as vegetarianism, smoking, alcohol consumption, stress and sexual activity. Most studies that report a relationship did not control for all confounders, while well-conducted studies report conflicting findings [2].

On the other hand, modern nutrition abounds with evidence that certain dietary practices contribute to nutrient adequacy and protection against diseases by influencing biological risk factors. This evidence forms the basis of authoritative dietary recommendations to prevent and treat disease. Fortunately, many of these practices form part of religious dietary rules and/or traditional (cultural) eating patterns.

Culture and Ethnicity

Culture is the total pattern of human behavior in thoughts, speech, actions and artifacts. It is the body of acquired knowledge, values, morals, beliefs, practices and customs, opinions, laws, traditions, religion, superstition and art, possessed and expressed by a designated group. It is: all human, nongenetic or nonmetabiological phenomena [1, 3]. Ethnicity is that part of our identity derived from membership, usually through birth, in a racial, religious, national, social or linguistic group or subgroup with its associated culture [3].

Culture is often characterized by ethnicity, traditional values and specific religious and spiritual practices. Culture influences attitudes to medical treatment, determines special meaning of medicines and diet (dietary preferences, food selection and preparation), childcare practices, power relationships within communities, household relationships, and many other everyday life practices.

The same religion can be found in different cultural groups and one cultural group may have subgroups or individuals with different religious beliefs.

Table 1. Religious dietary practices

Religion	Dietary practices	Background
Buddhism	Vegetarian diet (refrain from meat); moderation in all foods; fasting (monks after noon)	A religion about lifestyle; natural foods of the earth considered to be the most 'pure'
Christianity: (many different denominations)	Selective fasting and restrictions during holy days, slightly different in the different denominations	Bible: Old and New Testament: bread and wine at communion symbolic of Christ's body and blood shed for salvation of man
Eastern Orthodox	Selective fasting; restrictions on meat and fish	Bible: fasting and restrictions on holy days to increase spiritual progress
Protestant (different sub-groups)	Few restrictions of food or fasting; moderation in eating and drinking advised	Bible: God made all plants, fish and animals for mankind's husbandry and enjoyment, for use in moderation
Roman Catholic and related faiths	Fasting practiced; meat restricted on certain days	Bible: restrictions consistent with specified days on church calendar
Seventh-day adventist (Sabbatarians)	Vegetarianism advised; pork, alcohol, tea, and coffee prohibited and meat and fish avoided; fasting practiced	Bible: Sabbath on Saturday; dietary practices must honor and glorify God by practicing moderation
Mormonism (Church of Jesus Christ of the Latter Day Saints)	Alcohol and beverages containing caffeine prohibited; moderation in all foods; fasting practiced; meat to be eaten sparingly	Word of Wisdom; Book of Mormon; fasting is the discipline of self-control and honoring God; caffeine is addictive and leads to poor health
Hinduism	Fasting on specific days; beef prohibited; other meat and fish restricted or avoided; lacto-ovo-vegetarian	From the Vedic-Brahman civilization; the cow is sacred and cannot be eaten, but products (dairy) from the cow are pure and desirable; fasting promotes spiritual growth; respect for life is the basis for abstaining from meat and fish
Islam	Only 'halal' meat allowed; pork, certain birds and alcohol prohibited; tea, coffee and stimulants avoided; fasting on certain days (no food and drinks during daytime)	Halal meat (animals slaughtered according to religious prescription from the Qur'an (Koran); fasting has a cleansing effect of evil elements; correct eating is for good health and spiritual awareness
Judaism	'Kosher' laws guide eating; pork and non-fish sea foods, and meat and dairy in the same meal prohibited; leavened foods restricted during certain periods; fasting on certain days	Torah: Kosher practices prescribed; land animals without cloven hoofs and not chewing their cud (e.g. pig, hare, camel) are 'unclean' and forbidden; separate kitchen utensils for meat and dairy
Rastafarianism (Ital religion and diet)	Vegetarian (meat and fish restricted); added salt(s), preservatives and condiments restricted; alcohol, soft drinks, tea and coffee prohibited but herbal drinks allowed	A lifestyle based on individual meditation; pigs and shellfish are scavengers and not allowed; marijuana used for medicinal and medical purposes and seen as one of the herbs allowed

Dietary Practices of Different Religions and Cultures

Many religious dietary practices developed because of religious rules or ethnic heritage, often based on food hygiene and safety issues. In different religions, specific foods have different meanings, and certain foods, drinks and practices are either restricted to holy days or are general religious prescriptions. These include abstaining, fasting, restriction or totally forbidden foods. Table 1 gives a brief description of some dietary practices of a few religions.

In different parts of the world, many cultural groups and individuals follow diets based on traditions and foods (especially staples) that were available in the past. Examples are the Paleolithic diet (no starchy vegetables and grains, no dairy and no alcohol); carnivore diet (no carbohydrate-containing foods); omnivore diet (our typical 'modern Western' diet with a wide variety of plant and animal derived foods); Mediterranean diet (rich in vegetables, olive oil and fish); vegan and vegetarian diets (from total to selective restriction of animal-derived foods), as well as many traditional eating patterns [4, 5] of indigenous peoples all over the world.

It is useful to gain knowledge of dietary staples, any forbidden foods and practices, rituals, indigenous foods, traditional dishes, recipes, preparation methods and nutrient content of the diets of cultures in the HPs environment [5]. This information can help to analyze cultural influences on nutrient intakes and also for culture-sensitive dietary recommendations [5]. However, although some of these traditional diets, such as the hunter-gatherer diet followed by Australian aborigines in the past, are known to protect against cardiovascular and other diseases [6], they are not practical, accessible or acceptable any more.

Recommendations for Becoming Culturally Competent

(1) Be cautious about the cultural process. Be careful not to generalize, be condescending, biased and patronizing. Treat all patients and clients with respect, empathy, and interest. Culture is not restricted to people of color. Some people are not comfortable with an ethnic label; they want to be treated like 'everyone else'. Also, many immigrants from different cultures may be in a process of acculturation, adopting a new, and 'Westernized' culture and diet [7]. 'Remove' or ignore your own cultural and religious assumptions when communicating with patients with other cultures and religions. Show a willingness to understand theirs.

(2) Be aware of the different cultural values that influence decision making, compliance to dietary recommendations and health behaviors. These include inter alia people's relationship with nature (subjugating, submitting or in harmony), how the client sees disease (as punishment?) and the client's interpersonal relationships (vertical and authoritarian, horizontal and communal, egalitarian and sharing or individualistic). The client's time orientation (past, present or future) will determine actions taken towards health matters. The child-elder orientation will determine who is taking decisions in a family.

(3) Because of the diversity and wide variety in eating patterns, it is advised that HPs should assess cultural dietary practices of patients by asking appropriate and relevant questions before planning a dietary prescription and menus. This will ensure compliance to recommended diets.

(4) For these assessments, good communication skills are necessary. A few guidelines are:

- A hospital or other health setting may be experienced as being 'intrusive'. Approach the client with care and make sure you are speaking to the right person (for example in some cultures, in the case of a child, it may be the grandmother and not the parents).
- Some cultures regard formality of address as a sign of respect. Introduce yourself and ask the client how he or she would like to be addressed. This is also valid for 'touch'. Ask the client what is allowable.
- Ensure that the right 'distance' between you and the client is kept. People from some cultures prefer close proximity while others prefer more distance. This may even be applicable in the way the furniture in the interview/assessment room is arranged.

- The use of interpreters in the case of culture and language barriers may be helpful, but some may 'distort' the message based on their own knowledge or interpretation of cultural issues. The fact that the interview language is probably not the first language of the client may cause misunderstandings and 'crosstalk'. Therefore, gain knowledge of special meanings of specific words in the relevant culture.

(5) When interviewing or treating clients from religions different from your own, take account of the differences, be respectful but never try to influence the religious commitment of the client. It is unethical and inappropriate for HPs to depart from established, evidence-based practices into alternative medicine [2]. Using religious practices as part of treatment can do harm. However, there is no ethical problem for the HP and patient to discuss medical issues in context of a shared culture and faith.

(6) A good caring relationship may overcome cultural missteps and mistakes.

Conclusion

- Dietary assessments, advice and treatment of clients or patients from cultures and religions different from your own can be a challenge.
- But with goodwill, knowledge of and respect for dietary practices determined or influenced by religion, tradition, or a specific culture, barriers can be overcome to ensure compliance to dietary recommendations.

References

1 Gove PB (ed): Webster's Third New International Dictionary of the English Language. Cologne, Köneman, 1993, p 2662.

2 Sloan RP, Bagiella E, Powell T: Religion, spirituality, and medicine. Lancet 1999; 353:664–667.

3 Hartog J, Hartog EA: Cultural aspects of health and illness behavior in hospitals. West J Med 1983;139:910–916.

4 Kuhnlein HV, Recevuer O: Dietary change and traditional food systems of indigenous peoples. Ann Rev Nut 1996; 16:417–442.

5 Vorster HH, Oosthuizen W, Jerling JC, et al: The nutritional status of South Africans: a review of the literature from 1975–1996. Chapter 5: cultural influences on dietary patterns. Durban, Health Systems Trust, 1997, pp 29–30. http://www.healthlink.org.za/hst.

6 Naughton JM, O'Dea K, Sinclair A: Animal foods in traditional Australian aboriginal diets: polyunsaturated and low in fat. Lipids 1986;21:684–690.

7 Salant T, Lauderdale DS: Measuring culture: a critical review of acculturation and health in Asian immigrant populations. Soc Sci Med 2003;57:71–90.

Bier D, et al. (eds): Nutrition for the Primary Care Provider. World Rev Nutr Diet. Basel, Karger, 2015, vol 111, pp 87–93
DOI: 10.1159/000362304

Approach to the Patient and Differential Diagnosis

L. John Hoffer[a] Bruce R. Bistrian[b]

[a]Lady Davis Institute for Medical Research, Jewish General Hospital, McGill University, Montreal, Que., Canada;
[b]Beth Israel Deaconess Medical Center, Harvard Medical School, Boston, Mass., USA

Key Words

Protein-energy malnutrition · Micronutrient deficiency · Intestinal malabsorption · Inflammation · Weight loss · Cachexia · Starvation · Vitamins · Minerals

Key Messages

- Protein-energy malnutrition (PEM) ordinarily develops after a period of prolonged inadequate protein and energy consumption. The hallmarks of PEM are generalized muscle atrophy and subcutaneous adipose tissue depletion.
- Except for cachexia associated with chronic inflammatory, end-organ, and malignant diseases, the most common cause of weight loss in adults is depression. Chronic diseases, especially of the gastrointestinal tract, can negatively affect diet and nutrient absorption.
- Assessment of the severity of PEM and of the extent of systemic inflammation is important to determine when to begin invasive feeding (either by feeding tube or intravenously).
- The appearance of a vitamin or mineral deficiency in a normal adult eating a conventional diet suggests the possibility of a drug-nutrient interaction or an undiagnosed disease of the gastrointestinal system.
- It is important to identify the cause(s) of a diagnosed micronutrient deficiency in order to administer the appropriate treatment and to address the underlying disease.

Introduction

Primary care physicians encounter two general kinds of malnutrition, protein-energy malnutrition (PEM) and micronutrient (vitamin and mineral) deficiency.

PEM is the disease that results from chronic starvation or severe intestinal malabsorption. The clinical course of PEM is strongly influenced by systemic inflammation and coexisting muscle atrophy due to physical inactivity, a primary neuromuscular disease, or old age (sarcopenia). By definition, starving people do not consume (or absorb) enough food, so they are also at risk of micronutrient deficiencies.

With two important exceptions (vitamin D and iron), overt micronutrient deficiencies are rare in healthy adults whose body weight is maintained on a conventional diet. The development of a vitamin or mineral deficiency in such people strongly suggests the possibility of a drug-nutrient interaction or an as yet undiagnosed disease of the gastrointestinal system. Conversely, several chronic diseases affect diet and can impair nutrient absorption. People with these diseases are at risk of micronutrient deficiencies, even when their overall food intake is adequate and their body weight is normal.

Table 1. Characteristics of successfully adapted PEM

Metabolic and endocrine
Hypothermia
Secondary amenorrhea
Serum free thyroxin and TSH normal
Neurocardiovascular
Sinus bradycardia
Reduced cardiac output
Hypotension
Reduced sympathetic tone
Muscular and functional
Generalized muscle atrophy and weakness
Reduced myocardial mass
Ineffective cough
Reduced ventilatory response to hypoxia
Drug disposition
May be altered [9]
Immune function
Weakened body barriers due to skin thinning and ineffective cough
Reduced febrile response to infection
Normal humoral and cellular immunity in the absence of micronutrient deficiencies
Psychological abnormalities
Apathy
Anorexia

There are differences of opinion amongst experts as to the implications of subclinical deficiencies of vitamin D, omega-3 fatty acids, folic acid and cobalamin (vitamin B_{12}) with regard to cancer and cardiovascular disease risk, and age-related cognitive decline.

Protein-Energy Malnutrition

Also known also as 'hunger disease', PEM typically develops after a period of prolonged inadequate protein and energy consumption. The cardinal signs of PEM are generalized muscle atrophy and subcutaneous adipose tissue depletion. The pathologic features of PEM emerge when the body's protein reserve, skeletal muscle, has become depleted seriously enough to impair specific physiological functions (table 1). Metabolic adaptation strongly influences the clinical course and prognosis of PEM. Survival is common even in prolonged uncomplicated semi-starvation, thanks to an adaptive reduction in resting and total energy expenditure, which, together with the reduction in the body's metabolically active tissue mass, lowers energy expenditure enough to match the low rate of energy provision. Metabolic adaptation also increases the efficiency of dietary protein assimilation, and modifies endogenous protein turnover to reestablish whole body protein homeostasis despite the subnormal level of protein consumption. Successfully adapted PEM is sometimes referred to as adult 'marasmus,' a term borrowed from pediatric medicine, and more recently, as 'starvation-related malnutrition'. The metabolic response to systemic inflammatory disease, severe injury or severe infection amplifies body protein catabolism and prevents the adaptation to PEM, creating a potentially lethal condition. The terms 'adult kwashiorkor' and 'acute disease or injury-related malnutrition' are used to describe PEM that is induced or complicated by intense systemic inflammation. The terms 'cachexia' or 'chronic disease-related malnutrition' refer to partially adapted PEM in the context of chronic mild systemic inflammation, as occurs in inflammatory polyarthritis, advanced renal, liver, heart or pulmonary disease, and some cancers. PEM has a worse prognosis in the elderly, largely because their primary medical or surgical diseases tend to be more serious, and because sarcopenia has already reduced their body protein reserve [1–5].

PEM and sarcopenia are not uncommon in obese people. The diagnosis will be missed in these patients unless the physician specifically inquires about changes in food intake and body weight, and physically examines their muscles. At especially high risk are previously seriously obese people who have undergone gastric restriction surgery, or who have developed a serious chronic medical or surgical disease that induces

Table 2. Adapted and maladapted PEM

Feature	Adapted PEM	Maladapted PEM
BMI	reduced	normal or reduced
Muscle mass	reduced	reduced
Edema	usually absent	often present
Body weight	reduced but stable	tissue loss often masked by extracellular fluid accumulation
Drug disposition	may be altered	may be altered
Immune function	normal	impaired
Serum albumin	normal	reduced
C-reactive protein	normal	increased
Transthyretin	reduced	reduced

the cachexia syndrome. In such cases, the loss of muscle outstrips that of fat, and can reach a critical degree even in the presence of ample residual adipose tissue.

Diagnosis and Assessment of Protein-Energy Malnutrition

Several screening tools are available for identifying people who have PEM or are at high risk of developing it [4]. The simple and well-studied Malnutrition Universal Screening Tool (MUST) categorizes a patient's risk of 'malnutrition' (and directs the management response) as low, medium, or high, based on a MUST score of 0, 1 or 2. The MUST score is calculated as the sum of points awarded by considering body mass index (BMI, weight/height^2): >20, 18.5–20, or <18 (0, 1, or 2 points, respectively), history of involuntary weight loss: <5%, 5–10%, or >10% (0, 1, or 2 points, respectively), and acute illness or no food intake for >5 days (2 points; http://www.scottishintensivecare.org.uk/nutrition/docs/must.pdf).

Tools such as the MUST are valuable in high patient flow situations for they are easy for paramedical staff to use and draw attention to high-risk situations and overt cases of severe PEM. However, they cannot replace specific diagnosis and medical evaluation in the large grey zone that lies between adequate nutritional status and clinically important PEM.

The most useful way to diagnose PEM is in the classical medical-narrative tradition, which recognizes PEM as a pathophysiological entity with well-defined signs and symptoms, all of which are strongly modified by the patient's primary disease, the presence or absence of systemic inflammation, and the presence or absence of other causes of muscle atrophy (table 2). For example, it is entirely possible to have a BMI <18.5 but normal health. The MUST will correctly flag such a person for evaluation, which may disclose a naturally lean phenotype, constant body weight and normal appetite and diet. This person is healthy. Conversely, severe PEM is entirely possible in a person whose BMI is 30.

Importance of Identifying Protein-Energy Malnutrition and Systemic Inflammation

The principal reason for identifying PEM and determining the presence and extent of systemic inflammation is to determine when invasive feeding (either by feeding tube or intravenously) is helpful, and when to commence it. Well-adapted, moderately severe PEM (e.g. BMI approx.

17), as often occurs in anorexia nervosa, calls for careful monitoring and a serious, well-organized program to improve the patient's energy and protein intake by voluntary means, but it does not represent a medical emergency that requires invasive feeding, except when weight loss is continuing, electrolyte disturbances occur, and the potential for cardiac dysfunction is serious. By contrast, critically ill patients with severe closed head injury, major third-degree body burns, severe sepsis, pancreatitis or multiple injury syndromes require invasive nutritional support within the first 48 h even if they are well nourished for this therapy can improve their outcome by modulating systemic inflammation and mitigating body protein loss. When PEM is absent or only mild, and systemic inflammation is only moderate (as occurs after uncomplicated major abdominal surgery, mild systemic infections, and in chronic inflammatory conditions), invasive nutritional support can often be withheld for up to one week, as long as the resumption of normal food intake is anticipated in the near future. Patients with inflammatory disease and already existing moderate or severe PEM require earlier intervention [6].

Evaluation of Involuntary Weight Loss

Any patient who reports sustained involuntary weight loss requires careful evaluation. The evaluation should start by measuring body height and weight and seeking objective evidence that weight loss actually has occurred, and its extent. The most important question to ask early in the evaluation of such patients is whether their appetite and overall food intake are normal or decreased. Normal appetite and food intake in someone with important involuntary weight loss strongly suggests the possibility of uncontrolled diabetes mellitus, hyperthyroidism or malabsorption, and evidence to support or refute these diagnoses should be obtained. Patients with undiagnosed celiac disease commonly report abdominal bloating, but they may also be asymptomatic. Coexistent iron, folic acid, vitamin D or magnesium deficiency increases the likelihood of the diagnosis. Some patients present to their physician with osteomalacia or premature osteoporosis due to chronic vitamin D malabsorption.

Only rarely is an undiagnosed malignancy the cause of weight loss in the absence of symptoms or signs that point to serious disease, and especially if the complete blood count is normal. Renal cell cancer, painless cancer of the pancreas, and some types of lung cancer may present with serious constitutional symptoms and weight loss, but these rare diagnoses can usually be excluded by means of a careful physical examination, chest radiograph, urinalysis, and routine blood tests. The diagnosis of adrenocortical insufficiency should always be considered when a patient presents with weight loss, fatigue, postural hypotension, and nonspecific gastrointestinal symptoms [5].

Except for cachexia associated with chronic inflammatory, end-organ, and malignant diseases, the commonest cause of weight loss in adults is depression. Weight loss and depression are often exacerbated by social, economic and mechanical difficulties such as reduced mobility and impaired physical or sensory function, chewing or swallowing disorders, or ill-fitting dentures. Concurrent thiamine, folic acid, vitamin D or vitamin C deficiency can worsen the mood disturbance of a depressed person and further reduce their food intake in a vicious cycle. People suffering from dementia often demonstrate a disinclination to eat much food when their disease reaches the far-advanced stage. Because they have adapted PEM, these people actually require relatively little food. As long as their subnormal body weight remains relatively constant, there is no medical indication for invasive feeding. There is no good evidence that forced feeding improves either the length or quality of life at this stage of dementia, and some evidence

Table 3. Important drug- and diet-nutrient interactions

Anticonvulsant drugs	increased catabolism of folic acid, vitamin D, and possibly thiamine
Methotrexate	impaired folic acid utilization
High-dose loop diuretics	increased urinary thiamine excretion
Proton pump inhibitors	iron, folic acid and cobalamin malabsorption
Metformin	impaired cobalamin absorption
Aminoglycoside antibiotics	urinary magnesium wasting
Systemic glucocorticoid therapy	blocked vitamin D action
Certain cancer chemotherapeutic agents	magnesium, zinc deficiency
Excessive alcohol consumption	B vitamin malabsorption, urinary magnesium wasting
Cigarette smoking	increased vitamin C catabolism
Excessive consumption of tea, coffee or betel nuts	thiamine malabsorption
Grapefruit juice	inhibits intestinal CYP3A4, slowing metabolism of many commonly used drugs including (but not limited to) amiodarone, amlopidine, atorvastatin, budesonide, buspirone, carbamazepine, cisapride, cyclosporine, felodipine, lapatinib, lovastatin, nicardipine, nifedipine, nilotinib, simvastatin, sirolimus, tacrolimus, triazolam, and verapamil [10]
Vegan diet	inadequate cobalamin and zinc
Vegetable- and fruit-deficient diet	inadequate vitamin C, folic acid and carotenoid
Low-fat diet	reduced digestion and absorption of vitamins D and E
Protein-deficient diet	inadequate B vitamins and zinc
Seafood-free diet	inadequate long-chain omega-3 fatty acids
Sunlight avoidance	vitamin D deficiency

that it worsens both of them [7]. On the other hand, simple micronutrient supplementation is safe and rational in this setting since the paramount consideration at this time is quality of life, and several micronutrient deficiencies adversely affect mood.

Micronutrient Deficiencies

The important micronutrient deficiencies are explained in detail in other chapters in this textbook. This section provides a short list of practical tips and an overall diagnostic strategy for evaluating vitamin and mineral deficiencies.

Nutritional Anemias

The nutritional anemias comprise microcytic anemia (due to iron, and more rarely copper deficiency) and macrocytic megaloblastic anemia due to folic acid or cobalamin (vitamin B_{12}) deficiency. These topics are covered in detail elsewhere in this textbook.

Glossitis

Atrophic glossitis – a reddened tongue that is smooth in appearance because of atrophy of the filiform papillae – is a nonspecific inflammatory condition that is associated with iron, folic acid, cobalamin, niacin, or riboflavin deficiency.

Drug- and Diet-Nutrient Interactions

Several widely used drugs affect micronutrient metabolism or excretion and can cause micronutrient deficiency. Certain general dietary patterns are associated with an increased risk of specific micronutrient deficiencies. Examples of such interactions are provided in table 3.

When Should a Micronutrient Deficiency Be Investigated or Searched For?

In a classic article, Victor Herbert explained the 5 possible causes of any micronutrient deficiency: inadequate intake, impaired intestinal absorption, impaired metabolic utilization, increased excretion or catabolism, and increased metabolic requirement [8]. Herbert's scheme can be used to formulate two general dictums regarding micronutrients:

Rule 1: When a micronutrient deficiency is diagnosed but only one cause is apparent, search for the second cause.

Rule 2: When a patient has (or is at risk of) two independent causes of a micronutrient deficiency, it is appropriate to prescribe a suitable supplement, test for the pertinent biochemical deficiency, or both.

For example, women with a normal menstrual cycle and inadequate iron intake are frequently iron deficient, but no investigation is usually required since two causes are apparent. Iron deficiency in a man or nonmenstruating woman requires a search for the second cause (gastrointestinal bleeding, parasitic infection, or celiac disease). A patient with folic acid deficiency and a history of poor diet and chronic hemolytic anemia (which increases folic acid utilization), or poor diet and treatment with methotrexate or phenytoin (impaired utilization and increased catabolism, respectively) requires correction of the deficiency but no further investigation since two causes are apparent. On the other hand, a patient with isolated folic acid deficiency should be evaluated for a drug-nutrient interaction (including alcohol abuse), malabsorption, or hemolytic anemia. Given the high prevalence of vitamin D deficiency in the general population, any person prescribed phenytoin requires vitamin D supplementation (table 3).

Patients with fat maldigestion (pancreatic insufficiency, biliary cirrhosis, or cystic fibrosis) malabsorb the fat-soluble vitamins (vitamins A, D, E and K) even when receiving appropriate pancreatic enzyme replacement. Patients with generalized malabsorption (celiac disease or Crohn's disease involving the small intestine) malabsorb most micronutrients, especially vitamin A, certain B vitamins (including cobalamin), magnesium and zinc. Even a mild reduction in the consumption of these micronutrients places these patients at high risk of the corresponding deficiency diseases. People who have undergone a subtotal or total gastrectomy (including gastric restriction surgery for obesity) usually require lifelong supplementation with iron, folic acid, and cobalamin. Patients with chronic or severe inflammatory diarrhea require zinc supplementation to replace their fecal zinc losses.

Conclusions

- The hallmarks of PEM are generalized muscle atrophy and usually, but not always, subcutaneous adipose tissue depletion.
- The severity of PEM, intensity of systemic inflammation, and inability to voluntarily meet nutrient needs determine when artificial nutritional support is required.
- The cause of involuntary weight loss can almost always be identified from a careful history, physical examination, and routine tests as explained in this chapter.
- The appearance of a vitamin or mineral deficiency in a normal adult eating a conventional diet requires an explanation. The diagnosis can usually be made using the rules described in this chapter.
- Patients with diseases that increase their risk of specific vitamin or mineral deficiencies should be assessed with regard to these deficiencies and prescribed preventive supplements.

References

1 Hoffer LJ: Clinical nutrition: protein-energy malnutrition in the inpatient. CMAJ 2001;165:1345–1349.
2 Jensen GL, Mirtallo J, Compher C, et al: Adult starvation and disease-related malnutrition: a proposal for etiology-based diagnosis in the clinical practice setting from the International Consensus Guideline Committee. JPEN J Parenter Enteral Nutr 2010;34:156–159.
3 Macallan D: Infection and malnutrition. Medicine 2009;37:525–528.
4 Barker LA, Gout BS, Crowe TC: Hospital malnutrition: prevalence, identification and impact on patients and the healthcare system. Int J Environ Res Public Health 2011;8:514–527.
5 Bistrian BR: Nutritional assessment; in Goldman L, Schafer AI (eds): Goldman's Cecil Medicine. Philadelphia, Elsevier Saunders, 2012, pp 1384–1388.
6 Raynaud-Simon A, Revel-Delhom C, Hebuterne X, et al: Clinical practice guidelines from the French Health High Authority: nutritional support strategy in protein-energy malnutrition in the elderly. Clin Nutr 2011;30:312–319.
7 Hoffer LJ: Tube feeding in advanced dementia: the metabolic perspective. BMJ 2006;333:1214–1215.
8 Herbert V: The five possible causes of all nutrient deficiency: illustrated by deficiencies of vitamin B12. Am J Clin Nutr 1973;26:77–86.
9 Boullata JI: Drug disposition in obesity and protein-energy malnutrition. Proc Nutr Soc 2010;69:543–550.
10 Seden K, Dickinson L, Khoo S, Back D: Grapefruit-drug interactions. Drugs 2010;70:2373–2407.

Bier D, et al. (eds): Nutrition for the Primary Care Provider. World Rev Nutr Diet. Basel, Karger, 2015, vol 111, pp 94–99
DOI: 10.1159/000362305

Cardiovascular Disease

Ulf Risérus

Clinical Nutrition and Metabolism, Department of Public Health and Caring Sciences, Faculty of Medicine, Uppsala University, Uppsala, Sweden

Key Words

Cardiovascular disease · Dietary patterns · LDL cholesterol · HDL cholesterol · Triglycerides · Blood glucose

Key Messages

- The risk factors that drive cardiovascular disease (CVD) such as elevated LDL cholesterol and dyslipidemia, hypertension and impaired glucose tolerance, are largely influenced by diet and lifestyle habits.
- Prudent dietary patterns that can reduce CVD include the Mediterranean diet, the Dietary Approaches to Stop Hypertension diet, and other similar diets rich in fruits, vegetables, nuts, low-fat dairy, and plant oils.
- The type of fat, rather than the total amount of fat in the diet, appears to be most important for prevention and management of CVD. The majority of dietary fat should be unsaturated and derive from plant sources and fish.
- Similarly, favoring whole grains, fiber-rich cereals and raw fruits and vegetables above highly refined/processed carbohydrates has favorable cardiometabolic effects, including lowered postprandial glucose and insulin fluctuations, and lowered serum triglycerides.
- Improvement of dietary habits can have beneficial effects on most CVD risk factors, including hyperlipidemia, hyperglycemia and elevated blood pressure. Modification of dietary habits is a key intervention for reducing CVD-related mortality.

Introduction

The global burden of cardiovascular disease (CVD) is huge as it causes substantial mortality and morbidity in both developed and nondeveloped countries [1, 2]. CVD is the leading cause of death in most developed countries, representing 30% of all global deaths [1]. Notably, most of these cases could be prevented or postponed by lifestyle intervention [2, 3]. Together with smoking and sedentary lifestyle, an excess caloric intake and poor dietary quality are responsible for the majority of CVD deaths. An 'unhealthy' diet, i.e. a diet far from that currently recommended by international health organizations, has been estimated to account for approximately 30% of all acute myocardial infarctions [3]. Importantly, realistic dietary changes can reduce mortality rates

Table 1. Effects of recommended key foods on CVD risk factors

Foods to increase	Key nutrients(s)	Risk factor effects
Fruits and vegetables	fiber, vitamins/minerals, phenols	↓ LDL-C, ↓ BP, ↑ glycemic control, ↓ oxidative stress
Whole grains	fiber, B vitamins, minerals	↓ LDL-C, ↓ BP, ↑ glycemic control
Low-fat dairy	calcium, vitamin D, potassium	↓ BP
Legumes, soy	fiber, sterols, isoflavones	↓ LDL-C, ↑ HDL-C
Nuts, seeds	unsaturated fatty acids (omega-6 and -3), sterols	↓ LDL-C, ↓ oxidative stress, ↑ HDL-C
Seafood	unsaturated fatty acids (omega-3)	↓ TG, ↓ BP, ↓ heart rate, ↓ LDL-C, ↓ arrhythmic effect, ↓ inflammation
Vegetable oils	unsaturated fatty acids (omega-6 and -3)	↓LDL-C

Adapted and slightly modified from Flock and Kris-Etherton [5]. BP = Blood pressure; TG = triglycerides; LDL-C = LDL cholesterol; HDL-C = HDL cholesterol.

substantially [1, 2, 4, 5]. Apart from patients with diagnosed CVD, patients with type 2 diabetes and the metabolic syndrome are at high risk of CVD and can benefit from dietary intervention.

Pathophysiology

Atherosclerosis is a key driver of CVD, and the process is accelerated by modifiable risk CVD factors such as elevated LDL cholesterol and dyslipidemia, hypertension, impaired glucose tolerance and insulin resistance, endothelial dysfunction, inflammation and oxidative stress. In compliant patients, diet has favorable effects on most CVD risk factors, especially hyperlipidemia, hyperglycemia and elevated blood pressure (table 1). Successful secondary prevention of CVD by dietary interventions such as the Mediterranean diet may result in reduced coronary atherosclerosis/thrombosis and reduced risk of fatal complications such as sudden cardiac death and heart failure [4]. It is still uncertain which dietary components are responsible for the reduced CVD risk as the multifactorial effect is probably important. For example, long-chain n-3 fatty acids in fish have been suggested to have anti-arrhythmic effects, whereas plant-derived n-6 long-chain fatty acids lower serum LDL cholesterol. Consequently, fatty acids of both marine and vegetable origin should be included in a healthy diet to prevent CVD [2, 5]. Other dietary components could influence CVD risk by other mechanisms, e.g. reducing salt lowers blood pressure, and wholegrain foods rich in fiber improve blood lipids, and may possibly lower low-grade inflammation and endothelial dysfunction.

Changing Dietary Risk Patterns

High adherence to dietary patterns such as the 'Western diet' has been consistently associated with CVD in various populations [3, 6]. Such dietary patterns include foods high in animal fats, salt, red meats, added sugars, fried and processed foods, but are low in fruits, vegetables and fish. It is important to identify and interrupt such hazardous dietary habits in CVD patients as well as in individuals at high CVD risk. In both these groups, dietary change should be a major target for intervention in order to prevent CVD. To obtain optimal effect on CVD risk, the aim should always be to improve the overall dietary pattern [7], although small changes may also have a significant impact. Meaningful dietary changes include several substitutions, e.g. replacing fried foods with nonfried foods, limiting sugar-sweetened beverages (soft drinks and fruit juices), increasing fruits and vegetables and replacing butter with vegetable oils and soft margarines (free of trans-fatty acids) and replacing white bread with whole-grain bread high in fiber and preferably including some whole kernels.

Healthy Diet for Prevention and Treatment of CVD

In contrast to the Westernized dietary pattern associated with adverse CVD outcomes, there are food patterns consistently associated with reduced CVD [3, 6, 7]. Data from observational studies and randomized trials suggest that dietary changes reduce CVD risk factors as well as reduce the risk of recurrent myocardial infarction in secondary prevention trials [4, 8]. Dietary patterns that can reduce CVD and/or secondary prevention of CVD include the Mediterranean diet, the Dietary Approaches to Stop Hypertension (DASH) diet and other similar diets and food patterns currently recommended worldwide by health organizations and authorities [1–3, 6, 7]. The DASH diet is rich in fruits, vegetables, low-fat dairy, and reduced in saturated fats and cholesterol. The dietary composition of the Mediterranean diet and DASH is very similar, but the Mediterranean diet may be somewhat higher in unsaturated fat from vegetable oils and fish. Thus, these recommended diets are very similar in terms of the dietary pattern and food composition, and they all include a high intake of fruits, vegetables, legumes, vegetable oils, fish, low-fat milk products, but a low intake of red and processed meats, salty fast foods, bakery, sweets, refined carbohydrates and added sugars. These diets are suitable both for prevention and treatment of CVD. However, to achieve an optimal effect of treatment, dietary intervention of CVD may be slightly individualized based on the CVD risk profile, pathophysiology and lifestyle habits of the patients. For example, in a patient with obesity, type 2 diabetes or the metabolic syndrome, energy reduction in the diet should be specifically targeted to induce weight loss [9]. In clinical practice, it is usually not meaningful, nor is there any advantage in the implementation of dietary recommendations, to discuss relative proportions of macronutrients in a prescribed diet. Instead, practical advice on cooking, food preparation and healthy food choices should be exemplified and advocated to the patients [2, 7] (table 2).

Diet and Blood Lipids

In addition to blood pressure-lowering effects from avoidance of salty foods (table 2), hyperlipidemia is common and highly responsive to dietary changes and is thus a relevant target [10]. Total cholesterol, LDL cholesterol and triglycerides are risk factors closely linked to CVD, and at elevated concentrations they should be treated with dietary modification alone or in conjunction with lipid-lowering drugs if indicated [10].

In patients with elevated LDL cholesterol, an increased fiber intake and increased intake of unsaturated fats from vegetable oils and nuts are relevant interventions [5, 7, 10] (table 2). For example, replacing butter and high-fat dairy with canola oil or other vegetable oils, alone may decrease plasma LDL cholesterol as well as the total cholesterol to HDL cholesterol ratio by 10–20% in a few weeks. Notably, such lipid-lowering effects can be achieved without weight loss. Table 1 summarizes the effects of different dietary components on blood lipids and other risk factors.

Role of Dietary Fats

The type of fat, rather than the total amount of fat in the diet, appears to be most important for prevention as well as for the management of CVD [2]. Partial replacement of saturated fats from animal products with unsaturated fats from nontropical vegetable oils could alone have a small but clinically meaningful cardioprotective effect [2, 5, 7]. Such benefit has been mainly ascribed to reduced LDL cholesterol. Other potential beneficial effects of dietary fat modification have also been reported on blood pressure, insulin resistance, hepatic steatosis, and inflammation, but those data are less conclusive. It should be noted that in order to achieve a clinical benefit of saturated fat reduction, it is important that foods rich in saturated fat (e.g. butter and processed meats) are replaced with foods rich in polyunsaturated fat and/or fiber-rich unrefined carbohydrates [2]. If saturated fat instead is replaced by refined carbohydrates or added sugars, the benefit of reducing saturated fat may be abolished or even reversed. Regardless of the amount of total fat and carbohydrates in any given diet, the majority of the fat should be unsaturated from plant sources (e.g. vegetable oils, nuts and seeds) and fish. If the majority (approx. two thirds) of fat in a diet is unsaturated, cardiometabolic benefits can be observed also at total fat intakes above that usually recommended. Rapeseed (canola) oil and olive oil are oils that can be used frequently in dressings, cooking and baking, but other oils e.g. soybean oil and sunflower oil can also be used in diets with a regular intake of fatty fish. Omega-3 supplements (fish oil capsules) have been suggested to have cardioprotective effects in secondary prevention of CVD, although the evidence is not consistent. The most established metabolic effect of daily fish oil supplementation is lowering of serum triglycerides (approx. 5–25% reduction). Patients should however primarily be advised to consume fish

Table 2. Healthy food choices and preparation

Eat fresh and frozen vegetables and fruits without high-calorie sauces and added salt and sugars
Replace high-calorie foods with fruits and vegetables
Increase fiber intake by eating beans (legumes), whole-grain products, fruits, and vegetables
Use liquid vegetable oils (e.g. canola oil, olive oil, sunflower oil) or soft margarines in place of solid fats such as butter
Limit beverages and foods high in added sugars; common forms of added sugars are sucrose, glucose, fructose, maltose, dextrose, corn syrups, concentrated fruit juice, and honey
Choose foods made with whole grains rather than refined cereals; common forms of whole grains are whole wheat, oats/oatmeal, rye, barley, corn, brown rice, wild rice, buckwheat, triticale, bulgur (cracked wheat), millet, and quinoa
Cut back on pastries and high-calorie bakery products (e.g. muffins, buns, cookies, doughnuts)
Mainly select milk and dairy products that are low in fat
Reduce salt intake by comparing the sodium contents of similar products (e.g. different brands of tomato sauce and choosing products with less salt (e.g. unsalted nuts)
Choose versions of processed foods, including cereals and baked goods, that are reduced in salt
Limit the use of condiments (e.g. soy sauce, ketchup)
Use lean cuts of meat and remove skin from poultry before eating
Limit processed meats that are high in saturated fat and sodium
Grill, bake, or boil fish, meat, and poultry
Incorporate vegetable-based meat substitutes (e.g. beans and lentils) into favorite recipes
Encourage the consumption of whole vegetables and fruits in place of juices

Adapted and slightly modified with kind permission from Springer Science+Business Media from Gidding et al. [7].

2–3 times per week rather than taking omega-3 supplements. The latter may be an alternative for patients with myocardial infarction and/or high triglyceride levels, especially for those who do not eat fish for various reasons.

Role of Carbohydrates

Not only the type of fat, but also the type of carbohydrates plays a clear role in the management of CVD. Refined carbohydrates and foods high in added sugars could elevate both triglycerides and LDL cholesterol, and lower HDL cholesterol. They also cause more elevated blood glucose and insulin levels after ingestion as compared to nonrefined carbohydrates with lower glycemic index. With regard to carbohydrate-rich foods, a dietary substitution of whole grains, fiber-rich cereals and raw fruits and vegetables for highly refined/processed carbohydrates (e.g. white bread) and starches could have multiple favorable cardiometabolic effects including lowered postprandial glucose and insulin excursions and lowered serum triglycerides (table 1). Low-fat/high carbohydrate diets have been widely recommended for weight loss, but reducing the total amount of carbohydrates could be an alternative dietary approach to reduce total energy intake, resulting in weight loss and lowered CVD risk factors. A moderate decrease in carbohydrate amount (down to about 30–40 energy percent) has been examined in clinical studies with longer duration, and such diets produce similar weight loss and overall CVD risk reduction as conventional low-fat diets. Importantly, if a low-carbohydrate diet is to be used in obese patients to induce weight loss, it should be emphasized that the diet should be rich in unsaturated fats rather than high in saturated fats (e.g. vegetable oils, avocado, nuts and fish instead of butter and processed meat products) as well as protein from vegetable sources rather than solely from animals (e.g. lentils and beans instead of processed or red meat). Thus, to avoid potential long-term adverse effects on CVD risk (e.g. mediated by elevation of LDL cholesterol or endothelial function by high amounts of saturated or total fat), diets that are lower in carbohydrates but higher in protein and fat should consist of similar healthy foods as those recommended in any diet (table 2).

Conclusions

- Dietary goals in CVD prevention and treatment are to consume an overall healthy diet.
- Aim for a healthy body weight; aim for recommended levels of LDL cholesterol, HDL cholesterol, and triglycerides; aim for normal blood pressure and blood glucose level.
- Prescribe more fruits, vegetables, legumes (beans and lentils), whole grains, fish (2–3 times per week) and shellfish, unsalted nuts, dairy products (mainly low-fat), lean meats (preferably poultry), vegetable oils and soft margarines (free of trans-fats).
- This advice is appropriate in patients without as well as in patients with CVD.
- Limit fats and oils containing partially hydrogenated vegetable oils (e.g. sweets, fast food, processed foods), red meats and especially processed meats (e.g. sausages, bacon), sugar-sweetened beverages, sweets, grain-based desserts and bakery products.
- Moderate weight loss also reduces CVD risk factors of clinical significance. Reduce energy-dense foods high in fat, refined carbohydrates and added sugars (e.g. fried foods such as potato chips and French fries).
- A healthier eating pattern should always be given together with advice on how to increase physical activity and, if relevant, stop smoking.

References

1 Mendis S, Puska P, Norrving B (eds): Global Atlas on Cardiovascular Disease Prevention and Control. Geneva, WHO, 2011.

2 Mozaffarian D, Appel LJ, Van Horn L: Components of a cardioprotective diet: new insights. Circulation 2011;123: 2870–2891.

3 Iqbal R, Anand S, Ounpuu S, et al: Dietary patterns and the risk of acute myocardial infarction in 52 countries: results of the INTERHEART study. Circulation 2008;118:1929–1937.

4 de Lorgeril M, Salen P: Mediterranean diet in secondary prevention of CHD. Public Health Nutr 2011;14:2333–2337.

5 Flock MR, Kris-Etherton PM: Dietary guidelines for Americans 2010: implications for cardiovascular disease. Curr Atheroscler Rep 2011;13:499–507.

6 Mente A, de Koning L, Shannon HS, Anand SS: A systematic review of the evidence supporting a causal link between dietary factors and coronary heart disease. Arch Intern Med 2009;169:659–669.

7 Gidding SS, Lichtenstein AH, Faith MS, et al: Implementing American Heart Association pediatric and adult nutrition guidelines: a scientific statement from the American Heart Association Nutrition Committee of the Council on Nutrition, Physical Activity and Metabolism, Council on Cardiovascular Disease in the Young, Council on Arteriosclerosis, Thrombosis and Vascular Biology, Council on Cardiovascular Nursing, Council on Epidemiology and Prevention, and Council for High Blood Pressure Research. Circulation 2009; 119:1161–1175.

8 Esposito K, Marfella R, Ciotola M, et al: Effect of a Mediterranean-style diet on endothelial dysfunction and markers of vascular inflammation in the metabolic syndrome: a randomized trial. JAMA 2004;292:1440–1446.

9 Mann JI: Nutrition recommendations for the treatment and prevention of type 2 diabetes and the metabolic syndrome: an evidenced-based review. Nutr Rev 2006;64:422–427.

10 Reiner Z, Catapano AL, De Backer G, et al: ESC/EAS Guidelines for the management of dyslipidaemias. The Task Force for the management of dyslipidaemias of the European Society of Cardiology (ESC) and the European Atherosclerosis Society (EAS). Eur Heart J 2011;32: 1769–1818.

Bier D, et al. (eds): Nutrition for the Primary Care Provider. World Rev Nutr Diet. Basel, Karger, 2015, vol 111, pp 100–103
DOI: 10.1159/000362306

Hypertension

Rachael M. McLean

Departments of Preventive and Social Medicine and Human Nutrition, University of Otago, Dunedin, New Zealand

Key Words

Blood pressure · Hypertension · Sodium · Potassium · Body weight · Physical activity · Alcohol

Key Messages

- High blood pressure is a leading cause of death worldwide.
- Nutritional and other lifestyle interventions can have beneficial effects on blood pressure and cardiovascular disease risk.
- Lowering blood pressure is beneficial even in patients not generally considered to be hypertensive.
- The optimal nutritional approach to blood pressure control is a dietary pattern low in sodium, high in fresh fruit and vegetables and low-fat dairy products, and low in saturated fats.
- Maintaining a healthy body weight and limiting alcohol intake are also important for blood pressure control.

Introduction

High blood pressure, an important modifiable risk factor for cardiovascular and kidney disease, has been identified as the leading cause of death worldwide. The World Health Organization estimated that in 2004 high blood pressure was responsible for 7.5 million (or 12.8%) of deaths [1]. Observational studies of over one million adults show that systolic blood pressures above 115 mm Hg and diastolic blood pressures above 75 mm Hg are associated with increasing risk of coronary heart disease and stroke. In most populations, blood pressure rises with increasing age, with more than half of adults ≥60 years of age reported to have high blood pressure in high-income countries [2]. The American Heart Association classification of blood pressure for adults is outlined in table 1. Given the continuous relationship between increasing levels of blood pressure and risk of cardiovascular disease, the cutoff values given in table 1 are inevitably arbitrary. Any individual's blood pressure is determined by a combination of genetic and environmental influences. Nutritional factors are some of the most important environmental influences, although individual responses to specific dietary changes will vary.

Nutritional Determinants of Blood Pressure

Sodium

There is conclusive evidence from a range of studies of a positive association between dietary sodium intake and blood pressure. In the 1980s, the

Table 1. Classification of blood pressure for adults: Joint National Committee on Prevention, Detection, Evaluation, and Treatment of High Blood Pressure [12]

Blood pressure classification	SBP, mm Hg	DBP, mm Hg
Normal	<120	and <80
Prehypertension	120–139	or 80–89
Stage 1 hypertension	140–159	or 90–99
Stage 2 hypertension	≥160	or ≥100

SBP = Systolic blood pressure; DBP = diastolic blood pressure.

INTERSALT study of 52 populations in 32 countries demonstrated that a high-sodium diet was associated with higher blood pressure levels. INTERSALT also demonstrated that in populations that typically consume a low-sodium diet there was no rise in blood pressure with age, suggesting there is an adverse effect of long-term exposure to a high-sodium diet. Intervention studies have shown that reduction in dietary sodium results in significantly reduced blood pressure. Such changes in blood pressure can take up to 30 days to develop, but if sustained lead to long-term reductions in cardiovascular disease outcomes [3, 4]. A Cochrane systematic review and meta-analysis showed that a reduction of dietary sodium intake of around 1,700 mg/day would lead to an average reduction in blood pressure of 5/3 mm Hg (systolic/diastolic) for hypertensive and 2/1 mm Hg for normotensive adults. This might be expected to translate into reductions in mortality from stroke of up to 24%, and from coronary heart disease of up to 18% [5]. Some population groups (such as African-Americans) appear to be more salt sensitive than others with larger changes in blood pressure in response to changes in dietary sodium intake; however, there are no widely accepted criteria for identifying salt-sensitive individuals.

Few populations are able to achieve dietary sodium intakes consistent with dietary guidelines. The United States Department of Agriculture recommends maximum daily intake of 2,300 mg sodium for adults, with a more restricted intake in those at high risk of cardiovascular disease, i.e. 1,500 mg for middle-aged or older adults, African-Americans, and those who have hypertension, diabetes or chronic kidney disease [6]. This represents an appreciable reduction for populations consuming a typical Western style diet in which intakes are usually around 3,500 mg/day. In such diets, 90% of dietary sodium is consumed as salt (sodium chloride). Most (75–80%) is consumed as sodium within processed foods, with only around 10% added in the home in cooking or at the table [7]. Attempts to reduce dietary sodium in populations at large as well as in individuals need to involve not only limiting the use of salt and salty snacks in the home, but limiting the ingestion of processed foods known to contribute to sodium intake such as bread, processed meats, and processed soups and sauces. This requires better interpretation of sodium concentration information on food labels, and industry reformulation of processed foods to contain less sodium. Dietary sodium reduction at a population level is regarded as one of the most important public health nutrition approaches to reduce the risk of cardiovascular disease. Reducing dietary sodium has the potential to reduce blood pressure further even in people on blood pressure-lowering drugs.

Potassium

The INTERSALT study also demonstrated a negative association between dietary potassium and blood pressure, and further studies have suggested a potential interaction between dietary sodium and potassium and blood pressure. A meta-analysis of trials of potassium supplementation showed that potassium supplementation to a mean intake of 4.7 g/day (120 mmol/day) resulted in a mean reduction in systolic blood pressure of 3/2 mm Hg, with greater reductions in blood pressure shown in those individuals on a high-sodium diet [8]. Although these trials used potassium supplements, it is generally recommended that potassium intake be increased through di-

Table 2. Diet-related lifestyle recommendations to lower blood pressure

Lifestyle modification	Recommendation
Body weight	aim for a normal BMI (18.5–24.9)
Reduced sodium intake	limit dietary sodium intake to a maximum of 2,300 mg/day for adults, aiming for a maximum of 1,500 mg/day for high-risk individuals (equivalent to approximately 6 and 4 g of salt, respectively)
DASH-style dietary pattern	adopt a DASH-style diet: high in fresh fruit and vegetables (8–10 servings per day), high in dietary fiber and low-fat dairy products, and low in saturated fats
Moderation of alcohol intake	limit alcohol intake to no more than 1 standard drink per day for women or 2 standard drinks for men

etary change; consuming 8–10 servings of fruit and vegetables daily is recommended [9]. This way, individuals will obtain the added nutritional benefit of dietary fiber, and minimize any potential adverse effects of potassium supplementation in people with impaired renal function.

The Dietary Approaches to Stop Hypertension Diet
The Dietary Approaches to Stop Hypertension (DASH) Trial provides the best evidence of a successful nutritional intervention to reduce blood pressure. This randomized controlled trial showed that a diet high in fresh fruit and vegetables, dietary fiber, low-fat dairy products and low in saturated fat (the DASH diet) was associated with a significant decrease in blood pressure, compared with a 'typical American diet' even when daily sodium intake was similar in the two diets. When dietary sodium intake was altered, the low-sodium DASH diet was associated with a further reduction in mean blood pressure. Overall reduction in systolic/diastolic blood pressure was 9/5 mm Hg compared with the high-sodium control diet [3]. Several components of the DASH diet have the potential to beneficially influence blood pressure, but the combined effect justifies the recommendation of this dietary pattern.

Body Weight
As body weight increases, blood pressure increases. A meta-analysis of intervention trials showed that in overweight and obese people, a weight loss of 5.1 kg was associated with a decrease in blood pressure of 4/4 mm Hg [10]. Weight loss interventions that involved decreased energy intake decreased blood pressure even when dietary sodium intake remained constant. Maintaining body mass index (BMI) within the normal range (between 18.5 and 25) is regarded as a further important recommendation for helping to optimize blood pressure.

Alcohol
Observational studies and intervention trials show a positive association between blood pressure and alcohol intake above 3 standard drinks per day. A meta-analysis of intervention trials in those consuming alcohol showed that a reduction of alcohol consumption to below this level is associated with a mean reduction in blood pressure of 3/2 mm Hg [11].

Other Lifestyle-Related Factors
Increased physical activity has been shown to be associated with some reduction in blood pressure, independent of body weight or weight loss. A number of other individual dietary factors have been identified as having a possible beneficial effect on blood pressure, although in general the evidence is not strong enough to be included in current recommendations. These include vitamin C supplementation, increased calcium intake, increased magnesium intake and limiting consumption of caffeine and sugar-sweetened beverages. The best evidence remains to support an overall dietary approach, that of a low-sodium DASH-style dietary intervention, including advice to optimize BMI.

Recommendations

Based on the available evidence, the optimal nutritional approach to controlling blood pressure is to:

(1) Limit dietary sodium intake to a maximum of 2,300 mg/day for adults, aiming for a maximum of 1,500 mg/day for high-risk individuals.
(2) Adopt a DASH-style diet: high in fresh fruit and vegetables (8–10 servings per day), high in dietary fiber and low-fat dairy products, and low in saturated fats.
(3) Maintain a healthy body weight.
(4) Limit alcohol intake to no more than 1 standard drink per day for women or 2 standard drinks for men.

These recommendations are outlined in table 2.

Conclusions

- Nutritional approaches for the prevention and management of elevated blood pressure provide important opportunities to:
  - Decrease blood pressure (and therefore cardiovascular disease risk) in people with blood pressure greater than 115/75 mm Hg but not considered to require medication.
  - Delay or prevent the usual rise in blood pressure with increasing age.
  - Further decrease blood pressure in people on antihypertensive medication and minimize the need for multiple antihypertensive medications.
- The optimal nutritional approach to blood pressure control is to consume a low-sodium DASH-style diet, maintain a healthy body weight, and limit alcohol intake.

References

1 WHO: Global health risks: mortality and burden of disease attributable to selected major risks. Geneva, WHO, 2009.

2 Kearney PM, Whelton M, Reynolds K, et al: Global burden of hypertension: analysis of worldwide data. Lancet 2005;365: 217–223.

3 Sacks FM, Svetkey LP, Vollmer WM, et al: Effects on blood pressure of reduced dietary sodium and the Dietary Approaches to Stop Hypertension (DASH) diet. N Engl J Med 2001;344:3–10.

4 Cook NR, Cutler JA, Obarzanek E, al: Long term effects of dietary sodium reduction on cardiovascular disease outcomes: observational follow-up of the trials of hypertension prevention (TOHP). BMJ 2007;334:885–892.

5 He FJ, Li J, MacGregor GA: Effect of longer term modest salt reduction on blood pressure: Cochrane systematic review and meta-analysis of randomised trials. BMJ 2013;346:f1325.

6 US Department of Health and Human Services and US Department of Agriculture: Dietary Guidelines for Americans, 2010. Washington, US Department of Agriculture, 2010.

7 Medical Research Council Human Nutrition Research: Why 6g? A summary of the scientific evidence for the salt intake target. Cambridge, Medical Research Council, 2005.

8 Whelton PK, He J, Cutler JA, et al: Effects of oral potassium on blood pressure. JAMA 1997;277:1624–1632.

9 Appel LJ: ASH position paper: dietary approaches to lower blood pressure. J Clin Hypertens 2009;11:358–368.

10 Neter JE, Stam BE, Kok FJ, et al: Influence of weight reduction on blood pressure. Hypertension 2003;42:878–884.

11 Xin X, He J, Frontini MG, et al: Effects of alcohol reduction on blood pressure. Hypertension 2001;38:1112–1117.

12 Chobanian AV, Bakris GL, Black HR, et al: Seventh report of the Joint National Committee on Prevention, Detection, Evaluation, and Treatment of High Blood Pressure. Hypertension 2003;42: 1206–1252.

Bier D, et al. (eds): Nutrition for the Primary Care Provider. World Rev Nutr Diet. Basel, Karger, 2015, vol 111, pp 104–109
DOI: 10.1159/000362307

Obesity

Alice A. Gibson Kyra A. Sim Ian D. Caterson

The Boden Institute of Obesity, Nutrition, Exercise and Eating Disorders, The University of Sydney, Sydney, N.S.W., Australia

Key Words

Obesity · Body mass index · Obesity management · Weight loss · Lifestyle modifications · Adjunctive therapies

Key Messages

- Obesity management plans should incorporate both an active weight loss phase and a weight maintenance phase.
- A negative energy balance is essential for weight loss, but how such an energy deficit is to be achieved is dependent upon the individual. The major challenge for patients and healthcare providers is to maintain the weight management solutions over the long term.
- Lifestyle modifications, through alterations in diet, physical activity and behavior should be the main therapeutic approaches.
- The key strategies in behavioral therapy for weight control are self-monitoring, stimulus control, problem solving, contingency management, cognitive restructuring and social support.
- Adjunctive therapies, including very-low-energy diets, pharmacotherapy and bariatric surgery, may be considered for high-risk patients when lifestyle interventions have failed.

Introduction

Obesity is the result of a long-term positive energy balance. However, attributing obesity to excessive energy intake and insufficient physical activity is an oversimplification. The factors contributing to the disease state of obesity are complex due to an interaction between varying genetic or biological tendencies, and cultural and socioeconomic drivers of weight gain. Factors may act alone or in combination to modulate energy intake and/or expenditure and hence determine the likelihood of an individual becoming obese. The current 'obesogenic' environment is propelling the epidemic by providing an unfavorable situation that overwhelms sophisticated regulatory systems controlling appetite and maintaining energy balance [1].

Defining Obesity

Obesity is defined as an abnormal or excessive accumulation of adipose tissue in the body resulting in adverse effects on the health and well-being of

Fig. 1. Hierarchical approach to obesity management. All patients should receive lifestyle modification. Additional therapies can be considered as indicated. High risk: a WC ≥102 cm in men and ≥88 cm in women, or the presence of risk factors including type 2 diabetes/impaired glucose tolerance, hypertension, coronary heart disease, dyslipidemia, obstructive sleep apnea.

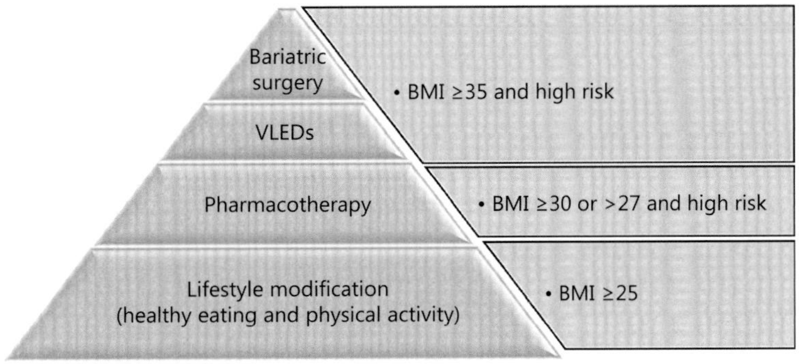

Table 1. Classification of overweight and obesity by cutpoints of BMI and WC (cm), and their related health risks

a BMI

Classification	BMI	Risk of comorbidities
Normal range	18.5–24.9	average
Overweight	≥25	
Preobese	25–29.9	increased
Obese class I	30–34.9	moderate
Obese class II	35–39.9	severe
Obese class III	≥40	very severe

b WC

Group	Increased risk	Substantial increased risk
Men	≥94	≥102
Women	≥80	≥88
Asian men	≥90	
Asian women	≥80	

Values are those suggested by the WHO [1].

the individual [1]. In clinical practice, a useful clinical definition of obesity is the body mass index (BMI) which gives a reasonable approximation of adiposity. BMI is derived by dividing an individual's weight (in kilograms) by height (in metres) squared (kg/m^2). Adults with a BMI between 25–29.9 are categorized as overweight or preobese and those with a BMI ≥30 as obese (table 1). The BMI cutoff points are however not applicable to all ethnic groups [2], extremes of age, muscularity and height.

Obesity is regarded as a disease in its own right [1] and is also a risk factor for a large number of noncommunicable, metabolic and mechanically induced disorders, the risk of which increases on a continuum with increasing adiposity. It is not only the amount, but also the distribution of adipose tissue which underlies the health risks and diseases associated with obesity. Waist circumference (WC), a surrogate marker of visceral fat, has been shown to be a more sensitive measure of long-term health risks (table 1) [1]. WC (really an abdominal circumference at a defined level) should be measured mid-way between the lowest rib and the upper border of the iliac crest.

Goals of Obesity Management

Any obesity management plan should be structured to include both an active weight loss phase and a weight maintenance phase. Modification of lifestyle, through dietary change, alterations in physical activity and behavior modification should be the main therapeutic approaches in the management of obesity (fig. 1). Effective weight management is defined as weight loss of 5–10% of body weight which is maintained for at least 2 years. Health benefits associated with this moderate weight loss include improvements in the following [3]:

- Glycemic control
- Dyslipidemia (particularly high triglyceride and low HDL cholesterol levels)
- Blood pressure
- Nonalcoholic fatty liver disease
- Sleep apnea
- All-cause mortality [4]
- The risk of heart disease, stroke and some cancers
- Psychological problems (social isolation and depression)
- Musculoskeletal problems, osteoarthritis
- Reproductive abnormalities, impaired fertility, polycystic ovaries.

Dietary Approaches

A negative energy balance is essential for weight loss. How such an energy deficit is achieved is dependent upon the individual. Weight loss is dynamic and needs to be reviewed on a regular basis. A prescribed energy deficit of 2–4 MJ/day (approx. 500–2,000 kcal) will lead to a steady rate of weight loss of 0.5–1 kg/week for a period until the body adapts and plateaus. There are dynamic physiological adaptations that manifest with weight loss; namely a reduced resting metabolic rate, increased appetite and decreased energy cost of physical activity [5, 6]. Dynamic models that allow prediction of how changes of diet or physical activity will translate into weight changes over time have been developed and are available online (http://bwsimulator.niddk.nih.gov/ [5] and http://www.pbrc.edu/research-and-faculty/calculators/weight-loss-predictor/ [7]). These models may be useful in clinical practice to establish a target energy intake for a patient, based on the desired weight loss outcome and duration. Furthermore, they can provide guidance on the energy intake necessary to maintain the new weight once it is reached.

The most important factor determining the success of any diet is the ability to maintain long-term adherence to the new lifestyle changes. It is better to prescribe a 'healthy eating plan' as opposed to a 'diet' as the word diet carries connotations of short-term adherence. Temporary changes will lead to temporary weight loss; if the predisposing factors remain, so too does the propensity for weight regain [8]. Any dietary advice for weight loss should ensure that it does not compromise micronutrient nutritional status. Table 2 gives an overview of common dietary approaches to weight loss, and all approaches are effective; the actual choice of eating intervention will depend on the needs or habits of the individual patient.

Physical Activity

Patients should be encouraged to increase daily physical activity to between 60 and 90 min each day. Additionally, it is important to encourage patients to reduce their 'inactivity' and to stand more. Pedometers may be useful to set daily or weekly targets, which can be gradually increased.

Behavior Modification

The main strategies in behavioral therapy for weight control are self-monitoring, stimulus control, problem solving, contingency management, cognitive restructuring and social support. There appears to be no evidence that any single behavioral strategy is superior to any other in terms of effects on weight loss or weight maintenance. Self-monitoring by recording food intake or exercise can help patients gain insight into their own habits and provides a useful starting point for developing a plan of action. The key to successful behavior change is frequent contact and support to ensure that lifestyle changes are sustained.

Table 2. Overview of common dietary approaches to weight loss

Dietary approach	Description	Reasoning
Low fat, high carbohydrate	<30% of energy from fat, or approx. 30 g/day for women and 40 g/day for men	fat is the most energy-dense macronutrient, so a reduction in fat intake will lead to a reduction in total energy intake
Low carbohydrate	<40% of energy from carbohydrate	depletion of glycogen stores leads to utilization of fat as an energy substrate (and rapid initial weight loss); circulating ketones thought to suppress appetite; decreased range of food choices may also lead to a decreased energy intake
High protein	>20% of energy from protein	increased satiety leading to reduced energy intake; higher thermic effect of food compared with carbohydrate and fat; preservation of lean body mass
Low GI	eating carbohydrate foods with a GI <55	consuming low-GI foods reduces hunger, which in turn leads to decreased food and energy intake; this, combined with the reduced anabolic effect of reduced insulin secretion, promotes weight loss
Portion control	decreasing portion of food eaten on each eating occasion; also includes using portion-controlled foods or meal replacements	people often eat what is offered and tend to overconsume if offered large portions; paying attention to portion size and actively choosing smaller portions will reduce energy intake

GI = Glycemic index.

Adjunctive Therapies

Adjunctive therapies, including very-low-energy diets (VLEDs), pharmacotherapy and bariatric surgery, may be considered for high-risk patients when lifestyle interventions have failed to achieve sufficient weight loss after a minimum of 3 months (fig. 1).

Very-Low-Energy Diet

VLEDs are nutritionally complete, formulated meals defined as diets providing <3.4 MJ/day, and are typically implemented between 8 and 16 weeks, but may be continued for as long as necessary. They usually supply a daily minimum of 50 g of carbohydrate and 50 g of high-quality protein, but must provide the recommended daily allowances of minerals, vitamins, trace elements and essential fatty acids. Most commonly used VLEDs are commercially prepared liquid or powder formulas, or bars. It is important that VLEDs are not misused. They are intended for those with a BMI >30 requiring significant weight loss, but should not be first-line treatment for moderate weight loss.

VLEDs are contraindicated for several specific patient groups (those with severe renal or hepatic disease, for example), though they may be used in those with diabetes, even type 1 diabetes, provided there is appropriate alteration in oral hypoglycemics (metformin may be continued) or insulin with regular blood sugar monitoring. They may, however, be considered as an option for adolescents with grade III obesity, or with a

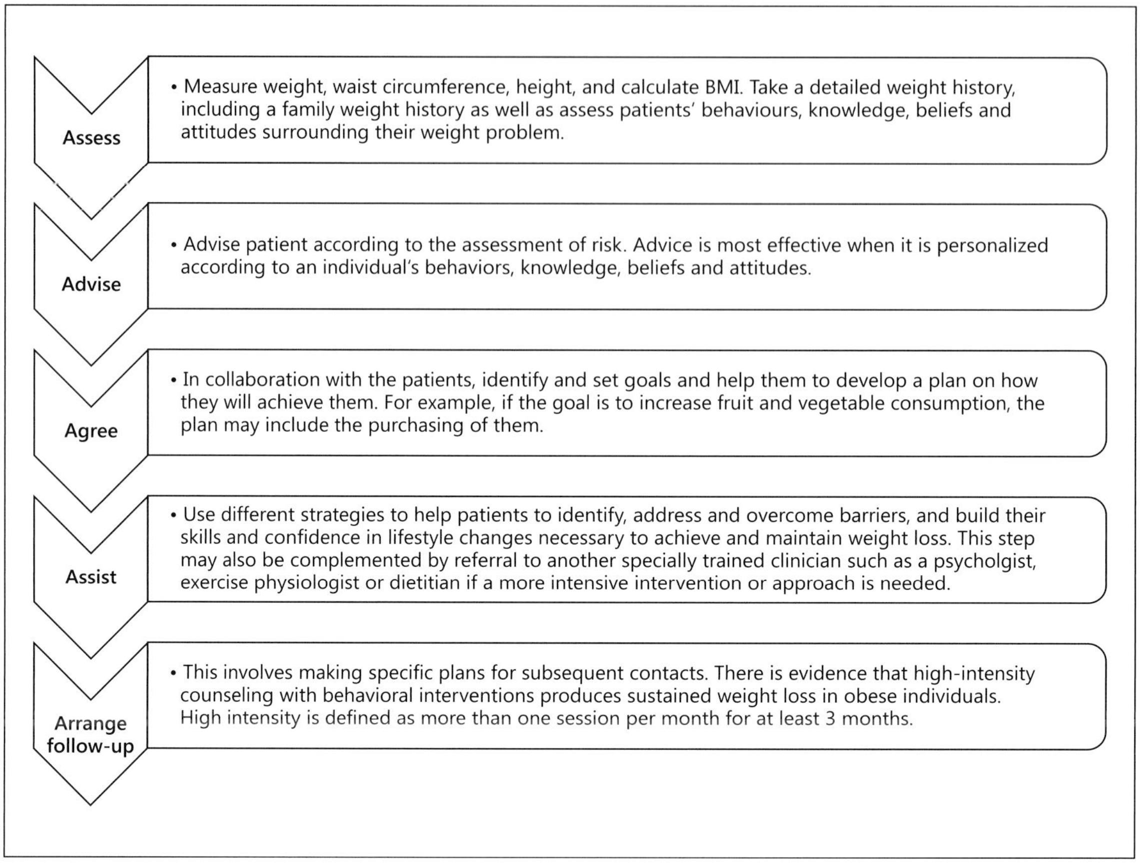

Fig. 2. The 5 As approach to weight management in the primary care setting. Concept adapted from Goldstein et al. [10].

BMI >35 with a severe comorbidity, under strict medical supervision and as an alternative to bariatric surgery. Commonly-reported side effects of some VLEDs include dry mouth, constipation or diarrhea, headache, dizziness, nausea, and cold intolerance. However, these are usually transient.

Pharmacotherapy

Pharmacologic agents indicated for the management of obesity are limited to phentermine for short-term weight loss and orlistat for longer-term weight loss. In the US, low-dose topiramate/phentermine combinations are available. Availability of these agents will depend on country-specific regulatory authorities.

Pharmacotherapy can augment the weight-reducing effects of lifestyle changes and can facilitate long-term maintenance of weight loss as well as the improvement in cardiometabolic risks. Pharmacotherapy should be considered as an adjunct to lifestyle modification for patients who have a BMI ≥30 or if lifestyle changes have failed to produce weight loss within 12 weeks. It should be used under appropriate medical supervision.

Bariatric Surgery

There are different techniques of bariatric surgery; gastric bypass, sleeve gastrectomy and laparoscopic gastric banding procedures are the most widely used. Bariatric surgical intervention combined with permanent lifestyle change is the most effective therapy for weight reduction in terms of the extent and duration of weight loss [9]. Surgery is indicated for patients with a BMI ≥40 or with a BMI ≥35 and medical comorbidities, and is best suited for well-motivated obese patients. Careful medical and nutritional supervision is necessary after surgery to prevent nutritional or digestive complications.

The 5 As Approach to Managing Obesity

The primary care setting provides an ideal opportunity for providing health behavior advice and counselling across multiple counselling sessions [10]. The 5 As approach (Assess, Advise, Agree, Assist, Arrange follow-up) can be used as a guide to structure weight management counselling (fig. 2).

Conclusions

- Obesity is a complex issue. Identifying patients who are overweight and obese, and particularly those with an increased WC, is essential for preventing obesity and its complications.
- Patients with obesity need to recognize it is a serious health problem and work collaboratively with primary healthcare providers and other healthcare professionals towards a weight management solution, understanding the long-term nature of the treatment.
- It is easy to simply tell patients that they need to eat better and exercise more to lose weight. The major challenge, however, is helping patients to achieve behavioral changes rather than just suggesting them.

References

1 WHO: Obesity: preventing and managing the global epidemic. World Health Organ Tech Rep Ser 2000;894:i–xii, 1–253.
2 WHO Expert Consultation: Appropriate body-mass index for Asian populations and its implications for policy and intervention strategies. Lancet 2004;363:157–163.
3 Goldstein DJ: Beneficial health effects of modest weight loss. Int J Obes Relat Metab Disord 1992;16:397–415.
4 Caterson ID, Finer N, Coutinho W, et al: Maintained intentional weight loss reduces cardiovascular outcomes: results from the Sibutramine Cardiovascular OUTcomes (SCOUT) trial. Diabetes Obes Metab 2012;14:523–530.
5 Hall KD, Sacks G, Chandramohan D, et al: Quantification of the effect of energy imbalance on bodyweight. Lancet 2011; 378:826–837.
6 Casazza K, Pate R, Allison DB: Myths, presumptions, and facts about obesity. N Engl J Med 2013;368:446–454.
7 Thomas DM, Martin CK, Heymsfield S, et al: A simple model predicting individual weight change in humans. J Biol Dyn 2011;5:579–599.
8 Wyatt HR, et al: Lessons from patients who have successfully maintained weight loss. Obes Manag 2005;1:56–61.
9 Sjöström L, Narbro K, Sjöström CD, et al: Effects of bariatric surgery on mortality in Swedish obese subjects. N Engl J Med 2007;357:741–752.
10 Goldstein MG, Whitlock EP, DePue J: Multiple behavioral risk factor interventions in primary care. Summary of research evidence. Am J Prev Med 2004; 27(suppl 2):61–79.

Bier D, et al. (eds): Nutrition for the Primary Care Provider. World Rev Nutr Diet. Basel, Karger, 2015, vol 111, pp 110–115
DOI: 10.1159/000362770

Diabetes Mellitus

Jim Mann

Department of Human Nutrition, University of Otago, Dunedin, New Zealand

Key Words

Type 2 diabetes · Lifestyle · Complications · Management · Prevention

Key Messages

- Rates of type 2 diabetes mellitus (T2DM) have reached epidemic proportions in many countries and are high throughout the world.
- In predisposed families or populations, genetic and lifestyle factors combine to result in the development of insulin resistance and T2DM.
- Excess body fatness appears to be the main driver of the increasing rates of T2DM.
- Decreasing energy-dense foods, increasing physical activity and achieving a body mass index as close as possible to the recommended range are the cornerstones of management and attempts to 'prevent' T2DM or reduce progression of prediabetes.
- A wide range of macronutrient intakes is acceptable with particular emphasis on the nature of carbohydrate- and fat-containing food choices.
- In some situations, inappropriate nutrition from the time of conception through to early life may result in epigenetic changes which increase subsequent risk of T2DM. Appropriate nutrition throughout the lifecycle may help to reduce the global epidemic.

Introduction

The term 'diabetes mellitus' describes a group of conditions characterized by raised blood glucose levels (hyperglycemia) resulting from an absolute or relative deficiency in insulin. Type 1 diabetes is characterized by destruction of the insulin-producing pancreatic islet β-cells, typically resulting from an autoimmune process. Insulin treatment is essential to maintain life. In type 2 diabetes mellitus (T2DM), a key abnormality is resistance to the action of insulin and in the early stages of the disease, insulin levels may actually be raised as the β-cells of the pancreas produce more insulin in an attempt to overcome insulin resistance. In many patients with T2DM, the insulin-producing β-cells may show a degree of failure at some stage during the course of the disease process. Patients with T2DM are initially treated with 'lifestyle modification' therapy. Oral hypoglycemic (blood glucose-lowering) agents may be added. Insulin may be required later. Impaired glucose tolerance, impaired fasting glucose and gestational diabetes (diabetes developing during pregnancy) may represent the earliest stages of T2DM and are often referred to as prediabetes.

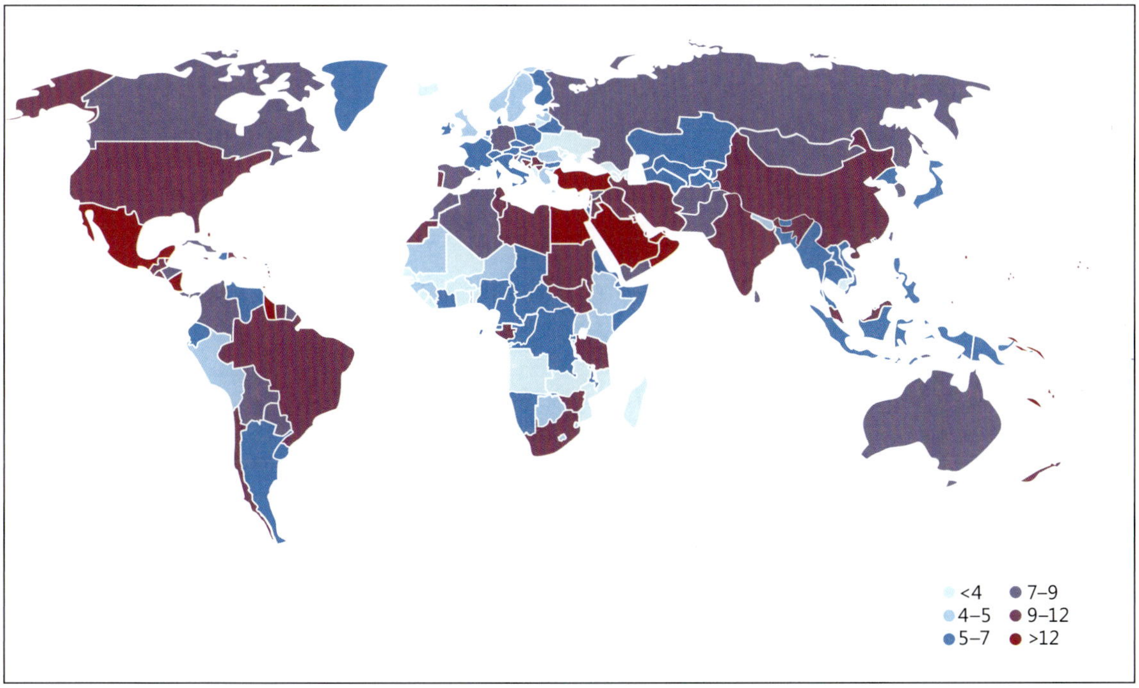

Fig. 1. Prevalence estimates (%) of diabetes in individuals aged 20–79 years (2013). Source: International Diabetes Federation [3].

Diabetes is believed to affect 8% of the world's adult population, with 382 million individuals having the condition. Rates are especially high in some indigenous populations which have undergone rapid acculturation (e.g. American Pima Indians, Polynesians, Melanesians and Australian Aboriginals) and other populations which have migrated, typically to countries of greater affluence (e.g. Asian Indian migrants to the UK and other countries). India and China have relatively high rates of diabetes and are two of the most populous countries in the world. Thus, China is the country with the highest number of people with diabetes, with a current figure of 98.4 million, followed by India with 65.1 million. If the current rates of growth continue unchecked, it has been estimated that by 2035, the total number of people with diabetes worldwide will exceed 592 million. In addition to those with diabetes, there are many with prediabetes. Thus, T2DM may be regarded as one of the major epidemics of the 21st century. Worldwide prevalence estimates of diabetes are shown in figure 1. The vast majority are affected by T2DM, and this chapter therefore considers the causes, management and possibilities for prevention of T2DM.

Lifestyle-Related Determinants of Type 2 Diabetes and Its Complications

The risk of developing T2DM is greatly increased when one or more close family members have the condition, although the precise mode of inheritance has not yet been resolved. It appears that, in predisposed populations or families, genetic and lifestyle factors combine to result in the development of insulin resistance and consequently, diabetes. The striking association between the risk of T2DM and increasing body fatness, particularly when the excess body fat is centrally distributed (i.e. in association with a high waist circumference), has been repeatedly reported in people of different ethnicities. Dietary attributes and lack of physical activity which contribute to the development of excess body fat also contribute to T2DM.

There have been several attempts to implicate individual foods or nutrients as causal or protective factors independently of any association they may have with overweight or obesity. It is likely that more than one of the attributes that characterize the Western lifestyle (excessive intakes of energy-dense foods; relatively low intakes of vegetables, fruits, and lightly processed cereal foods with intact cellular structure; inadequate physical activity) is likely to contribute to the etiology of T2DM. One very large prospective study has suggested that diets with a high glycemic load and low cereal fiber content increase the risk of T2DM. The glycemic load provides an indication of both glycemic index (GI) and quantity of carbohydrate. A high intake of saturated fatty acids may increase resistance to the action of insulin and therefore increase the risk of developing T2DM. Sugar does not appear to be an independent risk factor for T2DM, though high intakes of sugar-sweetened beverages have been associated with a subsequent increase in risk. Intrauterine growth retardation leading to babies born small for gestational age and prematurity have also been suggested as risk factors for the development T2DM in later life. This appears to be especially the case when rapid catch-up growth occurs in infancy and childhood (fetal programming or 'Barker' hypothesis). Cardiovascular disease is responsible for the greatest number of deaths and a large proportion of nonfatal illnesses in people with T2DM. Therefore, nutritional determinants of cardiovascular disease need to be taken into account when considering the nutritional management of people with diabetes. Several other complications of diabetes (e.g. retinopathy, nephropathy, and neuropathy) appear to be a result of hyperglycemia and other metabolic consequences of diabetes and hypertension. Diet plays a major role in their prevention and treatment, principally by helping to improve blood glucose control and lower blood pressure.

Nutritional Management of People with Diabetes

Dietary modification is the cornerstone of treatment for people with T2DM, and many who comply with dietary advice will show improvement in the metabolic abnormalities associated with this condition, possibly abrogating the need for oral medications and insulin. However, even when drug treatment is required, attention to diet may further improve blood glucose control and modify cardiovascular risk factors. The principles of treatment are summarized in table 1. These guidelines are based on the advice of the American Diabetes Association and the European Association for the Study of Diabetes. Much publicity has arisen from claims of the 'unique' benefits associated with Mediterranean, high-protein (e.g. Zone), high-fiber, low-carbohydrate, and even high-fat (e.g. Atkins) diets for people with diabetes. While the majority of experts would agree that a high-fat diet is undesirable in the long term, the consensus is that most dietary patterns would be acceptable for the majority of people with diabetes, provided they comply with the recommendations for energy and nutrients. No single dietary pattern has been shown to be associated with better long-term outcomes than any others.

The key recommendation for those who are overweight (BMI >25) is that calorie intake should be reduced and energy expenditure increased so that the BMI moves towards the recommended range (18.5–25). Prevention of weight regain is an important aim once weight loss has been achieved. For those who are overweight or obese, reducing energy-dense foods (those high in fats and added

Table 1. Key aspects of the current recommendations for diabetic diet and lifestyle

Parameter	Recommendations
EASD Nutrition Study Group	
Dietary energy and body weight	Achieve and/or maintain BMI of 18.5–25. Diet and exercise important.
Dietary fat	Saturated plus trans-unsaturated fatty acids: <10% total energy, <8% if low-density lipoprotein levels are raised. Polyunsaturated fatty acids: 6–10% total energy. Monounsaturated fatty acids: 10–20% total energy. Total fat: <35% total energy (if overweight <30%). Oily fish, soybean and rapeseed oil, nuts and green leafy vegetables to provide ω-3 fatty acids. Cholesterol: <300 g/day.
Carbohydrate	Total carbohydrate: 45–60% total energy, influenced by metabolic characteristics. Vegetables, fruits, legumes and cereal-derived foods preferred.
Dietary fiber and GI/load	Naturally occurring foods rich in dietary fiber are encouraged. Ideal dietary fiber intake should be more than 40 g/day (or 20 g/1,000 kcal/day), half soluble fiber (lesser amounts also beneficial). Five servings/day of fiber-rich vegetables and fruit and four or more servings of legumes/week help to provide minimum requirements. Cereal-based foods should be wholegrain and high in fiber. Carbohydrate-rich low-glycemic-index foods are suitable choices, provided other attributes are appropriate.
Sucrose and other free sugars	If desired and blood glucose levels are satisfactory, free sugars up to 50 g/day may be incorporated into the diet. Total free sugars should not exceed 10% of total energy (less for those who are overweight).
Protein	Protein should provide 10–20% total energy.
Vitamins, antioxidant nutrients, minerals and trace elements	Increase foods rich in tocopherols, carotenoids, vitamin C and flavonoids, trace elements and other vitamins. Fruits, vegetables, and wholegrains rather than supplements are recommended. Restrict salt to <6 g/day (<2.3 g sodium).
Alcohol	Up to 10 g/day for women and 20 g/day for men is acceptable for most people with diabetes who choose to drink alcohol. Special precautions apply to those on insulin or sulphonylureas, those who are overweight and those with hypertriglyceridemia.
Special 'diabetic' or functional foods and supplements	Nonalcoholic beverages sweetened with nonnutritive sweeteners are useful. Other special foods not encouraged.
Nonnutritive and hypocaloric sweeteners	No particular merit of fructose and other 'special' nutritive sweeteners over sucrose.
Families	Most recommendations suitable for the whole family.

Table 1 (continued)

Parameter	Recommendations
American Diabetes Association	
Dietary energy and body weight	Overweight and obese adults with T2DM should reduce energy intake while maintaining a healthy eating pattern. Modest weight loss may provide clinical benefit. Provide ongoing support to achieve lifestyle change.
Dietary fat	Fat quality more important than quantity. Amounts of saturated fat and trans fat and dietary cholesterol same as for general population. Mediterranean style, MUFA-rich eating pattern may benefit glycemic control and CVD risk, therefore effective alternative to lower fat, higher carbohydrate eating pattern. Foods rich in ω3. Supplements of ω3 not recommended.
Carbohydrate	No certainty regarding ideal amount, but total amount of carbohydrate and available insulin determine glycemic response after eating. Monitoring carbohydrate remains key to achieving glycemic control. Carbohydrate from vegetables, fruits, wholegrains, legumes and dairy products preferred to others, especially those containing added fats, sugars or sodium.
Dietary fiber and GI	Substituting low-glycemic-load foods for higher-glycemic-load foods may improve glycemic control. Consume at least the amount of fiber and wholegrains recommended for the general public.
Sucrose and other free sugars	Consumption should be minimized to avoid displacing nutrient-dense foods. Sugar-sweetened beverages should be limited or avoided to reduce risk for weight gain and worsening of cardiometabolic risk profile. Fructose in foods such as fruit may result in better glycemic control compared with isocaloric intake of sucrose or starch.
Protein	Intake should be individualized. Reducing protein below usual intakes not recommended.
Vitamins, antioxidant nutrients, minerals and trace elements	No clear evidence of benefit of supplementation in people who do not have deficiencies. Concern regarding long-term safety of supplementation with vitamins E and C and carotene and lack of evidence of efficacy. Sodium reduced to 2,300 mg/day, further individualized reduction with hypertension.
Families	Not applicable.

Sources: Mann et al. [1], American Diabetes Association [2] and Evert et al. [4].

sugars) and regular exercise are usually sufficient to achieve weight loss, prescription of precise energy requirements only being necessary for those unable to achieve the desired weight reduction. Even modest weight reduction (a loss of less than 10% body weight) in the overweight or obese improves insulin sensitivity, glycemic control and cardiovascular risk factors.

A wide range of macronutrient intakes is acceptable, the emphasis being on the nutritional attributes of food choices. To enhance glycemic control, the nature of carbohydrate is particularly important. Vegetables, legumes, intact fruits and manually processed wholegrain cereals are preferred choices. Rapidly digested carbohydrates (e.g. sugars, potatoes, rice, many types of breads and pastas) should be limited. The GI of carbohydrate-rich foods (e.g. breads, pastas) may provide a useful indication of their suitability. However, GI is unhelpful when considering energy-dense foods rich in fats and sugar. Such energy-dense foods typically have low GIs but should be severely restricted by most people with T2DM. The advice relating to dietary fat is based principally on the guidelines for reducing cardiovascular risk.

Potential for 'Preventing' Type 2 Diabetes

While the precise mechanisms by which genes and lifestyle interact to result in T2DM remain elusive, the geographic variation, rapid changes over time, and dietary patterns related to risk suggest that lifestyle modification might help to prevent, or at least delay, the onset of T2DM in predisposed individuals. Randomized controlled trials, first reported from Finland, the USA, and China and more recently from other countries, confirm that this is indeed the case. The lifestyle changes which might be expected to achieve the approximately 60% reduction in rates of progression from impaired glucose tolerance to T2DM demonstrated in the trials for periods of 10 years or more are similar to those recommended for treatment of T2DM. Achieving a weight loss of at least 5–7% initial body weight in those who are overweight or obese is a pivotal component of the 'prevention' program.

Conclusions

- Excess body fat is the main driver of T2DM. In some individuals, genetic and lifestyle factors also play a role in the development of insulin resistance and the onset of T2DM.
- Another contributing factor is inappropriate nutrition from conception to early life, which may increase an individual's subsequent risk of T2DM.
- Decreased intake of energy-dense foods, increasing physical activity and achieving the recommended body mass index are key aspects of the management of T2DM and for reducing the progression of prediabetes.
- Appropriate nutrition throughout the lifecycle may help to reduce this global epidemic.

References

1 Mann JI, De Leeuw I, Hermansen K, et al: Evidence-based nutritional approaches to the treatment and prevention of diabetes mellitus. Nutr Metab Cardiovasc Dis 2004;14:373–394.

2 American Diabetes Association: Clinical practice recommendations. Diabetes Care 2014;37(suppl 1):S1–S155.

3 International Diabetes Federation: IDF Diabetes Atlas, ed 6. Brussels, International Diabetes Federation, 2013. www.idf.org/diabetesatlas.

4 Evert AB, Boucher JL, Cypress M, et al: Nutrition therapy recommendations for the management of adults with diabetes. Diabetes Care 2014;37(suppl 1):S120–S543.

Bier D, et al. (eds): Nutrition for the Primary Care Provider. World Rev Nutr Diet. Basel, Karger, 2015, vol 111, pp 116–122
DOI: 10.1159/000362308

Obesity, Diabetes and the Asian Phenotype

Swati Bhardwaj[a–c] Anoop Misra[a–e]

[a]National Diabetes, Obesity and Cholesterol Diseases Foundation (N-DOC), SDA, [b]Diabetes Foundation (India), SDA, [c]Center of Nutrition and Metabolic Research (C-NET), [d]Fortis C-DOC Center of Excellence for Diabetes, Metabolic Diseases and Endocrinology, and [e]Center for Internal Medicine, Fortis Flt. Lt. Rajan Dhall Hospital, New Delhi, India

Key Words

Obesity · Metabolic syndrome · South Asians · Nutrition transition · Phenotype · Population-based prevention

Key Messages

- Rapid economic, demographic, and nutritional changes occurring in India and other south Asian countries contribute towards a sedentary lifestyle and imbalanced dietary profile, leading to a rise in obesity and the metabolic syndrome.
- Several phenotypic features may contribute to insulin resistance and the metabolic syndrome in South Asians: despite lower average body mass index (BMI) values, South Asians have a high percentage of body fat compared to Caucasians or Blacks, which is partly explained by body build, low muscularity, adaptation to chronic calorie deprivation, and ethnicity.
- Consequently, morbidities related to higher body fat (diabetes, hypertension, dyslipidemia, etc.) occur more frequently at lower BMI levels in Asians than in Caucasians.
- Other contributing factors are the nutrition transition, an increasingly sedentary lifestyle, and the rural-to-urban migration. These act in concert with genetic and phenotypic factors, resulting in obesity, insulin resistance, the metabolic syndrome, type 2 diabetes and cardiovascular disease.
- Health interventions required to prevent or reduce morbidity/mortality need to be addressed in both children and adults. Interventions should aim to increase physical activity and encourage healthier food patterns and health education.

Introduction

The prevalence of obesity and the metabolic syndrome is rapidly increasing in India and other south Asian countries, leading to increased morbidity and mortality due to type 2 diabetes mellitus (T2DM) and cardiovascular disease (CVD) [1]. Rapid economic, demographic, and nutritional changes are occurring in India and other neighboring South Asian countries, contributing towards a sedentary lifestyle and imbalanced dietary profile, further leading to obesity (fig. 1). Persistent obesity dysregulates metabolic processes including the action of insulin on glucose-lipid-free fatty acid metabolism, and severely af-

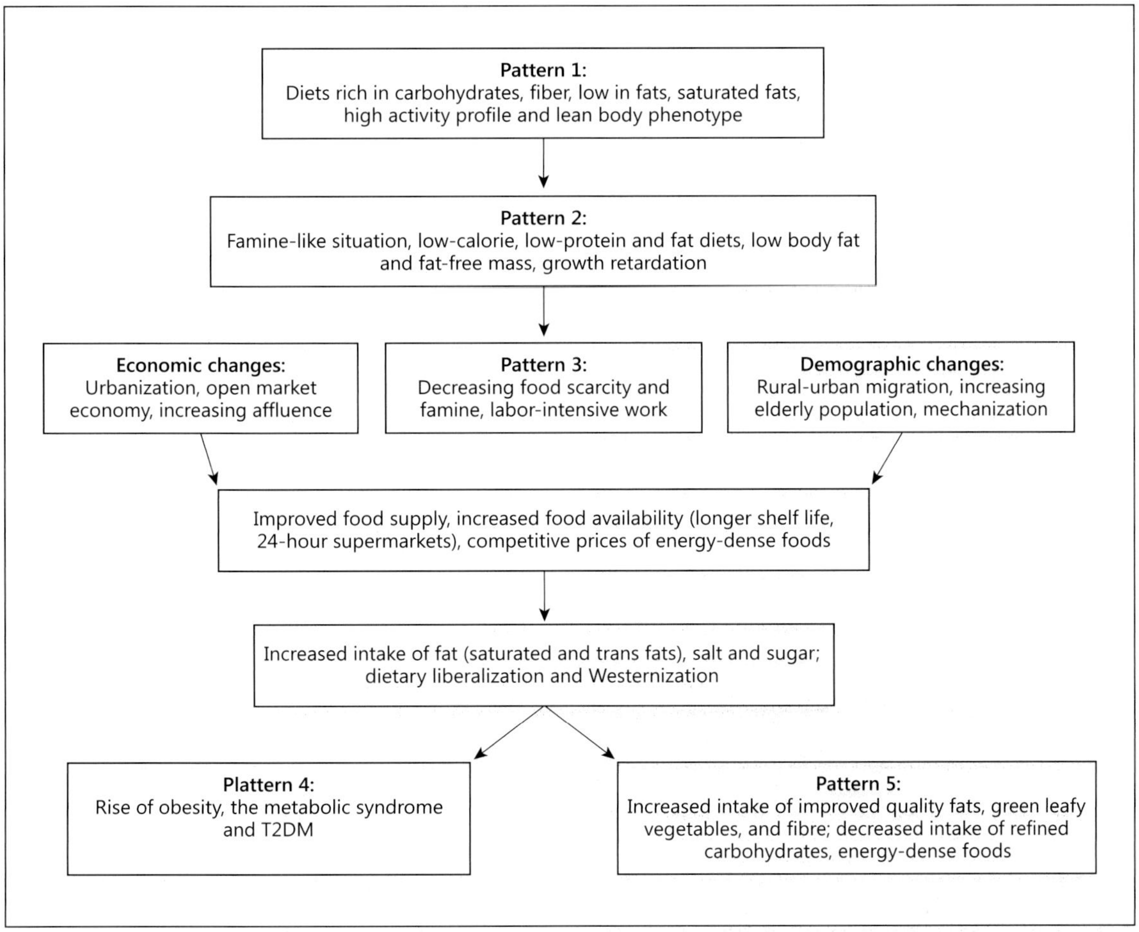

Fig. 1. Relationship between nutrition transition, urbanization, and the rise in obesity and the metabolic syndrome in developing countries. Pattern 3 may be seen at different rates of progression in different developing countries. Pattern 4 is likely to affect all socioeconomic strata. Adapted from Misra and Khurana [4].

fects other processes that regulate blood glucose, blood pressure, and lipids. Thus begin a cluster of conditions: dysglycemia, dyslipidemia, hypertension, and a procoagulant state, known as the metabolic syndrome. Data suggest that obesity and the metabolic syndrome are immediate precursors of T2DM and CVD [2]. A high prevalence of the metabolic syndrome and associated cardiovascular risk factors has been observed not only in urban South Asian/Asian-Indian adults and children but also in economically disadvantaged people residing in urban slums and rural areas. This increasing burden of obesity, the metabolic syndrome, T2DM, and CVD in South Asian countries has created an urgent need to strategize health policies and mass intervention programs to tackle nutrition and continue efforts to manage undernutrition. Clearly, these efforts require a thorough understanding of the factors influencing and driving obesity, the metabolic syndrome and T2DM in developing countries.

Table 1. Average values of various measures of obesity in South Asians/Asian Indians and other ethnic groups

Parameters	Asian-Indians				White Caucasians	Blacks	Mexican-Americans
	rural	urban slums	urban	migrant[1]			
BMI	19.6	20.9	22.4	24.7	26.3	28.5	25.7
Body fat, %	20.4	24.4	28.2	33.1	26.6	29.7	48.8
Waist circumference, cm	79.4	83.7	85.2	83.7	91.3	83.9	94.5
Waist-hip ratio	0.87	0.92	0.87	0.92	0.91	0.86	0.92

Adapted from Misra and Vikram [3]. [1] Migrant South Asians and Asian Indians.

Phenotypic Features of Obesity That May Contribute to Insulin Resistance and the Metabolic Syndrome in South Asians

The phenotype of obesity and body fat distribution are distinctive in South Asians. The average value of body mass index (BMI) in South Asians is lower than that seen in white Caucasians, Mexican-Americans and Blacks. However, BMI in Asian-Indians increases as they become affluent and urbanized (table 1). South Asians have a high percentage of body fat as compared to white Caucasians and Blacks, despite lower average BMI values (table 1), which is partly explained by body build (trunk-to-leg length ratio and slenderness), low muscularity, adaptation to chronic calorie deprivation, and ethnicity [3]. Importantly, morbidities related to higher body fat (diabetes, hypertension, dyslipidemia etc.) occur more frequently at lower BMI levels in Asians than in white Caucasians [4]. A high prevalence of abdominal obesity is seen in South Asians, and is also reported in Asian-Indians with BMI <25 [3]. Although the average waist circumference in South Asians appears to be lower, abdominal adiposity is significantly more than in white Caucasians. For example, intra-abdominal adipose tissue in South Asians is comparatively more than in Caucasians [5]. Furthermore, truncal subcutaneous adipose tissue (measured by subscapular and supra-iliac skinfold thickness) is thicker in South Asians than in white Caucasians (in both adults and children), which correlates better with insulin resistance than intra-abdominal adipose tissue. Fat deposition may occur at 'ectopic sites' and may have relevance to insulin resistance in Asian-Indians, e.g. intramyocellular lipids may be one such site. Another, and perhaps more important, ectopic site of fat deposition is the liver. Fat accumulation in liver (fatty liver) in the absence of significant alcohol intake (nonalcoholic fatty liver disease, NAFLD) is now recognized as a disease risk in overweight/obese subjects. NAFLD is strongly related to insulin resistance independent of obesity and abdominal adiposity. Limited data in South Asians suggest that approximately 25% of the urban population has NAFLD [6]. Furthermore, Asian-Indians have comparatively higher deposition of triglycerides in liver as compared to white Caucasians [7]. Overall, excess hepatic fat accumulation in Asian-Indians may be important in the genesis of insulin resistance, the metabolic syndrome and diabetes, and constitutes a prime area for research.

Fat deposition has also been reported in other sites of the body: 'buffalo hump' (excess fat deposition in dorsocervical region) and double chin (excess fat deposition under the chin). A Metabolic Syndrome Screening Score, including buffalo hump, double chin, age and gender, was generated based on these data and showed a sensitivity and specificity of 82 and 71%, respectively, in detecting metabolic syndrome [8].

Table 2. Cutoffs for obesity and abdominal obesity in Asian Indians vs. international criteria

Variable	Category	Consensus guidelines for Asian Indians[1]	Prevalent international criteria
Generalized obesity (BMI cutoffs)	normal	18.0–22.9	18.5–24.9[2]
	overweight	23.0–24.9	25.0–29.9[2]
	obesity	>25	>30
Abdominal obesity (waist circumference cutoffs in cm)	men	>90[3]	>102[4]
	women	>80[3]	>88[4]

Adapted from Misra and Khurana [9]. [1] From Consensus guidelines for Asian Indians [10]. [2]According to World Health Organization guidelines [11]. [3] Both as per Consensus Guidelines and the International Diabetes Federation (for Asian Indians) [12]. [4] According to Modified National Cholesterol Education Program, Adult Treatment Panel III guidelines [13].

Finally, South Asians could be termed as 'metabolically obese', though BMI levels may fall in the category of 'nonobese'. This phenomenon is partially explained by high body fat, high intraabdominal and subcutaneous fat, NAFLD, and fat deposition at other ectopic sites which contribute to insulin resistance, dyslipidemia, hyperglycemia, and excess procoagulant milieu in South Asians [5].

Definition of Generalized and Abdominal Obesity in Asian-Indians

The definitions of abdominal and generalized obesity are different in South Asians as compared to Caucasians, as indicated in table 2 [9].

Obesity, the Metabolic Syndrome and Type 2 Diabetes: Determinants and Correlates for South Asians/Asian-Indians

Diets

With the nutrition transition, consumption of traditional foods (low in saturated fat, SFA, low in simple sugars and high in fiber) has declined, and non-traditional energy-dense imbalanced foods ('fast-foods'; high in calories, carbohydrates, SFA, trans-fatty acid and low in fiber) are being increasingly consumed in India [5]. Higher intakes of carbohydrate, SFA, trans-fatty acid and n-6 PUFA, and lower intakes of n-3 PUFA and fiber, and a higher n-3:n-6 PUFA ratio have been reported in South Asians, as compared to other populations [5]. Furthermore, high dietary n-6 PUFA and SFA are significant independent predictors of fasting hyperinsulinaemia and high levels of C-reactive protein, respectively, in adolescent Asian-Indians. Specifically, in children and young individuals in North India, high intake of omega-6 PUFAs has been shown to correlate with fasting hyperinsulinemia [5]. High consumption of partially hydrogenated oils (Vanaspati) containing high amount of trans-fatty acid has been noted in India, particularly in socioeconomically disadvantaged populations.

Physical Activity

South Asians are more sedentary as compared to other ethnic groups [14]. Increasingly, sedentary lifestyle is attributed to increased mechanization in work places and household work. Leisure time

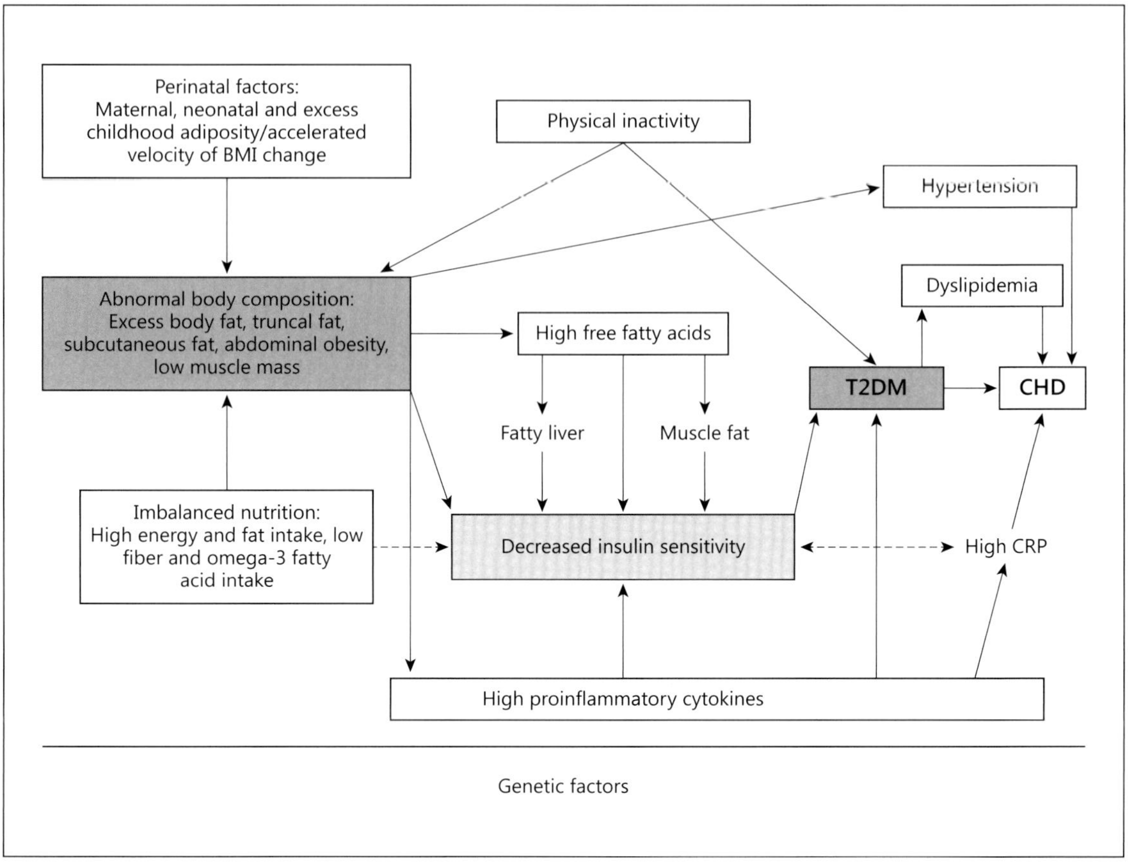

Fig. 2. Complex interactions of genetic, perinatal, nutritional and other acquired factors in the development of insulin resistance, T2DM and coronary heart disease in South Asians. CRP = C-reactive protein; CHD = coronary heart disease. Dashed lines represent weak relationships [20].

physical activities have also shifted from outdoor play to indoor entertainment (television and computer games) [4]. In a recent study done in South India, 79% of the industrial populations were demonstrated to follow a sedentary lifestyle [15].

Migration

The effect of migration on adiposity and diabetes has been discussed by us in a published review [16]. Migration (both intra- as well as intercountry) leads to significant stress due to the new environment, social, economic, and language disparities, job challenges and lack of social support, which may lead to metabolic derangements and diabetes. An adverse coronary risk profile was reported among rural-to-urban migrant populations living in urban slums in India [17].

Genetic versus Environmental Factors

A role of genetic predisposition in the development of obesity, the metabolic syndrome, dyslipidemia, and T2DM in Asian-Indians has been reported [18]. Adverse intrauterine environment has been reported to contribute to insulin resistance and the metabolic syndrome. Both fetal undernutrition (low birth weight, LBW) and over-nutrition increase the risk of future diabetes and adiposity in children in later life. LBW was associated with higher systolic blood pressure, fasting and postprandial hyperinsulinemia, subscapular/triceps skinfold ratio, plasma LDL, along with insulin resistance. Small and thin Indian newborns (weight 2.7 kg and ponderal index 2.4, calculated as kg/m^2) were shown to have poor muscle mass but higher adiposity for a given weight compared with white Caucasian babies. Furthermore, 'catch up' obesity seen in LBW offspring seems to be important for adult-onset insulin resistance and associated cardiovascular risk factors. Interestingly, normal to high folate levels coupled with low vitamin B_{12} levels in mothers predicted higher adiposity and insulin resistance in Indian babies [19]. These preliminary data need to be confirmed in further studies. The complex interplay of genetic, metabolic and environmental risk factors resulting in obesity insulin resistance, the metabolic syndrome, T2DM and coronary heart disease is shown in figure 2 [20].

Conclusions

- The prevalence of obesity, the metabolic syndrome and T2DM has shown a rapid rise in South Asian countries in the past few decades and has led to increased risk of CVD and consequent morbidity and mortality.
- The various factors responsible for increasing noncommunicable diseases are rapid nutrition transition, rural-to-urban migration, increasingly sedentary occupations and lifestyle, and maternal-fetal factors.
- Both genetic and environmental factors seem to contribute to this; however, the role of environment seems to be predominant.
- Health interventions required to prevent or reduce the morbidity/mortality need to be addressed in both children and adults. Interventions should be aimed at increasing the physical activity along with healthier food patterns and health education.
- Successful community-based intervention programs have been reported in developed countries, and a similar approach is required specifically in developing South Asian countries. Various other health strategies consisting of individual and community initiatives, backed up by governmental and legislative efforts, would also help in minimizing the increasing prevalence of obesity and the metabolic syndrome in developing countries (see box).

Box. Community intervention programs for childhood obesity in India

Community-based interventions are aimed at generating awareness and providing a conductive environment for children to follow a healthy lifestyle (balanced diet and increased physical activity) and promote healthy food alternatives. In India, we have initiated comprehensive programs aiming at childhood obesity, namely 'CHETNA' (Hindi for 'The Awareness'; Children Health Education through Nutrition and Health Awareness program), which was carried out in New Delhi, and 'MARG' (Hindi for 'The Path'; Medical Education for Children/Adolescents for Realistic Prevention of Obesity and Diabetes and for Healthy Ageing), carried out in 15 cities of North India covering nearly 700,000 children. Under these programs, children are given nutritional and physical activity education with the help of lectures, leaflets, debates and skits. These comprehensive programs initiated on a large scale for the first time in South Asia are aimed to impart education regarding healthy lifestyle not only to children, but also to teachers and parents. The 'MARG' program is the first large-scale community intervention project in South Asia which focuses 100% on primary prevention of not only diabetes, but noncommunicable diseases in general.

References

1 Misra A, Khurana L: The metabolic syndrome in South Asians: epidemiology, determinants, and prevention. Metab Syndr Relat Disord 2009;7:497–514.

2 Third Report of the National Cholesterol Education Program (NCEP) Expert Panel on Detection, Evaluation, and Treatment of High Blood Cholesterol in Adults (Adult Treatment Panel III): final report. Circulation 2002;106:3143–3421.

3 Misra A, Vikram NK: Insulin resistance syndrome (metabolic syndrome) and obesity in Asian Indians: evidence and implications. Nutrition 2004;20:482–491.

4 Misra A, Khurana L: Obesity and the metabolic syndrome in developing countries. J Clin Endocrinol Metab 2008;93(suppl 1):S9–S30.

5 Misra A, Khurana L, Isharwal S, Bhardwaj S: South Asian diets and insulin resistance. Br J Nutr 2008:1–9.

6 Sharma R, Sinha S, Danishad KA, et al: Investigation of hepatic gluconeogenesis pathway in non-diabetic Asian Indians with non-alcoholic fatty liver disease using in vivo (31P) phosphorus magnetic resonance spectroscopy. Atherosclerosis 2009;203:291–297.

7 Petersen KF, Dufour S, Feng J, et al: Increased prevalence of insulin resistance and nonalcoholic fatty liver disease in Asian-Indian men. Proc Natl Acad Sci USA 2006;103:18273–18277.

8 Misra A, Jaiswal A, Shakti D, et al: Novel phenotypic markers and screening score for the metabolic syndrome in adult Asian Indians. Diabetes Res Clin Pract 2008;79:1–5.

9 Misra A, Khurana L: Obesity-related non-communicable diseases: South Asians vs White Caucasians. Int J Obes (Lond) 2011;35:167–187.

10 Misra A, Chowbey PK, Makkar BM, et al: Consensus statement for diagnosis of obesity, abdominal obesity and the metabolic syndrome for Asian Indians and recommendations for physical activity, medical and surgical management. J Assoc Physicians India 2009;57:163–170.

11 WHO: Obesity and overweight. http://www.who.int/mediacentre/factsheets/fs311/en/ (accessed May 2013).

12 International Diabetes Federation: IDF worldwide definition of the metabolic syndrome. http://www.idf.org/webdata/docs/MetS_def_update2006.pdf (accessed May 2013).

13 Grundy SM, Brewer HB Jr, Cleeman JI, et al: Definition of metabolic syndrome: report of the National Heart, Lung, and Blood Institute/American Heart Association conference on scientific issues related to definition. Circulation 2004;109:433–438.

14 Bedi US, Singh S, Syed A, et al: Coronary artery disease in South Asians: an emerging risk group. Cardiol Rev 2006;14:74–80.

15 Mohan V, Deepa M, Farooq S, et al: Surveillance for risk factors of cardiovascular disease among an industrial population in southern India. Natl Med J India 2008;21:8–13.

16 Misra A, Ganda OP: Migration and its impact on adiposity and type 2 diabetes. Nutrition 2007;23:696–708.

17 Misra A, Vikram NK, Pandey RM, et al: Hyperhomocysteinemia, and low intakes of folic acid and vitamin B_{12} in urban North India. Eur J Nutr 2002;41:68–77.

18 Misra A, Nishanth S, Pasha ST, et al: Relationship of Xba1 and EcoR1 polymorphisms of apolipoprotein-B gene to dyslipidemia and obesity in Asian Indians in North India. Indian Heart J 2001;53:177–183.

19 Yajnik CS, Deshmukh US: Maternal nutrition, intrauterine programming and consequential risks in the offspring. Rev Endocr Metab Disord 2008;9:203–211.

20 Misra A, Bhardwaj S: Obesity and the metabolic syndrome in developing countries: focus on South Asians; in Black RE, Singhal A, Uauy R (eds): International Nutrition: Achieving Millennium Goals and Beyond. Nestle Nutr Inst Workshop Ser. Vevey, Nestec/Basel, Karger, 2014, vol 78, pp 133–140.

Bier D, et al. (eds): Nutrition for the Primary Care Provider. World Rev Nutr Diet. Basel, Karger, 2015, vol 111, pp 123–129
DOI: 10.1159/000362309

Cancer Prevention and Treatment

Timothy Key

Cancer Epidemiology Unit, Nuffield Department of Population Health, University of Oxford, Oxford, UK

Key Words

Cancer · Obesity · Alcohol · Meat · Dietary fiber · Fruit and vegetables

Key Messages

- Nutritional factors and alcohol may be responsible for around 30% of cancers in developed countries.
- Overweight/obesity increases the risk for cancers of the esophagus (adenocarcinoma), colorectum, breast (postmenopausal), endometrium, and kidney.
- Alcohol causes cancers of the oral cavity, pharynx, larynx, esophagus, colorectum, liver, and breast.
- High intakes of red and processed meat and low intakes of dietary fiber probably increase the risk for colorectal cancer.
- Healthy diets should provide adequate amounts of all nutrients and of fruit and vegetables.
- For patients being treated for cancer, diets should provide adequate amounts of all nutrients, and obesity should be avoided.

Introduction

Worldwide, there are nearly 13 million new cases of cancer and 8 million deaths from cancer each year [1]. The most commonly diagnosed are cancers of the lung, breast and colorectum. The most common causes of cancer death are lung, stomach and liver cancers (fig. 1). The most important cause of cancer in developed countries is tobacco, which causes around 30% of cancer deaths. Other important causes of cancer are reproductive and hormonal factors, infections, occupational exposures, ionizing radiation, pollution and ultraviolet radiation [2]. Dietary factors, including obesity, are estimated to cause around 25% of cancer deaths in developed countries, and alcohol causes about 6% of cancer deaths.

Evidence on the effects of nutrition on cancer risk comes from observational epidemiological studies, randomized trials, clinical studies and laboratory research. The strongest evidence comes from randomized trials, but these trials need to be very large and few have been performed. The majority of direct evidence on the associations of diet with cancer risk comes from observational studies; these need to be interpreted carefully because measurements of long-term diet are only moderately accurate and because differences in particular dietary factors can be confounded by other aspects of diet, as well as by smoking and other lifestyle factors.

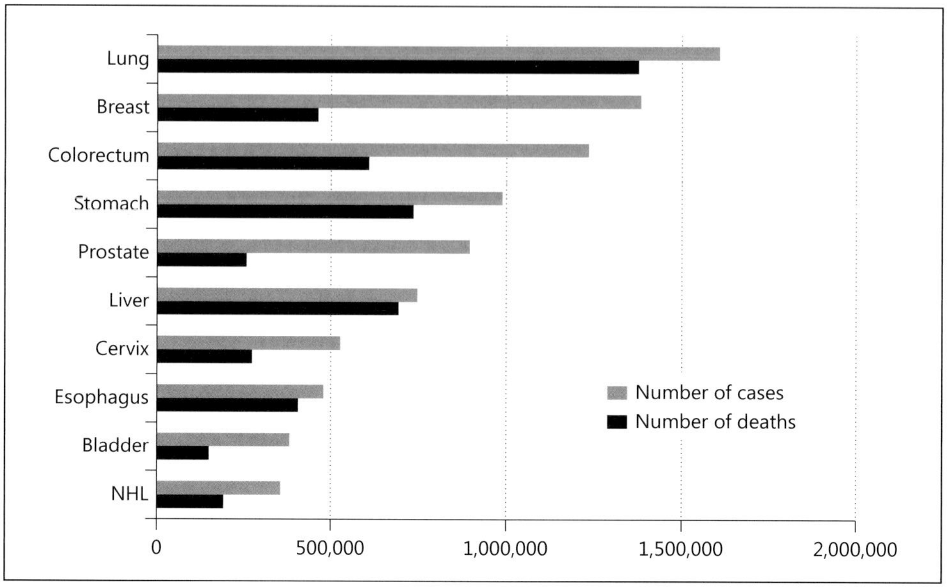

Fig. 1. The ten most common cancers in the world; estimates for 2008. NHL = Non-Hodgkin lymphoma. Data from GLOBOCAN 2008 [1].

Mechanisms for Dietary and Nutritional Factors Predisposing to or Protecting from Cancer

Dietary factors may be associated with cancer development in various ways (table 1). The most obvious is the ingestion of dietary carcinogens or precarcinogens, but there are currently only two established examples which are clearly related to cancer in humans, both largely restricted to particular populations in developing countries. It therefore seems that the major effects of dietary and nutritional factors on cancer risk are through less direct means, such as by affecting hormone levels and thus cell behavior [2].

Cancers of the Esophagus, Oral Cavity and Pharynx

Cancer of the esophagus is the eighth most common cancer in the world; incidence rates are over a hundred times higher in parts of central Asia, China and southern Africa than in most parts of Europe, North America and West Africa. Cancers of the oral cavity and pharynx are less common, but share several etiological factors with cancer of the esophagus. In developed countries the main risk factors for this group of cancers are alcohol and tobacco, and up to 75% of these cancers are attributable to these two lifestyle factors [3–5]. There is also evidence that consuming drinks and foods at a very high temperature probably increases the risk for these cancers. Obesity is an established risk factor specifically for adenocarcinoma (but not squamous cell carcinoma) of the esophagus, increasing the risk by over 2-fold [6]. In some developing countries, a substantial proportion of these cancers may be due to micronutrient deficiencies related to a restricted diet that is low in fruit and vegetables and animal products; the relative roles of various micronutrients are not clear, but deficiencies of riboflavin, folate, vitamin C and zinc may be involved [7, 8]. One type of cancer within this classification, nasopharyngeal cancer, is rela-

Table 1. Dietary and nutritional factors which may influence cancer risk

Factor	Examples and possible mechanisms
Dietary carcinogens	aflatoxin; mutagens in Chinese-style salted fish; possibly *N*-nitroso compounds formed from dietary nitrites
Alcohol	may act through conversion to acetaldehyde which is mutagenic, as a co-carcinogen that increases the absorption of other carcinogens, or by mucosal damage, hormonal changes, inflammation and impaired immunity
Energy balance	excess energy causing obesity and hormonal changes such as increased estrogens which stimulate cell division; may increase inflammation
Dietary fiber	effects on large intestine: dilutes gut contents, reduces transit time through the colon, may reduce absorption of carcinogens, ferments to short-chain fatty acids which may promote differentiation and lower pH thus inhibiting production of carcinogenic secondary bile acids; may also influence endogenous hormones
Vitamins and minerals	deficiency may damage tissues; deficiency, e.g. of folate, may lead to abnormal DNA methylation; no evidence that levels above those needed to prevent deficiency have any benefit, and might be detrimental
Possible plant anti-carcinogens	many hypothesized beneficial effects, but none is established to be important

tively common in parts of Southeast Asia and is associated with a high intake of Chinese-style salted fish, especially during early childhood, as well as with infection with the Epstein-Barr virus [2, 5].

Stomach Cancer

Stomach cancer is the fourth most common cancer [1]. Until about 1980, stomach cancer was the most common cause of cancer death in the world, but incidence rates have fallen dramatically in Western countries since the middle of the 20th century, and stomach cancer is now much less common in Europe and North America than in Asia. Infection with the bacterium *Helicobacter pylori* is an established risk factor [2, 4]. Diet is thought to be important in the etiology of this disease, and dietary changes are implicated in the recent decline in stomach cancer incidence and mortality rates in many countries. Substantial evidence suggests that the risk of stomach cancer is increased by high intakes of some traditionally preserved salted foods, especially meats and pickles, and salt itself, and that risk is decreased by adequate intakes of fruit and vegetables, perhaps due to their vitamin C content [2, 7, 8].

Colorectal Cancer

Colorectal cancer is the third most common cancer. Incidence rates are approximately 10-fold higher in developed than in developing countries [1]. Diet-related factors may account for up to 80% of the between-country differences in rates of colorectal cancer. The best established dietary-related risk factors are overweight/obesity and alcohol, but these factors do not explain all of the large variation in rates between countries, and it is likely that some aspects of a Western diet are a major determinant of risk [3, 7]. It has proved difficult to identify which aspects of diet are most important, but there is now substantial evidence that high intakes of red and processed meat and low intakes of dietary fiber probably increase risk [7, 8]. Further research is needed to clarify these relationships and to determine whether other nutritional factors such as fruit and vegetables, folic acid and vitamin D also modify risk.

Liver Cancer

Liver cancer is the sixth most common cancer. Approximately 75% of cases of liver cancer occur in developing countries, and liver cancer rates vary over 20-fold between countries, being much higher in sub-Saharan Africa and Southeast Asia than in Europe and North America. The major risk factor is chronic infection with hepatitis B virus, and to a lesser extent, hepatitis C virus [2, 4]. Ingestion of foods contaminated with the mycotoxin aflatoxin is an important risk factor among people in developing countries with active hepatitis virus infection [2, 3]. Excessive alcohol consumption is the main diet-related risk factor for liver cancer in Western countries, probably via the development of cirrhosis and alcoholic hepatitis [2, 3, 5].

Pancreatic Cancer

Cancer of the pancreas is more common in Western countries than in developing countries. Smoking increases the risk by about 3-fold. Overweight/obesity increases the risk, but this association is relatively small with some inconsistencies in the evidence, and no associations with dietary intakes have been conclusively demonstrated [2, 7, 8].

Lung Cancer

Lung cancer is the most common cancer in the world and was estimated to account for almost 1.4 million deaths in 2008. Heavy smoking increases the risk by around 30-fold, and smoking causes over 80% of lung cancers in Western countries [2]. Many observational studies have found a weak inverse association between consumption of fruits, vegetables and related nutrients and lung cancer risk, but this apparent relationship may be due to residual confounding by smoking, since smokers generally consume less fruit and vegetables than nonsmokers [7].

Breast Cancer

Breast cancer is the second most common cancer in the world, and accounts for 23% of cancers in women. Incidence rates are about four times higher in Western countries than in less developed countries. Much of this international variation is due to differences in reproductive factors such as age at menarche, parity, age at birth and breastfeeding, but differences in diet may also contribute [7]. Obesity increases breast cancer risk in postmenopausal women by around 50%, probably by increasing serum concentrations of estradiol. The only other established dietary risk factor for breast cancer is alcohol, with about a 10% increase in risk for an average of one alcoholic drink every day [5, 7]. There has been much interest in the hypothesis that a high fat intake increases breast cancer risk, but the extensive data now available have not confirmed this hypothesis. The results of studies of other dietary factors including meat, dairy products, fruit, vegetables and fiber are inconclusive.

Endometrial Cancer

The highest incidence rates of endometrial cancer occur in Western countries. Risk is about 3-fold higher in obese women than lean women. As with breast cancer, the effect of obesity in postmenopausal women on the risk for endometrial cancer is probably mediated by the increase in serum concentrations of estrogens [7].

Cervical Cancer

Cancer of the cervix is the seventh most common cancer in the world, and it is the third most common cancer in women. The highest rates are in sub-Saharan Africa, Central and South America, and Southeast Asia. The major cause of cervical cancer is infection with certain subtypes of the human papillomavirus, and there is no strong evidence that nutritional factors affect risk [2, 7, 8].

Prostate Cancer

Prostate cancer is the fifth most common cancer in the world and the second most common in men. Prostate cancer incidence rates are strongly affected by diagnostic practices and therefore difficult to interpret, but mortality rates are less affected by diagnostic practices and are about ten times higher in North America and Europe than in Asia. Little is known about the etiology of prostate cancer. Diets high in red meat, dairy products and animal fat have frequently been implicated, but the data overall are inconclusive. A recent large trial showed no benefit of supplementation with selenium and/or vitamin E [9]. Prospective studies have shown that risk is positively associated with high levels of insulin-like growth factor-1, and more research is needed to explore whether dietary factors such as animal protein may influence risk through insulin-like growth factor-1 [7].

Bladder Cancer

Cancer of the bladder is the ninth most common cancer in the world. Tobacco smoking increases the risk for bladder cancer, accounting for between a third to two thirds of all bladder cancers, and there is no strong evidence that nutritional factors affect risk [2, 8].

Kidney Cancer

Obesity is an established risk factor for cancer of the kidney, increasing the risk by at least 50% and accounting for up to 30% of kidney cancers in both men and women [3, 6]. There are only limited data on the possible role of diet in the etiology of kidney cancer.

Nutritional Factors in Cancer Treatment

The effects of nutrition on the progress of cancer after diagnosis are particularly difficult to study. Observational studies are hard to interpret because the diet of patients can be strongly linked to the stage of their cancer, their overall health, and the type of treatment. Randomized controlled trials are therefore needed to provide reliable evidence, but are difficult to conduct and few have been performed. The available evidence suggests that obesity has an adverse effect on prognosis among patients with colorectal cancer and breast cancer, and therefore that avoidance of obesity may improve survival [8, 10]. Trials have not shown that supplements of micronutrients have benefits.

Patients with cancer have a serious disease, and their medical treatment may include surgery, radiation, toxic chemotherapy and hormonal therapy. Both the disease itself and the treatment may cause nutritional stress and adversely affect appetite. For these patients, adequate nutritional support is of great importance.

Conclusions

- The most important known effects of nutrition and related factors on cancer risk are the adverse effects of obesity and alcohol (table 2).
- Obesity increases the risk for cancers of the esophagus (adenocarcinoma), colorectum, breast (postmenopausal), endometrium and

Table 2. Diet, nutrition and cancer: summary

Increase risk	Decrease risk
Convincing Evidence	
Overweight and obesity	
esophagus (adenocarcinoma)	
colorectum	
breast (postmenopausal women)	
endometrium	
kidney	
Alcohol	
oral cavity	
pharynx	
larynx	
esophagus	
colorectum	
liver	
breast	
Aflatoxin	
liver	
Chinese-style salted fish	
nasopharynx	
Probable Evidence	
Preserved meat and red meat	Fruits and vegetables
colorectum	oral cavity
Salt-preserved foods and salt	esophagus
stomach	stomach
Very hot (thermally) drinks and food	colorectum
oral cavity	Dietary fiber
pharynx	colorectum
esophagus	

kidney; alcohol causes cancers of the oral cavity, pharynx, larynx, esophagus, colorectum, liver, and breast.

- In particular populations, aflatoxin in moldy foods causes liver cancer, and Chinese-style salted fish causes nasopharyngeal cancer; these risk factors are prevalent in some populations but are absent in many parts of the world.
- The majority of the evidence suggests that high intakes of red and processed meat probably increase the risk for colorectal cancer, and that high intakes of salt-preserved foods and salt probably increase the risk for stomach cancer.
- High intakes of dietary fiber probably reduce the risk of colorectal cancer, and adequate intakes of fruit and vegetables may reduce the risk for cancers of the gastrointestinal tract.
- Very hot drinks and foods probably increase the risk for cancers of the oral cavity, pharynx and esophagus. Further research is needed to clarify these relationships.

References

1 Ferlay J, Shin HR, Bray F, et al: GLOBOCAN 2008 v1.2, Cancer Incidence and Mortality Worldwide: IARC CancerBase No 10. Lyon, International Agency for Research on Cancer, 2010. http://globocan.iarc.fr (accessed 9th May 2012).

2 Swerdlow AJ, Peto R, Doll RS: 6.1 Epidemiology of cancer; in Warrell DA, Cox TM, Firth JD (eds): Oxford Textbook of Medicine, ed 5. Oxford, Oxford University Press, 2010. http://otm.oxfordmedicine.com/cgi/content/full/med-9780199204854-chapter-0601 (accessed 9th May 2012).

3 Tomatis L, Aitio A, Day NE, et al (eds): Cancer: Causes, Occurrence and Control. Lyon, International Agency for Research on Cancer, 1990.

4 Boyle P, Levin B (eds): World Cancer Report 2008. Lyon, International Agency for Research on Cancer, 2008.

5 Secretan B, Straif K, Baan R, et al: A review of human carcinogens – part E: tobacco, areca nut, alcohol, coal smoke, and salted fish. Lancet Oncol 2009;10:1033–1034.

6 Renehan AG, Tyson M, Egger M, et al: Body-mass index and incidence of cancer: a systematic review and meta-analysis of prospective observational studies. Lancet 2008;371:569–578.

7 Key TJ, Allen NE, Spencer EA, Travis RC: The effect of diet on risk of cancer. Lancet 2002;360:861–868.

8 World Cancer Research Fund/American Institute for Cancer Research: Food, Nutrition, Physical Activity, and the Prevention of Cancer: a Global Perspective. Washington, American Institute for Cancer Research, 2007.

9 Lippman SM, Klein EA, Goodman PJ, et al: Effect of selenium and vitamin E on risk of prostate cancer and other cancers: the selenium and vitamin E cancer prevention trial (SELECT). JAMA 2009;301:39–51.

10 Davies NJ, Batehup L, Thomas R: The role of diet and physical activity in breast, colorectal, and prostate cancer survivorship: a review of the literature. Br J Cancer 2011;105(suppl 1):S52–S73.

Bier D, et al. (eds): Nutrition for the Primary Care Provider. World Rev Nutr Diet. Basel, Karger, 2015, vol 111, pp 130–135
DOI: 10.1159/000362310

Nutritional Management in HIV/AIDS Infection

Averalda E. van Graan

Centre of Excellence for Nutrition, North-West University, Potchefstroom, South Africa

Key Words

HIV · AIDS · Nutritional management · Nutritional assessment · Wasting · Nutrients

Key Messages

- Nutritional support is one of the most immediate and critical needs of people living with HIV and AIDS, and nutritional management is integral to the care and management of the disease.
- The virus and its associated conditions and symptoms negatively influence nutritional status through decreased intake, increased requirements, and malabsorption, resulting in malnutrition. Adequate nutrient intakes are therefore essential.
- Comprehensive nutritional assessments should be performed regularly to ensure optimal nutritional intervention.
- Optimal nutrition could assist to maintain lean body mass, reduce the severity of HIV-associated symptoms, support antiretroviral therapy, and improve quality of life.
- ESPEN guidelines state energy requirements to be increased by 20–30% during the recovery phase after opportunistic infections. The guidelines recommend protein intake of 1.2 g/kg in stable phases of the disease and 1.5 g/kg/day during episodes of acute illness.
- In general, there is conflicting evidence on the optimal protocols for nutrition support of these patients. Nutritional recommendations are guidelines only, and should always be viewed on a case-by-case basis alongside the individual patient's clinical presentation.

Introduction

HIV remains one of the leading causes of mortality in the world, with 1.5 million adults succumbing to the disease and 30.1 million adults living with the disease in 2010 [1]. These numbers are testament to the magnitude of the burden the HIV pandemic continues to place on the international community [2]. Nutritional support is often identified as one of the most immediate and critical needs of people living with HIV and AIDS (PLWHA) [3], and nutritional management is integral to the care and treatment of the disease [4]. HIV and nutrition are inextricably interrelated, and the well-known vicious cycle of malnutrition and HIV eloquently illustrates the relationship between the virus, impairment of the immune system, increased susceptibility to infection, increased nutritional needs, and poor nutrition [5]. While many developing countries are still struggling to increase antiretroviral therapy (ART) coverage, for many PLWHA the disease has become a long-term chronic condition. Nutritional care providers now manage severe wasting, tuberculosis, cancer, renal failure, hepatic disease and chronic complications related to highly active ART (HAART) [6]. Nutrition support and intervention strategies thus vary from nutrition education, supplementation to enteral and parental nutrition, to assist in symptom management, support medication therapy, improve resistance against opportunistic infections (OI), complications, and to increase quality of life [7].

Pathophysiology in a Nutshell

The HIV retrovirus possesses the reverse transcriptase enzyme, which enables viral RNA to be transcribed to proviral DNA. The infection begins with the attachment of HIV virions to the cell surface of CD4+ T-lymphocytes via an interaction between gp120, CCR5 and CXCR4, chemokine coreceptors, which enables viral entry into the cells. Glycoprotein 41 binds with cell chemokines, leading to receptor fusion, uncoating of viral RNA and the production of DNA copies from both RNA templates by the polymerase enzyme. A double-stranded, unintegrated strand of DNA is inserted into the host cell genome by the enzyme integrase [8]. When the provirus is activated, the DNA is converted back to RNA, transported outside the nucleus and translated into new HIV proteins and enzymes. The protease enzyme cleaves the long protein strands into smaller strands, incorporates it into HIV particles together with enzymes and the viral RNA, which are then released from the host cell [9].

Table 1. Effect of common HIV symptoms and conditions on nutritional intake, requirements, absorption and losses

Decreased intake
Loss of appetite
Nausea
Dysphagia
Analgesia
Taste changes
Candidiasis
Changes in mental condition
Lack of access to food
GI tract discomfort
Absorption
Malabsorption
GI ulcers and lesions
Diarrhea
Increased requirements
Fever, night sweats
Weight loss
Wasting
Opportunistic infections
Cancers
Losses
Vomiting
Diarrhea

Nutritional Status and HIV Infection

In HIV infection, poor nutritional status is associated with disease progression, as well as increased morbidity and mortality. The virus, its commonly related conditions and symptoms negatively influence nutritional status [6] through decreased intake, increased requirements, malabsorption and losses, which result in malnutrition (table 1). Malnutrition in HIV often manifests as weight, muscle and adipose tissue loss, vitamin and mineral deficiencies, and abnormal biochemical parameters [4, 6]. The era of HAART has in addition brought new challenges such as hyperlipidemia and lipodystrophy. Due to the heterogeneity of possible clinical presentations of the disease, nutritional assessment becomes an important step in the nutritional management of HIV infection.

Table 2. Nutritional management in HIV

Assessment	**Nutritional requirements and management**

Anthropometry
Critical
  Weight
  Height
  BMI
Additional
  Waist circumference
  Mid-upper arm circumference
Determine nutritional risk
  Body composition
	Energy
	Asymptomatic: +10%
	Symptomatic (opportunistic infection): no additions (WG); +20–50% (ESPEN)

Biochemistry
Markers that can be used in addition to routine blood biochemistry
  Serum albumin
  Lipid profile
  Random blood glucose
  Serum ferritin
  Folate
  Vitamins B_{12} and D
  CD4 and viral load
	Protein
	12–15% of energy; 0.8 g/kg (WG)
	1.2 g/kg (stable phase); 1.5 g/kg (acute illness) (ESPEN)

Clinical
In addition to standard nutrition-focused clinical examination
  Weight change
  Dehydration
  GI tract symptoms
  Functional capacity
  Lipodystrophy
	Vitamins and minerals
	1× RDA

Dietary
Diet history (usual intake, 24-hour recall, frequency)
Lifestyle (smoking, exercise, alcohol use)
Medication use (adverse effects, nutrient-medication interaction)
Socioeconomic factors (food availability, food safety, food preparation)
Complementary and alternative therapies
	Implementation
	In following order
	  Normal food intake, dietary modulation and nutritional counselling (basic nutrition, food safety, medication-nutrient interactions, medication adverse effects[1], timing considerations)
	  Oral nutritional supplements
	  Tube feeding
	  Parenteral nutrition

Adapted from references [4, 7, 10, 12, 13].
[1] Common: nausea, vomiting, diarrhea, taste alterations, loss of appetite, anemia, low vitamin B_{12}, copper, zinc, hyperlipidemia.

Nutritional Assessment

A comprehensive nutritional assessment [4] should be performed regularly to ensure optimal nutritional intervention. A complete nutritional assessment entails anthropometric, biochemical, clinical and dietary intake assessment, and includes the timely collection of appropriate data, which should be analyzed and interpreted alongside evidence-based standards, bearing in mind the effects, co-morbidities and treatment of HIV infection [7].

Anthropometric Measurements

Weight loss, wasting, obesity, and lipodystrophy are common in HIV patients. The etiology of HIV-associated wasting is multifactorial and alterations in protein metabolism and body protein turnover has been well documented. Underlying nutritional status, dietary intake, the severity of the inflammatory response and disease are factors affecting the rate of weight loss. During cycles of repeated OI, weight loss and recovery, adipose tissue seems to be preferentially repleted, while loss in lean body mass is increased during episodes of OI [6]. ART is associated with many adverse effects and metabolic abnormalities such as HIV-associated lipodystrophy syndrome, which is characterized by lipoatrophy in the extremities and face and lipohypertrophy in the abdominal and dorsocervical region, and breast hypertrophy [4, 6]. Measurements of body weight, dimensions, composition and calculation of BMI can be used to identify wasting and assess lean body mass and body fat [7]. Several anthropometry methods exist; however, in clinical practice anthropometric measurements usually include the measurements listed in table 2 [7, 10].

Biochemical Assessment

The HI virus, coinciding with OI, immune dysfunction, hormonal changes, and HAART is associated with alterations in metabolism and endocrine function [7]. Abnormalities include lactic acidosis, glucose intolerance, insulin resistance, and hyperlipidemia. These disorders and ART are associated with increased risk of cardiovascular disease, which together with classical risk factors account for 25% of the risk. Bone disease in this population is multifactorial and associated with the virus, HAART and traditional osteoporosis risk factors [2, 11]. Altered levels of nutrition-related markers have been well documented in HIV infection, and biochemical assessment provides additional information regarding nutritional status. Nutrition-related biochemical values listed in table 2 are seen as indicators of nutritional status in disease complications and prognosis. Alterations in nutrition-related biochemical values should be interpreted with caution as these values could also reflect inflammatory responses and or altered metabolism [7].

Clinical Assessment

Clinical assessment entails obtaining a medical history of the patient and performing a nutrition-focused physical examination. A medical history can provide insight into comorbidities that could have nutritional implications [7]. Clinical parameters that should be assessed in conjunction with a general nutrition-focused physical examination are listed in table 2. Other key areas to assess include determining the presence of comorbid conditions, OI, and factors related to nutritional requirements [7, 12].

Dietary Assessment

Dietary assessment is done to examine eating patterns, identify nutrient intake imbalances and identify factors influencing the ability to achieve adequate intakes. Food-drug interactions, nutrient supplements, complementary and alternative therapies, potential medication-nutrition-related side effects, lifestyle patterns, and socioeconomic factors should form part of the dietary assessment [4, 7]. A diet history is the best means to obtain dietary intake information and can be assessed by the methods listed in table 2 [4]. Nutritional assessment plays an important role to ensure optimal nutrition intervention in the nutritional care of PLWHA.

Nutritional Goals

Overarching nutritional goals include the following:
- Maintain and improve body weight
- Maintain and restore lean body mass
- Manage disease symptoms
- Manage metabolic abnormalities
- Maintain and correct nutrient deficiencies
- Support medication therapy [4, 7].

Nutritional Requirements

For PLWHA, vigilance is needed to ensure dietary adequacy, particularly in areas of high food insecurity or poor dietary diversity [2]. Adequate nutrient intakes are essential, as optimal nutrition could assist to maintain LBM, reduce the severity of HIV-associated symptoms, support ART and improve quality of life [4]. Nutritional interventions for PLWHA include food-based supplement interventions, oral supplements with specific nutrients, enteral or total parental therapy and appetite stimulants [13]. A working group (WG) on nutritional care in HIV infection recently reviewed existing evidence to support the development of new WHO guidelines [2], which in some categories differ from the previous recommendations and ESPEN guidelines for HIV.

Energy Requirements

The WG reports an increased energy intake of 10% in asymptomatic HIV infection in normal-weight individuals with untreated HIV [2, 14]. Data in asymptomatic HIV-infected patients on ART and HIV wasting are less consistent, with some reporting increased requirements <10% and others reporting decreased requirements. Energy expenditure in HIV with secondary infection is reported to be decreased, and previous recommendations for increased energy intake of 30% now have limited supporting evidence. No recommendations for HIV lipodystrophy have been made despite evidence indicating an increase in energy expenditure [2, 15]. This leaves nutritional care providers with no clear guidelines regarding the latter two groups. However, ESPEN guidelines state energy requirements to be increased by 20–30% during the recovery phase after OI [14].

Macronutrient Requirements

The WG recommends macronutrients to be consumed at amounts of the RDA and adjusted in line with energy adjustments. On protein intake, the WG reports that no evidence exists to support increased or no increase in protein intake. Data were insufficient to support recommendations on the amount or type of fat in HIV infection [2]. ESPEN guidelines, however, recommend protein intake of 1.2 g/kg in stable phases of the disease and 1.5 g/kg/day during episodes of acute illness [14]. Nutrition monitoring is thus important and is the best indication of the adequacy of intake for weight maintenance or gain [10].

Micronutrient Requirements

Recommendations on micronutrients remained unchanged at one RDA or a routine multivitamin supplement, as the WG report insufficient evidence to change the recommendations. Sufficient evidence exists to comment on the potential harm of higher doses of selected micronutrients such as vitamin A, zinc and multiple micronutrient supplements in some populations [2]. A Cochrane review reports zinc supplementation to be safe, but suggests that further evidence is needed to establish the benefits of vitamin A supplementation in adults [16]. It is thus clear that further investigation is warranted regarding the nutritional requirements in HIV infection as shortcomings in knowledge exist.

Nutritional Management

Nutrition support in HIV infection has not been adequately investigated, resulting in a lack of evidence to demonstrate improved clinical outcomes [14] and thus little guidance for evidence-based practice. A review on macronutrient interventions concluded that supplementation improved energy and protein intake, but did not have an effect on weight, fat mass, fat-free mass, disease progression, and complications leading to death [17]. Micronutrient supplementation is recommended at one RDA or a routine multivitamin [2]. The choice of mode of nutrition support is based on expert opinion only [14].

Conclusions

- The HI virus, coinciding OI, immune dysfunction, hormonal changes, ART and medication side effects, influences nutritional requirements and management.
- Nutritional assessment involves anthropometric, biochemical, clinical and dietary assessment.
- Nutritional recommendations are guidelines, and should always be considered in conjunction with the individual patient's clinical presentation.
- Nutrition support entails providing adequate nutrients through food intake, nutritional counseling, oral nutritional supplements, tube feeding and parenteral nutrition.

References

1 WHO: HIV/AIDS fact sheet. November 2011. http://www.who.int/mediacentre/factsheets/fs360/en/index.html.
2 Raiten DJ, Mulligan K, Papathakis P, Wanke C: Executive summary – nutritional care of HIV-infected adolescents and adults, including pregnant and lactating women: what do we know, what do we do, and where do we go from here. Am J Clin Nutr 2011;94(suppl):1667S–1676S.
3 WHO: Executive summary of a scientific review. Consultation on nutrition and HIV/AIDS in Africa: evidence, lessons and recommendations for action. Durban, April 2005. http://www.who.int/nutrition/topics/Executive%20Summary%20WHO.pdf.
4 Dong KR, Imai CM: Medical nutrition therapy for HIV and AIDS; in Mahan KL, Escott-Stump S, Raymond JL: Krause's Food and Nutrition Care Process. Missouri, Elsevier Saunders, 2011, pp 864–881.
5 FANTA project: Nutrition and HIV/AIDS: a training manual nutritional management of HIV/AIDS related symptoms. FANTA, RCQHC and the linkages project; 2003. http://www.fantaproject.org/focus/preservice.html.
6 Pribram V: Introduction to nutrition and HIV; in Pribram V (ed): Nutrition and HIV. Chichester, Wiley-Blackwell, 2011, pp 18–31.
7 American Dietetic Association: Position of the American Dietetic Association: nutrition intervention and human immunodeficiency virus infection. J Am Diet Assoc 2010;110:1105–1119.
8 Kumar P, Clark M: Infectious diseases, tropical medicine and sexually transmitted diseases; in Kumar P, Clark M (eds): Clinical Medicine. Edinburgh, WB Saunders, 2002, pp 21–151.
9 Welz T, Samarawickrama A, Pribram V, et al: Introduction to human immunodeficiency virus; in Pribram V (ed): Nutrition and HIV. Chichester, Wiley-Blackwell, 2011, pp 3–17.
10 Pribram V: Decreased nutritional status and nutritional interventions for people living with HIV; in Pribram V (ed): Nutrition and HIV. Chichester, Wiley-Blackwell, 2011, pp 107–131.
11 Fitch K, Grinspoon S: Nutritional and metabolic correlates of cardiovascular and bone disease in HIV-infected patients. Am J Clin Nutr 2011;94(suppl):1721S–178S.
12 Woodman S, Sutcliffe M, McDonald A: Nutritional screening and assessment; in Pribram V (ed): Nutrition and HIV. Chichester, Wiley-Blackwell, 2011, pp 132–156.
13 Nagata JM, Cohen CR, Young SL, et al: Descriptive characteristics and health outcomes of the food by prescription nutrition supplementation program for adults living with HIV in Nyanza Province, Kenya. PLoS One 2014;9:e91403.
14 Ockenga J, Grimble R, Jonkers-Schuitema C, et al: ESPEN guidelines on enteral nutrition: wasting in HIV and other chronic infectious diseases. Clin Nutr 2006;25:319–329.
15 Kosmiski L: Energy expenditure in HIV infection. Am J Clin Nutr 2011;94(suppl):1677S–1682S.
16 Irlam JH, Visser MME, Rollins NN, Siegfried N: Micronutrient supplementation in children and adults with HIV infection. Cochrane Database Syst Rev 2010;CD003650.
17 Mahlungulu S, Grobler LA, Visser ME, Volmink J: Nutritional interventions for reducing morbidity and mortality in people with HIV. Cochrane Database Syst Rev 2007;CD004536.

Bier D, et al. (eds): Nutrition for the Primary Care Provider. World Rev Nutr Diet. Basel, Karger, 2015, vol 111, pp 136–140
DOI: 10.1159/000362311

Osteoporosis

Saira Adeel Vin Tangpricha

Division of Endocrinology, Metabolism and Lipids, Department of Medicine, Emory University School of Medicine, Atlanta, Ga., USA

Key Words

Vitamin D · Calcium · Osteoporosis

Key Messages

- Vitamin D and calcium play an important role in bone physiology.
- A 10-year risk for fracture can be calculated by the FRAX tool and can assist physicians to determine which patients should receive pharmacologic therapy for osteoporosis.
- Several effective therapies have been approved for the treatment of osteoporosis in patients with a high risk of fracture.

Introduction

Osteoporosis is a systemic skeletal disorder characterized by decreased bone mass and deterioration of the bone microarchitecture leading to decreased bone strength and increased risk of fractures [1]. Osteoporosis occurs more commonly in elderly individuals; however, secondary causes of osteoporosis can be found in younger individuals. Attainment of peak bone mass during adolescence and early adulthood is important for the prevention of osteoporosis. The quality and quantity of bone are influenced by a number of factors but are regulated by two key cells: the osteoblasts which function as the bone-forming cells and osteoclasts which function as the bone-resorbing cells. The balance between the number and activity of these cells determines the rate of bone loss in adults. Vitamin D maintains adequate calcium and phosphorus homeostasis for adequate mineralization of bone. A number of other nutrients may play a role in skeletal health. Screening for osteoporosis is currently performed by dual-energy X-ray absorptiometry (DEXA). Individuals at highest risk of fracture should be offered pharmacologic therapy based on a number of risk factors for future fracture.

Physiology

The skeleton is a dynamic organ undergoing constant renewal and is replaced every 10 years [2]. Osteoblast cells are responsible for the laying down of new bone by producing an extracellular matrix consisting of collagen and other proteins.

The osteoblast cells in bone promote the deposition of a hydroxyapatite crystal which is composed of calcium and phosphorus, providing strength and rigidity for the bone. The skeleton provides not only the structural support for the human body but is also a storage organ for calcium and phosphorus, which is regulated by two key calciotropic hormones, parathyroid hormone and fibroblast growth factor-23. The osteoclast cells in bone resorb the extracellular matrix for release of calcium and phosphorus back into the extracellular fluid and circulation, and remove old bone for deposition of new bone.

Bone resorption and formation are tightly regulated by two key proteins: receptor activator of nuclear factor κ-B ligand (RANKL) and osteoprotegerin. RANKL is a pro-osteoclast maturation protein which promotes maturation of osteoclasts to increase bone resorption. Osteoprotegerin is a decoy receptor that blocks the signaling of RANKL on osteoclasts. The ratio of RANKL/osteoprotegerin is one of the factors that determines the rate of bone turnover and has been a target for novel osteoporosis therapies.

Calcium and Phosphorus

Calcium and phosphorus are the key minerals for the formation of the hydroxyapatite crystals in bone. Inadequate intake of calcium and phosphorus from the diet can result in rickets in children and osteomalacia in adults. Decreased calcium intake will result in increased parathyroid hormone secretion from the parathyroid glands to increase mobilization of calcium from the bone, increase reabsorption of calcium from the kidneys, and to convert circulating 25-hydroxyvitamin D [25(OH)D] to more hormonally active 1,25-dihydroxyvitamin D to increase intestinal absorption of calcium.

The Institute of Medicine (IOM) recommends 1,000–1,300 mg of calcium daily for most children and adults [3]. Foods rich in calcium include dairy products such as milk, cheese, and yogurt and some vegetables such as kale and turnip greens. Most common calcium supplements contain either calcium carbonate or calcium citrate. It is important to note that the total amount of calcium available in these supplements is listed as the 'elemental calcium'.

Several recent studies have raised concerns about potential increased risk of cardiovascular mortality with the use of calcium supplements to prevent and treat osteoporosis. Michaëlsson and colleagues [4] demonstrated in a prospective cohort of over 60,000 women that intake of more than 1,400 mg of calcium from diet and supplements was associated with increased risk of cardiovascular and all-cause mortality. The risk was more pronounced in women with high dietary and supplemental calcium use. Three recent cohort studies [5–7] and a meta-analysis of 15 trials [8] have reported similar findings in increased risk of cardiovascular disease with calcium supplement use. This is in contrast to a prospective cohort study of 35,000 postmenopausal women demonstrating increased risk of cardiovascular disease mortality with low calcium intake (<700 mg daily) compared to high calcium intake (1,400 mg daily) [9]. The secondary analysis of 1,460 elderly women randomized to 1,200 mg of calcium or placebo found no difference in the risk of cardiovascular mortality [10]. The issue of whether calcium supplementation results in increased cardiovascular disease risk clearly requires further investigation. Physicians should take a detailed dietary calcium intake history from their patients with osteoporosis and prescribe calcium supplements only when dietary calcium intake does not meet the recommendations of the IOM guidelines.

Low phosphorus intake is a rare cause of osteomalacia given that phosphorus is ubiquitous in most foods. Most clinical causes of low phosphorus causing poor skeletal mineralization result from genetic diseases of phosphorus wasting such as X-linked hypophosphatemic rickets or acquired diseases such as oncogenic osteomalacia.

Vitamin D

Vitamin D is important for optimal absorption of calcium from the intestines. Vitamin D belongs to the steroid family of hormones. Vitamin D can be synthesized in the skin upon exposure to UVB radiation from the sun or obtained from the diet from limited foods. Vitamin D circulates to the liver and is hydroxylated to 25(OH)D, the vitamin D metabolite used to determine vitamin D status. 25(OH)D circulates to the kidney and is hydroxylated in the 1 position to form 1,25-dihydroxyvitamin D, which is the hormonally active metabolite of vitamin D that enhances intestinal absorption of calcium.

There has been some debate over the amount of dietary vitamin D required and the level of serum 25(OH)D required for optimal skeletal health. The IOM recommends between 600–800 IU of vitamin D for most adults. However, vitamin D requirements may vary according to season, latitude, adiposity, and skin tone. The Endocrine Society recommends 1,500–2,000 IU of vitamin D for those individuals at risk for vitamin D deficiency including osteoporosis. They further recommend that a target serum 25(OH)D level should be at least 30 ng/ml for patients with osteoporosis [11].

Estrogens and Phytoestrogens

Estrogen therapy has been shown to prevent postmenopausal bone loss and reduce fracture risk [12]. Data from the Women's Health Initiative showed increased incidence of breast cancer, coronary artery disease, stroke and venous thromboembolism with estrogen-progestin therapy and increased risk of thromboembolism and stroke with estrogen therapy alone [12]. In light of these data, even though it has been FDA approved for the prevention of postmenopausal osteoporosis, estrogen is not recommended as first-line therapy. There is conflicting evidence regarding the effect of phytoestrogens on bone mineral density, and precise dietary recommendations are currently not available [13].

Vitamin K

Vitamin K is involved in the carboxylation of osteocalcin, thereby allowing it to bind to hydroxyapatite in bone. Some data suggest that vitamin K supplementation (>45 mg/day given as menaquinone-4) may decrease bone loss and fracture risk, but other studies have not confirmed this benefit [14].

Vitamin A

Both insufficient as well as excessive vitamin A intake has been associated with detrimental effects on bone health [15]. The Iowa Women's Health Study showed an increased fracture risk associated with supplemental but not dietary vitamin A intake, but this effect was not dose dependent [16].

Vitamin C

Some but not all studies found a positive association between vitamin C intake and bone mineral density but other factors such as estrogen/hormonal therapy, calcium intake and smoking may be contributory factors [14].

Magnesium

Magnesium is an essential nutrient that is required for adequate calcium metabolism. Studies have found a positive correlation between magnesium intake and bone mineral density in men as well as both premenopausal and postmenopausal women [17].

Diagnosis and Treatment of Osteoporosis

Osteoporosis is diagnosed by DEXA or clinically with history of a low-trauma fracture [18, 19]. The National Osteoporosis Foundation and the US Preventative Services Task Force recommends a screening DEXA of the hip and lumbar spine for all postmenopausal women 65 years and older [19, 20]. The National Osteoporosis Foundation also recommends a screening DEXA in men above the age of 70 and in men and women above the age of 50 who have risk factors for osteoporosis (e.g. early menopause, hypogonadism, glucocorticoid use). An individual is diagnosed to have osteoporosis when the bone mineral density of the hip or spine falls less than –2.5 standard deviations below the mean of a young healthy sex-matched population (T score <–2.5). Individuals are considered to have low bone mineral density when the bone mineral density falls between –1.0 and –2.5 standard deviations compared to a young healthy sex-matched population (T score >–2.5 and ≤1.0).

The DEXA of the hip and spine are very important predictors of future fractures; however, there are many other risk factors for a future fracture that are not taken into account by the DEXA alone including age, gender, previous history of fracture, medical comorbidities, family history, and history of alcohol and tobacco use. Recently, the WHO released an online fracture risk assessment tool named FRAX™ which takes into account several risk factors for fracture and provides a 10-year risk score for fracture [21]. The National Osteoporosis Foundation recommends pharmacologic treatment of all individuals with hip or vertebral fractures, a femoral neck, total hip or lumbar spine T score of ≤–2.5, or a FRAX 10-year risk score indicating ≥3% risk of a hip fracture or ≥20% risk of any major osteoporosis fracture in individuals with low bone mass (T score between –1.0 and –2.5) [20].

Along with the DEXA measurement, a careful history and physical examination should be performed to determine if there is an underlying etiology for osteoporosis [22]. Some common causes to consider include early menopause (women), hypogonadism (men), glucocorticoid excess (due to intake or Cushing's syndrome), increased alcohol consumption, hyperthyroidism, hyperparathyroidism, hypercalciuria, insufficient vitamin D or calcium intake or chronic malabsorption (due to celiac disease, inflammatory bowel disease, short gut syndrome, etc.). Less common causes include multiple myeloma and genetic disorders of collagen including Ehlers-Danlos syndrome and osteogenesis imperfecta.

Several effective pharmacologic agents are available for the treatment of osteoporosis. These include oral and intravenous bisphosphonates, anabolic agents such as teriparatide (Forteo®) and biologic agents such as denosumab (anti-RANKL antibody) [23]. The bisphosphonates and denosumab reduce osteoclast formation and maturation, resulting in reduced bone resorption. The mechanism of how intermittent teriparatide works as an anabolic bone agent is unclear, but it appears to favor increased osteoblast over osteoclast formation and function [24].

Conclusions

- Osteoporosis is a disease that increases the risk of fragility fracture in men and women. Evaluation of potential secondary causes of osteoporosis and modification of contributing risk factors for continued bone loss is the first step in the management of patients with osteoporosis.
- Adequate vitamin D and calcium nutrition and addressing modifiable risk factors remain the cornerstone of therapy for prevention and treatment of osteoporosis.
- Lifestyle changes including increased physical activity, fall prevention, and decreased consumption of alcohol and smoking cessation are also important in counseling patients with osteoporosis.

- Screening individuals at highest risk with DEXA still remains the gold standard for diagnosing men and women with osteoporosis.
- Pharmacologic therapy should be prescribed to those with increased risk of fracture based on past history of fractures, family history, DEXA results, and the presence of secondary causes of accelerated bone loss.

References

1 Kanis JA: Assessment of fracture risk and its application to screening for postmenopausal osteoporosis: synopsis of a WHO report. WHO Study Group. Osteoporos Int 1994;4:368–381.

2 Manolagas SC: Birth and death of bone cells: basic regulatory mechanisms and implications for the pathogenesis and treatment of osteoporosis. Endocr Rev 2000;21:115–137.

3 Institute of Medicine: Dietary reference intakes for calcium and vitamin D. Washington, The National Academies Press, 2011, pp 260–262.

4 Michaëlsson K, Melhus H, Warensjö Lemming E, Wolk A, Byberg L: Long term calcium intake and rates of all cause and cardiovascular mortality: community based prospective longitudinal cohort study. BMJ 2013;346:f228.

5 Bolland MJ, Avenell A, Baron JA, et al: Effect of calcium supplements on risk of myocardial infarction and cardiovascular events: meta-analysis. BMJ 2010; 341:c3691.

6 Bolland MJ, Grey A, Avenell A, et al: Calcium supplements with or without vitamin D and risk of cardiovascular events: reanalysis of the Women's Health Initiative limited access dataset and meta-analysis. BMJ 2010;342:d2040.

7 Bolland MJ, Barber PA, Doughty RN, et al: Vascular events in healthy older women receiving calcium supplementation: randomized controlled trial. BMJ 2008;336:262–266.

8 Bolland MJ, Avenell A, Baron JA, et al: Effect of calcium supplements on risk of myocardial infarction and cardiovascular events: meta-analysis. BMJ 2010; 341:c3691.

9 Bostick RM, Kushi LH, Wu Y, et al: Relation of calcium, vitamin D, and dairy food intake to ischemic heart disease mortality among postmenopausal women. Am J Epidemiol 1999;149:151–161.

10 Lewis JR, Calver J, Zhu K, et al: Calcium supplementation and the risks of atherosclerotic vascular disease in older women: results of a 5-year RCT and a 4.5-year follow-up. J Bone Miner Res 2011;26:35–41.

11 Holick MF, Binkley NC, Bischoff-Ferrari HA, et al: Evaluation, treatment, and prevention of vitamin D deficiency: an Endocrine Society clinical practice guideline. J Clin Endocrinol Metab 2011; 96:1911–1930.

12 Rossouw JE, Anderson GL, Prentice RL, et al: Risks and benefits of estrogen plus progestin in healthy postmenopausal women: principal results From the Women's Health Initiative randomized controlled trial. JAMA 2002;288:321.

13 Lagari VS, Levis S: Phytoestrogens and bone health. Curr Opin Endocrinol Diabetes Obes 2010;17:546–553.

14 Ahmadieh H, Arabi A: Vitamins and bone health: beyond calcium and vitamin D. Nutr Rev 2011;69:584–598.

15 Promislow JHE, Goodman-Gruen D, Slymen DJ, Barrett-Conner E: Retinol intake and bone mineral density in the elderly: the Rancho Bernardo Study. J Bone Miner Res 2002;17:1349–1358.

16 Lim LS, Harnack LJ, Lazovich D, Folsom AR: Vitamin A intake and the risk of hip fracture in postmenopausal women: the Iowa Women's Health Study. Osteoporos Int 2004;15:552–559.

17 Ryder KM, Shorr RI, Bush AJ, et al: Magnesium intake from food and supplements is associated with bone mineral density in healthy older white subjects. J Am Geriatr Soc 2005;53:1875–1880.

18 Kanis JA, Melton LJ 3rd, Christiansen C, et al: The diagnosis of osteoporosis. J Bone Miner Res 1994;9:1137–1141.

19 US Preventive Services Task Force: Screening for osteoporosis in postmenopausal women: recommendations and rationale. Ann Intern Med 2002;137: 526–528.

20 National Osteoporosis Foundation: Clinician's Guide to Prevention and Treatment of Osteoporosis. Washington, National Osteoporosis Foundation, 2010.

21 Kanis JA, Oden A, Johansson H, et al: FRAX and its applications to clinical practice. Bone 2009;44:734–743.

22 Hudec SM, Camacho PM: Secondary causes of osteoporosis. Endocr Pract 2013;19:120–128.

23 Murad MH, Drake MT, Mullan RJ, et al: Clinical review. Comparative effectiveness of drug treatments to prevent fragility fractures: a systematic review and network meta-analysis. J Clin Endocrinol Metab 2012;97:1871–1880.

24 Bodenner D, Redman C, Riggs A: Teriparatide in the management of osteoporosis. Clin Interv Aging 2007;2:499–507.

Bier D, et al. (eds): Nutrition for the Primary Care Provider. World Rev Nutr Diet. Basel, Karger, 2015, vol 111, pp 141–145
DOI: 10.1159/000362312

Nutrition Support in Gastrointestinal Disease

James S. Scolapio   Donna J. Smith

Division of Gastroenterology, University of Florida, Jacksonville, Fla., USA

Key Words

Total enteral nutrition · Total parenteral nutrition · Inflammatory bowel disease · Short bowel syndrome

Key Messages

- When to begin total enteral nutrition (TEN) or total parenteral nutrition (TPN) is based on a patient's nutritional state and disease severity.
- Nutrition support is typically started when a patient is unable to attain adequate oral intake for longer than 10 days.
- TEN and TPN should supply approximately 25–30 kcal/kg/day.
- TEN should be the method of choice for nutrition support as TPN is associated with metabolic complications including hyperglycemia.
- Early enteral nutrition (within 48 h of admission) is preferred to TPN in patients with severe acute pancreatitis.
- Small, frequent, low-fat, low-fiber meals are first line of therapy in patients with gastroparesis.
- Micronutrient deficiencies are common in patients with inflammatory bowel disease and should be replaced accordingly.
- Patients with short bowel syndrome with a colonic remnant benefit from a high-complex carbohydrate diet low in oxalate.

Introduction

This review focuses on the nutrition support of hospitalized patients with gastrointestinal disease that require nutrition support with either total enteral nutrition (TEN) or total parenteral nutrition (TPN). When to begin nutrition support, how to deliver the formula, the type of formula and the nutritional treatment for specific gastrointestinal disease states are discussed below.

When to Provide Nutrition Support

The physician's primary role includes taking a complete medical history and physical examination to determine how best to manage the patient's nutritional needs including enteral access for the gastroenterologist. It is also the physician's responsibility to be knowledgeable of the current nutrition literature and published guidelines and how these relate to the patient's specific gastrointestinal disease process.

No single laboratory test can assess the presence or severity of malnutrition. The medical history including questions about nutrition intake and weight change along with a focused physical examination are probably the best tools for determining a patient's nutrition status, i.e. normal or severely malnourished. The subjective global assessment classification score for patients has been shown to correlate with more sophisticated laboratory tests [1]. Patients are given the following scores: 'A' normal nutrition reserves, i.e. no weight loss history and no signs of muscle or fat wasting on physical examination; 'B' less than 10% weight loss over the previous 6 months with some evidence of muscle or fat wasting, and 'C' greater than 10% weight loss over the previous 6 months with little or no oral intake of food over the previous 2 weeks. Patients scored C usually have obvious muscle and fat wasting upon physical examination and are considered at high risk of having severe malnutrition.

In most patients who receive a score of A or B, the physician should wait 10–14 days before administering TEN or TPN. Usually, the patient's underlying medical problem that prohibited the adequate intake of food is corrected within this time period. Patients with severe malnutrition (score C) probably derive the most benefit from either TEN or TPN [2].

The second factor for considering *when* to feed a patient is his/her disease severity. An example would be a patient with severe pancreatitis who is scored A or B in whom it may take over 2 weeks to regain the ability to take adequate oral nutrition; in this case, starting TEN or TPN earlier than 14 days would be appropriate and recommended. Patients scored C should have TEN or TPN started within 48 h of hospitalization.

TPN versus TEN

If a patient cannot ingest an adequate amount of food by mouth, then TEN (nasogastric or nasoenteric tube feeding) or TPN will be necessary [3, 4]. Percutaneous gastrostomy and percutaneous jejunostomy feeding tubes should only be considered in those patients that you suspect will require TEN for more than 4 weeks' duration. A gastroenterologist plays a key role in providing enteral access for a patient. In patients requiring short-term nutrition support, defined as less than 30 days, nasogastric or nasoenteric placement of a 10- to 12-Fr polyurethane tube is appropriate. Smaller tubes have a higher occurrence of occlusion. Larger tubes, i.e. 16 Fr, may inhibit LES (lower esophageal sphincter) function, thereby increasing the risk of aspiration of gastric contents and may cause significant nasal irritation. In patients at risk of gastric aspiration (i.e. delayed gastric emptying, high gastric residuals, supine position) nasoenteric feeding should be used. Feeding distal to the ligament of Treitz reduces the risk of gastric regurgitation and pulmonary aspiration. Before starting the tube feeding, correct tube position should be confirmed by X-ray. Percutaneous endoscopic gastrostomy tubes should be used when patient recovery is anticipated to take more than 30 days. Contradictions to long-term placement devices may include both mechanical and ethical end of life issues. A speech/swallow pathologist should assess a patient's swallow function before placement of a long-term device, to prevent inappropriate placement.

TPN should only be used in those patients in whom TEN is not possible. This may be the result of a mechanical intestinal obstruction, intestinal fistula, or medical illness that does not allow safe passage of a feeding tube. TPN is associated with complications including catheter sepsis and risk of hyperglycemia.

Formula Selection

A dietician and pharmacist can be very helpful when designing the appropriate enteral or parenteral feeding formula. If a patient is not obtaining adequate oral nutrition, then TEN or TPN formula should be calculated to provide approximately 25–30 kcal/kg/day [3]. The nutrient mix or ratio should contain approximately 30% of the total calories as lipid, protein should provide 1.0–1.5 g/kg/day, and the remaining macronutrient should be given as carbohydrate. Patients should obtain their goal rate of nutrition infusion over a 48- to 72-hour period.

Tube feeding can be infused one of three ways: bolus syringe infusion, gravity infusion or by continuous pump feeding [3]. Bolus and gravity feeding are also referred to as intermittent feeding. Small bowel feeding should be done by continuous pump delivery to reduce gastrointestinal intolerance such as abdominal cramping and diarrhea. Infusion rates greater than 120 ml/h may result in gastrointestinal bloating and diarrhea. If a patient cannot tolerate the higher infusion rate, a calorically dense formula can be used. In patients at risk of aspiration of gastric contents, using a continuous pump infusion may minimize the risk of aspiration. Feeding should be started at 20 ml per hour and advanced to the target rate over a 48-hour period. Intermittent gastric feeding involves a larger volume per feeding than controlled continuous feeding using a pump. With gravity feeding, starting with one can of formula (approx. 240 ml) administered over 1 h and advancing to the target number of feedings (4× per day) and volume (1–2 cans per feeding) is recommended. Bolus or syringe feeding is not encouraged in most hospitalized patients. Cyclic continuous feeding, i.e. 10–12 h during sleep may help stimulate appetite and oral intake during the day while supplying necessary supplemental calories. Certain medications (Dilantin®, ciprofloxacin, and Sinemet®) may bind to the formula and result in reduced absorption. Spacing of medications an hour before or after feeding is recommended. Feeding tubes should routinely be flushed with at least 20–30 ml of additional water every 4 h during continuous feeding and before and after intermittent feedings and medication delivery to prevent tube occlusion.

TEN formulas usually contain 1 kcal per milliliter of formula and approximately 44 g of protein per 1 liter of formula. Elemental and semi-elemental formulas have small-peptide proteins, which are easier to absorb, as well as less total fat compared to traditional polymeric formulas. Most of the polymeric formulas are isotonic and therefore dilution with water during infusion is not necessary. Enteral formulas contain approximately 84% free water, and the remaining daily fluid needs of the patient, which is approximately 30 ml/kg/day, are given as tube flushes using regular tap water. Typically in the hospital setting, tube feeds are administered via a 24-hour pump infusion.

Standard polymeric formulas should be used in the majority of patients [3]. Most formulas contain 1 kcal per ml of fluid, 44 g of protein per liter, and approximately 30% lipid. These formulas are lactose and gluten free. Formulas do not require dilution with water before infusion.

Specific Gastrointestinal Disease Management

Acute Pancreatitis

It had been standard practice to administer TPN to all patients with severe pancreatitis, assuming that this would rest the pancreas compared to stimulation of pancreatic enzyme secretion using enteral feeding. However, a study has questioned the wisdom of this practice [4]. In fact, acute severe pancreatitis is an example where enteral nutrition appears more favorable than TPN [4]. Although there are no data to suggest enteral nutrition improves clinical outcome (faster resolution of pancreatitis) compared to nil per os and i.v. fluids, the data would suggest enteral nutrition is associated with less infectious complications, improved inflammatory response and improved APACHE II scores compared to TPN [4]. Nasojejunal feeding, using either a polymeric formula or semi-elemental formula, administered within 48 h of hospitalization, appears beneficial compared to TPN.

Gastroparesis

The diagnosis of gastroparesis is based on the combination of symptoms of early satiety and delay of gastric emptying of a solid phase meal. Markedly uncontrolled glucose levels may aggravate symptoms of gastroparesis and delay gastric emptying. Glycemic control should be optimized, and medications that induce delayed gastric emptying should be stopped when possible. Oral nutrition is preferable for nutrition and hydration, using small, frequent low-fat, low-fiber meals. If patients are unable to tolerate solid foods, then homogenized or liquid meals are recommended. If oral intake is insufficient, then jejunal feeding should be pursued. Metoclopramide is the first line of prokinetic therapy and should be administered in the lowest effective dose because of potential side effects. Gastric electric stimulation may be considered for compassionate treatment in patients with refractory symptoms [5]. Completion gastrectomy should only be considered in patients with severe refractory symptoms. Acupuncture can be considered as an alternative therapy [5].

Inflammatory Bowel Disease

High dietary fats and meats are associated with an increased risk of inflammatory bowel disease. Among the various dietary interventions, none have shown significant clinical efficacy. A meta-analysis of 16 prospective randomized trials in Crohn's patients reported that the frequency of clinical remission of small bowel disease after treatment with steroids was 80%, compared with 60% after treatment with an elemental or polymeric diet alone [6, 7]. Pooled data of studies comparing polymeric (standard formulas) and elemental formulas showed no advantage with elemental formulas (65 vs. 61% remission rates). Published studies do not support the concept that improved nutrition status coupled with 'bowel rest' improves clinical remission rate and avoids the need for colectomy in chronic ulcerative colitis and Crohn's colitis patients. Patients with active inflammatory bowel disease may be deficient in micronutrients such as vitamin D and iron. Micronutrient levels in the blood should be checked and replaced accordingly. The use of preoperative TPN appears to only benefit those patients with severe malnutrition.

Short Bowel Syndrome

Short bowel syndrome and the need for TPN usually results when a patient has had a surgical resection with less than 150 cm of small intestine remaining [8]. Short bowel results from intestinal vascular events, larger resections for Crohn's disease and other intestinal disorders such as volvulus and adhesive disease. TPN is usually required until intestinal adaptation occurs. The type of oral diet given to a patient with short bowel syndrome depends on whether part of the colon is remaining. Those patients with a colonic remnant benefit from a high complex carbohydrate diet low in fat. Likewise, patients should be placed on a low-oxalate diet. Those patients without a colonic remnant do not require a specific diet and are encouraged to eat small frequent meals throughout the day. Antidiarrheal medications are also helpful in slowing gastrointestinal transit, thus promoting fluid and nutrient absorption. Trophic factors including growth hormone and glucagon-like peptide-2 (GLP-2) have been FDA approved in a select group of patients with short bowel syndrome. Intestinal transplant is also a treatment option in a select group of patients with short bowel syndrome. This would include those patients with pending end-stage liver disease from TPN, loss of venous access and recurrent catheter infections.

Conclusions

- Following the recommendations of peer-reviewed published guidelines is recommended in treating patients with gastrointestinal disease who require nutritional support.

- TPN or TEN should only be used in those patients who cannot obtain adequate oral nutrition and hydration.
- Although nutrition support is usually begun on day 10 of inadequate oral nutrition, patients with severe acute pancreatitis appear to benefit when TEN is started within 48 h of hospital admission.
- Patients with IBD and SBS may have significant micronutrient deficiencies, and replacement is usually recommended.
- Newer therapies for gastroparesis include electrical stimulation (pacemaker) and acupuncture. Novel trophic factors including glucagon-like peptide-2 have been approved for the nutritional treatment of short bowel syndrome.

References

1 Detsky AS, Baker JP, Mendelson RA, et al: Evaluating the accuracy of nutritional assessment techniques applied to hospitalized patients: methodology and comparisons. JPEN J Parenter Enteral Nutr 1984;8:153–159.

2 Mueller C, Compher C, Ellen D, et al: A.S.P.E.N. clinical guidelines: nutrition screening, assessment, and intervention in adults. JPEN J Parenter Enteral Nutr 2011;35:16–24.

3 Bankhead R, Boullata J, Brantley S, et al: Enteral nutrition practice recommendations. JPEN J Parenter Enteral Nutr 2009;33:122–167.

4 Kalfarentoz F, Kehagias J, Mead N, et al: Enteral nutrition is superior to parenteral nutrition in severe acute pancreatitis: results of a randomized prospective trial. Br J Surg 1997;84:1665–1669.

5 Camilleri M, Parkman H, Shafi M, et al: Clinical guideline: management of gastroparesis. Am J Gastroenterol 2012;373: 1–20.

6 Yamamoto T: Nutrition and diet in inflammatory bowel disease. Curr Opin Gastroenterol 2013;29:216–221.

7 Messori A, Trallori G, D'Albasio G, et al: Defined formula diets versus steroids in the treatment of active Crohn's disease. A meta-analysis. Scand J Gastroenterology 1996;31:267–272.

8 Scolapio JS: Current update in short bowel syndrome. Curr Opin Gastroenterol 2004;20:143–145.

Bier D, et al. (eds): Nutrition for the Primary Care Provider. World Rev Nutr Diet. Basel, Karger, 2015, vol 111, pp 146–150
DOI: 10.1159/000362314

Liver Diseases

Jonathan Obert Matt Cave Luis Marsano

University of Louisville and Robley Rex VAMC, Louisville, Ky., USA

Key Words

Liver disease · Nutrition · Cirrhosis · Nonalcoholic fatty liver disease · Alcoholic liver disease

Key Messages

- Nutrition is an important aspect of the successful treatment of liver disease. Nutritional regimens should be tailored to the specific needs of patients with each category of liver disease.
- Patients with cirrhosis should be given high-calorie diets (35–40 kcal/kg/day) along with multivitamin and mineral supplements to overcome their hypermetabolic state and reverse malnutrition. Protein restriction should be avoided in these patients.
- For nonalcoholic fatty liver disease, the first line of treatment is lifestyle modification, including decreased caloric intake, increased exercise, and the addition of beneficial foods. Slow weight reduction has also shown to have beneficial effects.
- Patients with alcoholic liver disease (alcoholic hepatitis) often suffer from protein and micronutrient deficiencies. The key micronutrients for these patients include thiamine, zinc, magnesium, selenium, vitamin E, riboflavin, vitamin A, vitamin D, and folate.

Introduction

Liver disease is ubiquitous in America, and all primary care providers will likely encounter patients with different types of liver disease frequently throughout their careers. Nutrition is an important part of successfully treating liver disease, but is often overlooked or misunderstood. Liver disease is a broad term that can be used to describe anything that causes damage to the liver, ranging from an acute alcoholic hepatitis all the way to cirrhosis. Whatever process is causing liver disease, one important aspect of treatment is nutrition. The nutritional treatment of many causes of liver diseases is similar, but each cause of liver disease has an optimal nutritional regimen that will benefit that patient. The objective of this chapter is to act as a reference guide for some of the most common types of liver disease.

Cirrhosis

Malnutrition is often overlooked in patients with cirrhosis. The causes of malnutrition are multiple, and include: (a) a hypermetabolic state with increased nutritional needs (>110% of expected), (b) decreased glycogen storing capacity that causes the patient to go into 'starvation mode' after a few hours of fasting, leading to consumption of his own muscular mass as a source of energy, (c) anorexia and dysgeusia, often manifestations of the low-grade endotoxemia and proinflammatory state that develops due to increased intestinal permeability, (d) gastrointestinal disorders such as delayed gastric emptying that often trigger nausea, abnormal small intestine motility with associated bacterial overgrowth and maldigestion, and decreased bile salts in patients with cholestasis causing fat malabsorption and constipation, (e) medical interventions and diagnostic studies that require preprocedure fasting, and (f) prescription of unpalatable very low-sodium diets in order to control fluid retention, and inappropriate low-protein diets to control hepatic encephalopathy.

Patients with cirrhosis, unless they are obese, require high-calorie diets with 35–40 kcal/kg/day to overcome their hypermetabolic state and reverse their malnutrition. Current evidence indicates that protein restriction should be avoided because it does not help in preventing hepatic encephalopathy, and worsens protein-calorie malnutrition [1]. In prospective, randomized studies in patients with overt hepatic encephalopathy, normal protein intake is superior to protein restriction to control the disorder [2]. The diet should be divided into frequent small meals to prevent the onset of the 'starvation mode'. Cirrhotic patients should receive 1.2–1.5 g of protein per kg of weight [1]. A reasonable feeding protocol that is commonly utilized is to give 3 meals, 3 snacks, and a bedtime supplement with approximately 500–750 kcal and 26–30 g of protein. Most of the protein is provided in the 3 meals and bedtime supplement. The supplement at bedtime is critical because it has been demonstrated to increase lean body mass (in contrast, supplements given during the day did not improve muscular mass) [1].

Because the majority of patients with decompensated cirrhosis have 'covert' (minimal or grade 1) hepatic encephalopathy, it is a good idea to give 'probiotic yogurt' (with live cultures) as two of the snacks because they have been shown to help control mild hepatic encephalopathy.

Patients with obesity still require the frequent meals, bedtime supplement, and 1.5 g protein per kg; however, in order to control weight, they can have a daily calorie restriction of 500 kcal subtracted from their calculated or measured caloric needs.

Daily multivitamins and minerals supplements may correct undiagnosed micronutrient deficiencies. Zinc deficiency is common and can worsen dysgeusia, hepatic encephalopathy, and exaggerate intestinal permeability; 50 mg/day of elemental zinc is usually enough to correct this deficiency. Leg cramps are common in cirrhotics, especially if they are receiving diuretics. Leg cramps interfere with sleep and have a negative effect on quality of life. Supplementation with calcium, magnesium and zinc controls leg cramps in most cirrhotics.

Once the patient has fluid retention (edema and/or ascites), sodium restriction is recommended in order to minimize the use of diuretics that can lead to renal dysfunction. The best proven sodium restriction is 2 g/day sodium. Fluid restriction is not needed, unless the patient has significant hyponatremia (below 126 or 128 mEq/l).

Nonalcoholic Fatty Liver Disease

Nonalcoholic fatty liver disease (NAFLD) is the term given to all liver disorders that develop due to abnormal fat deposition in the liver in the absence of alcohol consumption. Nonalcoholic fatty liver is the term used when inflammation is not present, and nonalcoholic steatohepatitis (NASH) is used when inflammation and fibrosis are present, and, in some instances, NASH can lead to cirrhosis [3]. NASH is thought to be the cause of up to three fourths of all cryptogenic cirrhosis [3]. The Western diet has led to an increased prevalence of NAFLD in the United States. High fructose intake has been found to be an independent risk factor for NAFLD and the increased use of high fructose corn syrup over the past few decades has been associated with a dramatic increase in NAFLD in the United States. It is estimated that nearly 12% of total energy intake in Americans is from fructose [3].

Nutrition in NAFLD

The first line of treatment for NAFLD is lifestyle modification, including decreased caloric intake, increased exercise, and possibly the addition of known beneficial foods. Slow weight reduction, avoiding a ketotic state, has been proven beneficial in decreasing liver enzymes, decreasing the amount of hepatic fatty infiltration, and reducing progression of fibrosis and inflammation that can lead to cirrhosis [4]. A diet that is a net negative of 500 calories daily (compared with the patient's metabolic needs) is a reasonable goal for slow weight reduction and improved outcome with NAFLD. Although slow weight reduction is the primary goal in treating NAFLD, studies have compared different diets and the one that seems most beneficial is the Mediterranean diet [4]. The increased cost of the Mediterranean diet makes compliance more of an issue, especially in patients with lower socioeconomic status. Regular coffee as a source of caffeine consumption has been shown to reduce the risk of fibrosis in patients with NASH [5]. An exact amount of coffee or caffeine has not been studied, but it has been shown that drinking coffee with a caffeine consumption of up to 350 mg is possibly protective against NASH [5]. Another study has determined that caffeine independently has protective effects against the development of NAFLD [6]. Modest alcohol consumption (defined as ≤2 drinks/day in men and ≤1 drinks/day in women) has been found to be protective against the development of NASH when NAFLD has already been diagnosed [7]. Antioxidant therapy has become a popular topic as a potential therapy for NASH, and evidence for vitamin E treatment is promising. In nondiabetic adults with proven NASH, the AASLD guidelines recommend using vitamin E (800 IU/day) [8].

Alcoholic Liver Disease

Alcoholic liver disease (ALD) is due in part to oxidative stress in the liver. Alcohol is metabolized by the liver into acetaldehyde which can cause liver toxicity [2]. Alcohol alters the metabolic pathways in the liver and, with induction of cytochrome P4502E, there is increased oxidative stress in the liver.

It is well known that patients with alcoholic hepatitis are malnourished. The deficiency is not always caloric, but is often due to protein and micronutrient deficiencies. There is a direct correlation between nutrition and mortality in alcoholic hepatitis. One study has shown that patients who were able to consume over 3,000 kcal/day had nearly zero mortality, whereas patients who were unable to tolerate over 1,000 kcal/day had a greater than 80% 6-month mortality [2]. Steroids have been shown to be beneficial in alcoholic hepatitis, but enteral nutrition has been shown to be as beneficial as steroids in improving short-term mortality and to be superior to steroids in improving one-year mortality [2].

It is very important to supplement micronutrients in ALD. Thiamine is often deficient and must be supplemented before enteral feeding is initiated. Overlooking thiamine supplementation can cause Wernicke's encephalopathy, which is a serious complication of refeeding before supplementing with thiamine. Thiamine should be supplemented daily in all patients with ALD to correct baseline deficiency. Other micronutrients that are also deficient in ALD include zinc, magnesium, selenium, vitamin E, riboflavin, vitamin A, vitamin D, and folate [2]. These can all be supplemented using a daily multivitamin with minerals and adding 50 mg/day of zinc. Monitoring for signs of refeeding syndrome is important in alcoholic hepatitis as patients are often severely malnourished. It is important to closely monitor potassium, magnesium, and phosphorus in these patients after enteral nutrition is initiated, and to replace deficits immediately.

Conclusions

- Due to the prevalence of liver disease and the importance of nutrition in the treatment of those with liver disease, a reference guide would be beneficial to all physicians.
- Malnutrition is often a complication of liver disease, and it is important to recognize it. Frequent feeding with no protein restriction as well as high protein snacks before bed are important in treating chronic liver disease.
- Although coffee, caffeine, and vitamin E have been shown to be beneficial and/or protective in patients with NAFLD, the primary goal in treating this disease should be slow weight loss with diet and exercise.
- Micronutrients should never be overlooked in patients with any form of liver disease, and providing multivitamins with minerals is a good way to correct many of these deficiencies.
- Implementing the nutritional strategies outlined in this chapter will benefit patients with liver disease and hopefully serve as a quick reference guide for physicians (table 1).

Table 1. Summary of nutritional treatment regimens for patients with liver disease

Liver disease	Calories	Protein	Micronutrients	Distribution of meals and precautions	Supplements
Cirrhosis	35–40 kcal/kg in frequent small feedings	1.2–1.5 g/kg BW/day	– 2 g Na diet/day if ascites – zinc 50 mg/day – calcium – magnesium – multivitamin with minerals – water restriction in serum Na <126 mEq/l	– 3 meals + 3 snacks + bedtime supplement – watch for refeeding syndrome	– bedtime supplement with 500–750 kcal and 26–30 g of protein
NAFLD and NASH	net negative 500 kcal/day if patient is over-weight	1.2–1.5 g/kg BW/day – Mediterranean diet is ideal	– vitamin E 800 IU/day	avoid high-fructose corn syrup	– caffeine/coffee – modest alcohol (<2 drinks/day for males and <1 for females) is okay
Alcoholic hepatitis	>3,000 calories/day is optimal 35–40 kcal/kg is reasonable	1.2–1.5 g/kg BW/day	– thiamine initially – potassium prn – magnesium prn – phosphorus prn – multivitamin with minerals – zinc	– 3 meals + 3 snacks + bedtime supplement – watch for refeeding syndrome	– bedtime supplement with 500–750 kcal and 26–30 g of protein

References

1 Plauth M, Cabre E, Riggio O, et al: ESPEN Guidelines on Enteral Nutrition: liver disease. Clin Nutr 2006;25:285–294.

2 Beier J, Landes S, Mohammad M, McClain C: Nutrition in liver disorders and the role of alcohol; in Ross AC, Caballero B, Cousins RJ, et al (ed): Modern Nutrition in Health and Disease. Philadelphia, Lippincott Williams & Wilkins, 2012, pp 1115–1125.

3 Naniwadekar AS: Nutritional recommendations for patients with non-alcoholic fatty liver disease: an evidence based review. Nutr Issues Gastroenterol 2010;82:8–16.

4 Mahady SE, George J: Management of nonalcoholic steatohepatitis: an evidence-based approach. Clin Liver Dis 2012;16:631–645.

5 Molloy JW, Calcagno CJ, Williams CD, et al: Association of coffee and caffeine consumption with fatty liver disease, nonalcoholic steatohepatitis, and degree of hepatic fibrosis. Hepatology 2012;55:429.

6 Biredinc A, Stepanova M, Pawloski L, Younossi ZM: Caffeine is protective in patients with non-alcoholic fatty liver disease. Aliment Pharmacol Ther 2012;35:76–82.

7 Dunn W, Sanyal AJ, Brunt EM, et al: Modest alcohol consumption is associated with decreased prevalence of steatohepatitis in patients with non-alcoholic fatty liver disease (NAFLD). J Hepatol 2012;57:384–391.

8 Al-Busafi A, Bhat M, Wong P, et al: Antioxidant therapy in nonalcoholic steatohepatitis. Hepat Res Treat 2012;2012:947575.

Bier D, et al. (eds): Nutrition for the Primary Care Provider. World Rev Nutr Diet. Basel, Karger, 2015, vol 111, pp 151–163
DOI: 10.1159/000362315

Neurological Disorders

Neeraj Kumar

Department of Neurology, Mayo Clinic, Rochester, Minn., USA

Key Words

Nervous system · B-group vitamins · Thiamine · Folate · Niacin · Copper · Vitamin D · Vitamin E

Key Messages

- The B-group vitamins (vitamin B_{12}, thiamine, folate, niacin, pyridoxine), copper, vitamin D, and vitamin E are important for optimal functioning of the nervous system.
- Vitamin B_{12} deficiency is mainly seen in patients with intrinsic factor-related malabsorption such as in pernicious anemia. Treatment consists of a short course of daily or weekly therapy, often followed by monthly maintenance therapy.
- There are multiple causes of thiamine deficiency. High-risk patients should receive parenteral thiamine prior to any administration of glucose or parenteral nutrition.
- Daily folate supplements are recommended in women of childbearing age as prophylaxis against fetal neural tube defects. Higher doses are needed in patients with malabsorption.
- Niacin deficiency is mainly seen in populations dependent on corn as the primary carbohydrate source, as well as in alcoholism. Deficiencies can be treated with oral or intramuscular nicotinic acid.
- Vitamin D deficiency is due to inadequate sun exposure or malabsorption, affecting bone growth and mineralization. 400 IU of vitamin D per day is adequate to prevent deficiency in individuals with minimal sun exposure, but larger doses may be required in individuals with signs of clinical deficiency.
- Vitamin E deficiency is rare, although it sometimes occurs in patients with chronic cholestasis and pancreatic insufficiency. Treatment may require the use of larger oral doses, intramuscular administration or a water-miscible product (d-α-tocopherol glycol).

Introduction

Deficiency diseases such as kwashiorkor and marasmus are endemic in underdeveloped countries. Individuals at risk in developed countries include the poor and homeless, the elderly, patients on prolonged or inadequate parenteral nutrition, individuals with food fads or eating disorders like anorexia nervosa and bulimia, those suffering from malnutrition secondary to chronic alcoholism, and patients with pernicious anemia or disorders that result in malabsorption like sprue, celiac disease, bacterial overgrowth, hepatobiliary or pancreatic disease, inflammatory bowel disease, and ileal resection. Of particular concern in the developed world is the epidemic of obesity. The rising rates of bariatric surgery have been accompanied by neurological complications related to nutrient deficiencies.

The references cited in this chapter include recent review articles. The accompanying table 1 supplements the text.

Vitamin B_{12}

The two active forms of vitamin B_{12} (B_{12}) [1–4] are methylcobalamin and adenosylcobalamin. Methylcobalamin is a cofactor for a cytosolic enzyme, methionine synthase, in a methyl transfer reaction which converts homocysteine to methionine. Methionine is adenosylated to S-adenosylmethionine, a methyl group donor required for biologic methylation reactions involving proteins, neurotransmitters, and phospholipids. Methionine also facilitates the formation of formyltetrahydrofolate which is involved in purine synthesis. During the process of methionine formation, methyltetrahydrofolate donates the methyl group and is converted into tetrahydrofolate, a precursor for purine and pyrimidine synthesis. Impaired DNA synthesis could interfere with oligodendrocyte growth and myelin production. Adenosylcobalamin is a cofactor for L-methylmalonyl coenzyme A mutase which catalyzes the conversion of L-methylmalonyl coenzyme A to succinyl coenzyme A in an isomerization reaction. Accumulation of methylmalonate may provide abnormal substrates for fatty acid synthesis.

Causes of Deficiency

The majority of patients with clinically expressed B_{12} deficiency have intrinsic factor-related malabsorption such as that seen in pernicious anemia. B_{12} deficiency is particularly common in the elderly and is most likely due to the high incidence of atrophic gastritis and achlorhydria-induced food B_{12} malabsorption. Food-bound B_{12} malabsorption is rarely associated with clinically significant deficiency. B_{12} deficiency is commonly seen following gastric surgery (bariatric surgery or gastrectomy). Other causes of B_{12} deficiency include conditions associated with malabsorption. Even in the presence of severe malabsorption, 2–5 years may pass before B_{12} deficiency develops.

Clinical Significance

The best-characterized neurological manifestation of B_{12} deficiency is a myelopathy that has commonly been referred to as subacute combined degeneration. The neurological features typically include a spastic paraparesis, extensor plantar response, and impaired perception of position and vibration. Accompanying optic nerve or peripheral nerve involvement may be present. Neuropsychiatric manifestations include decreased memory, personality change, and rarely, delirium. Clinical, electrophysiological, and pathological involvement of the peripheral nervous system has been described with B_{12} deficiency. Clues to possible B_{12} deficiency in a patient with polyneuropathy included a subacute onset of symptoms, findings suggestive of an associated myelopathy, onset of symptoms in the hands, macrocytic red blood cells, and the presence of a risk factor for B_{12} deficiency. Subclinical B_{12} deficiency refers to biochemical evidence of B_{12} deficiency in the absence of hematological or neurological manifestations. The incidence of cryptogenic polyneuropathy, cognitive impairment, and B_{12} deficiency increase with age, and the latter may be a chance occurrence rather than causative.

Investigations

Serum B_{12} determination has been the mainstay for evaluating B_{12} status. Elevated levels of serum methylmalonic acid and plasma total homocysteine are useful as ancillary diagnostic tests. The specificity of methylmalonic acid is superior to that of plasma homocysteine. Though plasma total homocysteine is a very sensitive indicator of

Table 1. Summary of the sources, causes of deficiency, neurological significance, laboratory tests, and treatment for deficiency states related to B12, thiamine, folate, niacin, pyridoxine, copper, vitamin D, and vitamin E deficiency

Nutrient	Sources	Major causes of deficiency	Neurological significance	Laboratory tests or imaging	Treatment	Additional comments
B_{12}	meats, egg, milk, fortified cereals, legumes	pernicious anemia, elderly (due to atrophic gastritis and food B_{12} malabsorption), gastric surgery, acid reduction therapy, gastrointestinal disease, nitrous oxide toxicity, rarely strict vegetarianism, often unknown	myelopathy or myeloneuropathy, peripheral neuropathy, neuropsychiatric manifestations, optic neuropathy, autonomic dysfunction	serum B_{12}, serum methylmalonic acid, plasma total homocystine, hematological tests (anemia, macrocytosis, neutrophil hypersegmentation), serum gastrin, intrinsic factor and parietal cell antibodies, increased signal on T2-weighted MRI involving dorsal column	intramuscular B_{12} 1,000 mg daily for 5 days and monthly	even in the presence of severe malabsorption, 2–5 years may pass before B_{12} deficiency develops
Thiamine	enriched, fortified, or whole-grain products, organ meats	recurrent vomiting, gastric surgery, alcoholism; increased demand (critically ill, hyperthyroidism, malignancy, systemic infection) with marginal nutritional status (decreased intake or absorption) alongside increased glucose intake	beriberi (dry, wet, infantile), Wernicke encephalopathy, Korsakoff syndrome	urinary thiamine, serum thiamine, erythrocyte transketolase activation assay, red blood cell thiamine diphosphate	50–300 mg a day of thiamine (intravenous, intramuscular, oral); higher doses may be required in Wernicke encephalopathy	at-risk patients should receive parenteral thiamine prior to administration of glucose or parenteral nutrition
Folate	in virtually all foods (spinach, yeast, peanuts, liver, beans, broccoli, grains and cereals fortified with folic acid)	alcoholism, gastrointestinal disease, folate antagonists (e.g. methotrexate, trimethoprim), errors of folate metabolism; folate deficiency generally coexists with other nutrient deficiencies	neurological manifestations are rare and indistinguishable from those due to B_{12} deficiency	serum folate, red blood cell folate, plasma total homocysteine	oral folate 1 mg three times a day followed by a maintenance dose of 1 mg/day; for acutely ill patients 1–5 mg/day (parenteral)	clinically significant depletion of body folate stores may be seen in weeks/months; higher requirements in pregnancy, lactation, methotrexate toxicity
Niacin	meat, fish, poultry, enriched bread, fortified cereals	corn as primary carbohydrate source, alcoholism, malabsorption, carcinoid and Hartnup syndrome	encephalopathy (peripheral neuropathy)	erythrocyte nicotinamide adenine dinucleotide, urinary excretion of methylated niacin metabolites	25–50 mg of nicotinic acid (intramuscular, oral) three times a day	deficiency state often unaccompanied by gastrointestinal or dermatologic manifestations

Table 1 (continued)

Nutrient	Sources	Major causes of deficiency	Neurological significance	Laboratory tests or imaging	Treatment	Additional comments
Pyridoxine	meat, fish, eggs, soybeans, nuts, dairy products	B_6 antagonists (INH, hydralazine, penicillamine), alcoholism, gastrointestinal disease	infantile seizures, peripheral neuropathy	plasma pyridoxal phosphate	50–100 mg of pyridoxine daily (oral); pyridoxine supplementation in patients on isoniazid	pure sensory neuropathy with toxicity
Copper	organ meats, seafood, nuts, mushroom, cocoa, chocolate, beans, whole-grain products	gastric surgery, zinc toxicity, gastrointestinal disease, total parenteral nutrition and enteral feeding	myelopathy or myeloneuropathy	serum and urinary copper, serum ceruloplasmin, serum and urinary zinc, hematological parameters (anemia, neutropenia, vacuolated myeloid precursors, ringed sideroblasts, iron-containing plasma cells), increased signal on T2-weighted MRI involving dorsal column	oral elemental copper: 8 mg/day for a week, 6 mg/day for the second week, 4 mg/day for the third week and 2 mg/day thereafter	zinc toxicity may result from excess use of zinc supplements or zinc-containing denture creams
Vitamin D	sunlight, liver, eggs, dairy products (often supplemented with vitamin D)	inadequate sunlight exposure, dietary insufficiency, malabsorption, gastric surgery, older antiepileptic drugs, disease involving the pancreas, liver or kidney	myopathy, myalgias	serum 25(OH) vitamin D, calcium and phosphorus, parathormone, radiologic changes of rickets or osteomalacia	50,000 IU of vitamin D weekly; 400 IU of vitamin D per day for maintenance	some studies suggest inverse association between vitamin D intake and levels, and risk of multiple sclerosis
Vitamin E	vegetable oils (sunflower and olive), leafy vegetables, fruits, meats, nuts, unprocessed cereal grains	chronic cholestasis (particularly in children), pancreatic insufficiency, gastrointestinal disease, ataxia with vitamin E deficiency, homozygous hypobetalipoproteinemia, abetalipoproteinemia, chylomicron retention disease	spinocerebellar syndrome with peripheral neuropathy, ophthalmoplegia, pigmentary retinopathy	serum vitamin E, ratio of serum α-tocopherol to sum of serum cholesterol and triglycerides	vitamin E ranging from 200 mg/day to 200 mg/kg/day (oral, intramuscular); supplementation of bile salts in some patients	vitamin E deficiency is virtually never the consequence of a dietary inadequacy; neurological findings are rare in vitamin E-deficient adults with chronic cholestasis

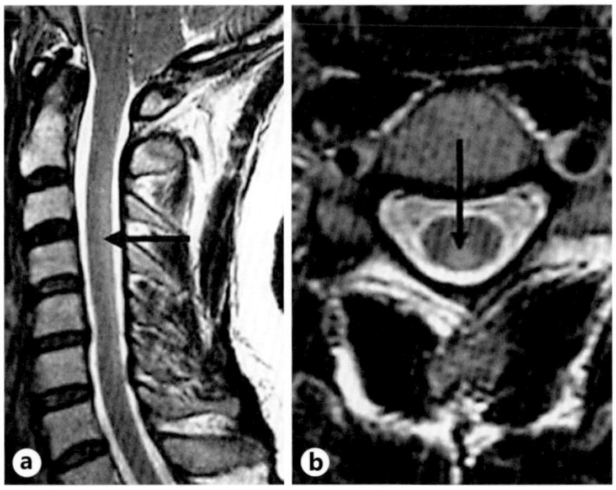

Fig. 1. MRI showing increased signal involving the cervical dorsal column. Sagittal (**a**) and axial (**b**) T2-weighted MRI showing increased signal in the paramedian aspect of the dorsal cervical cord (arrows). The signal change involves the dorsal columns. This can be seen in patients with a myelopathy due to B_{12} or copper deficiency.

B_{12} deficiency, its major limitation is its poor specificity. Hematologic manifestations of B_{12} deficiency include anemia, macrocytosis, neutrophil hypersegmentation, and megaloblastic bone marrow changes. Anti-intrinsic factor antibodies are specific (over 95%) but lack sensitivity and are found in approximately 60% of patients with pernicious anemia. Patients with pernicious anemia may also have an elevated serum gastrin level. Elevated gastrin levels are a marker for hypochlorhydria or achlorhydria. Electrophysiologic abnormalities include nerve conduction studies suggestive of a sensorimotor axonopathy, and abnormalities on somatosensory and visual evoked potentials. MRI abnormalities include a signal change in the posterior and lateral columns and subcortical white matter (fig. 1).

Management
The goals of treatment are to reverse the signs and symptoms of deficiency, replete body stores, ascertain the cause of deficiency, and monitor response to therapy. A short course of daily or weekly therapy is often followed by monthly maintenance therapy. If the oral dose is large enough, even patients with an absorption defect may respond to oral B_{12}. Patients with pernicious anemia have a higher risk of gastric cancer and carcinoids and therefore should get an endoscopy. Patients with pernicious anemia also have a higher frequency of thyroid disease and iron deficiency and should be screened for these conditions.

Response to treatment may relate to the extent of involvement and delay in starting treatment. Response of the neurological manifestations is often slow and incomplete. Response of the hematologic derangements is prompt and complete. Methylmalonic acid and homocystine are more reliable ways for monitoring response to therapy than B_{12} levels.

Thiamine

Thiamine [3–5] functions as a coenzyme in the metabolism of carbohydrates, lipids, and branched-chain amino acids. It has a role in energy production in adenosine triphosphate synthesis, in myelin sheath maintenance, and in neurotransmitter production. Following cellular uptake, thiamine is phosphorylated into thiamine diphosphate, the metabolically active form that is involved in several enzyme systems. Thiamine diphosphate is a cofactor for pyruvate dehydrogenase, α-ketoglutarate dehydrogenase, and transketolase. Pyruvate dehydrogenase and α-ketoglutarate dehydrogenase are involved in the tricarboxylic acid cycle in oxidative decarboxylation of α-ketoacids such as pyruvate and α-ketoglutarate to acetyl coenzyme A and succinate, respectively. Transketolase transfers activated aldehydes in the hexose monophosphate shunt (pentose-phosphate pathway) in the generation of nicotinamide adenine dinucleotide phosphate for reductive biosynthesis.

Causes of Deficiency

Thiamine deficiency can result from reduced intake or reduced absorption or increased metabolic requirement or increased losses or defective transport. Often, multiple contributing factors coexist. Thiamine requirements increase in children, during pregnancy and lactation, and with vigorous exercise. Disorders such as systemic infections, malignancy, and hyperthyroidism are also associated with an increased metabolic demand. Relative thiamine deficiency may be seen in high-risk patients during periods of high carbohydrate intake as is seen with nasogastric feeding, total parenteral nutrition, or intravenous hyperalimentation. In these circumstances, a high percentage of calories are derived from glucose, and the amount of corresponding thiamine replacement is inadequate. This is particularly common when there is preceding starvation or where several days of intravenous nutrition without adequate vitamin replacement are followed by oral food intake. The well-recognized clinical setting for thiamine deficiency is alcoholism. Thiamine deficiency is being increasingly identified outside the context of alcoholism. Early neurological complications following bariatric surgery are frequently related to thiamine deficiency. Due to a short half-life and absence of significant storage amounts, a continuous dietary supply of thiamine is necessary. A thiamine-deficient diet may result in manifestations of thiamine deficiency in a few days.

Clinical Significance

Thiamine deficiency affects the central nervous system, peripheral nervous system, and cardiovascular system in varying combinations. Cardiac involvement may manifest as high-output or low-output cardiac failure. The best-characterized neurological disorders related to thiamine deficiency are beriberi, Wernicke encephalopathy, and Korsakoff syndrome (Korsakoff psychosis). Wernicke encephalopathy or Korsakoff syndrome may be associated with a peripheral neuropathy. Wernicke encephalopathy often results from severe, short-term thiamine deficiency, whereas peripheral neuropathy is more often a consequence of prolonged mild to moderate thiamine deficiency. Dry beriberi is characterized by a sensorimotor, distal, axonal peripheral neuropathy often associated with calf cramps, muscle tenderness, and burning feet. Autonomic neuropathy may be present. A rapid progression of the neuropathy may mimic Guillain-Barré syndrome. Pedal edema may be seen due to coexisting wet beriberi. The symptoms of subclinical thiamine deficiency are often vague and nonspecific and include fatigue, irritability, headaches, and lethargy.

The clinical features of Wernicke encephalopathy include a subacute onset of the classic triad of ocular abnormalities, gait ataxia, and mental status changes. The onset may be gradual, the classic triad is frequently absent, one or more components of the triad may be seen later in the course, and some patients may not have any of the manifestations related to the classic triad. Reliance on the classic triad, not recognizing thiamine deficiency outside the context of alcoholism, nonspecific or poorly recognized signs and symptoms all result in missing the diagnosis. Ocular abnormalities include nystagmus (horizontal more common than vertical), ophthalmoparesis (commonly involving the lateral recti), and conjugate gaze palsies (usually horizontal). Gait and trunk ataxia is a consequence of cerebellar and vestibular dysfunction. A coexisting chronic peripheral or acute neuropathy may be an additional contributing factor for the gait difficulty. Mental status changes are the most constant component of the disease and include inability to concentrate, apathy, confusion, delirium, frank psychosis, and coma. It is important to recognize that the intoxicated patient who does not recover fully may be suffering from Wernicke encephalopathy.

About 80% of patients with Wernicke encephalopathy who survive develop Korsakoff syndrome. Korsakoff syndrome is an amnestic-confabulatory syndrome characterized by severe anterograde and retrograde amnesia that follows Wernicke encephalopathy; Korsakoff syndrome emerges as ocular manifestations and encephalopathy subside. In Korsakoff syndrome, memory is disproportionately impaired relative to other aspects of cognitive function.

Investigations

Urinary thiamine excretion and serum thiamine levels may be decreased in thiamine deficiency but do not accurately reflect tissue concentrations and are not reliable indicators of thiamine status. A normal serum thiamine level does not exclude Wernicke encephalopathy. The preferred tests are the erythrocyte transketolase activation assay or measurement of thiamine diphosphate in red blood cell hemolysates.

MRI is the imaging modality of choice. Typical MRI findings include increased T2 or proton density or FLAIR signal in the paraventricular regions. Involved areas include the thalamus, hypothalamus, mammillary body, periaqueductal midbrain, tectal plate, pons, fourth ventricle floor, medulla, midline cerebellum, and, rarely, in the splenium of the corpus callosum or basal ganglia structures. Mammillary body enhancement on MR has been reported as being the only imaging abnormality in Wernicke encephalopathy. The signal abnormalities resolve with treatment, but shrunken mamillary bodies may persist as sequelae. Additional findings in the chronic stages include dilated aqueduct and third ventricles with atrophy of the midbrain tegmentum, paramedian thalamic nuclei, mamillary bodies, and frontal lobes.

Management

Intravenous glucose infusion in patients with thiamine deficiency may consume the available thiamine and precipitate an acute Wernicke encephalopathy. At-risk patients should receive parenteral thiamine prior to administration of glucose or parenteral nutrition. Patients suspected of having beriberi or Wernicke encephalopathy should promptly receive parenteral thiamine. A commonly used thiamine replacement regimen is 100 mg intravenously every 8 h. Higher doses may be required in Wernicke encephalopathy, particularly when Wernicke encephalopathy occurs in the setting of alcoholism. Long-term oral maintenance with 50–100 mg thiamine is commonly employed. Wernicke encephalopathy often develops in a predisposed individual because of increased metabolic demands related to coexisting conditions like an infection which requires independent attention.

In wet beriberi, a rapid improvement is seen with clearing of symptoms within days. Improvement in motor and sensory symptoms takes weeks or months. Response in Wernicke encephalopathy is variable. Ocular signs improve in a few hours. A fine horizontal nystagmus may persist. Improvement is gait ataxia and memory is variable and often delayed. Mental status improves over days or weeks. Prompt treatment of Wernicke encephalopathy prevents the development of Korsakoff syndrome. Korsakoff syndrome does not respond to thiamine therapy.

Folic Acid

Folate [2–4] functions as a coenzyme or cosubstrate by modifying, accepting, or transferring one-carbon moieties in single-carbon reactions involved in the metabolism of nucleic and amino acids. The biologically active folates are in the tetrahydrofolate form. Methyltetrahydrofolate is the predominant folate and is required for the B_{12}-dependent remethylation of homocysteine to methionine. Methylation of deoxyuridylate to thymidylate is mediated by methylene tetrahydrofolate. Impairment of this reaction results in accumulation of uracil which replaces the decreased thymine in nucleoprotein synthesis and initiates the process that leads to megaloblastic anemia.

Causes of Deficiency

Folate deficiency rarely exists in the pure state. It is often associated with conditions that affect other nutrients. Hence, attribution of neurological manifestations to folate deficiency requires exclusion of other potential causes. Populations at increased risk of folate deficiency include alcoholics, premature infants, and adolescents. Increased folate requirements are seen in pregnancy, lactation, and chronic hemolytic anemia. Folate deficiency may be seen with small bowel disorders associated with malabsorption. Folate absorption may be decreased in conditions associated with reduced gastric secretions such as gastric surgery, atrophic gastritis, acid-suppressive therapy, and acid neutralization by treatment of pancreatic insufficiency. Drugs such as aminopterin, methotrexate, pyrimethamine, trimethoprim, and triamterene act as folate antagonists and produce folate deficiency by inhibiting dihydrofolate reductase. Serum folate falls within 3 weeks after decrease in folate intake or absorption, red blood cell folate declines weeks later, and clinically significant depletion of folate stores may be seen within months. Clinical features of folate deficiency occur more rapidly with low stores or coexisting alcoholism.

Clinical Significance

Theoretically, folate deficiency could cause the same deficits as those seen with B_{12} deficiency because of its importance in the production of methionine, S-adenosylmethionine, and tetrahydrofolate. For unclear reasons, neurological manifestations like those seen in B_{12} deficiency are rare in folate deficiency. The myeloneuropathy or neuropathy or megaloblastic anemia seen in association with folate deficiency is indistinguishable from B_{12} deficiency.

Folate deficiency has been associated with affective disorders. In recent years, there has been some evidence suggesting that chronic folate deficiency may increase the risk of cardiovascular disease, cerebrovascular disease, peripheral vascular disease, venous thrombosis, and may cause cognitive impairment. The precise significance of these observations awaits further studies. Folate deficiency causes increased frequency of neural tube defects in babies born to folate-deficient mothers.

Investigations

Plasma homocysteine levels have been shown to be elevated in a majority of patients with clinically significant folate deficiency. Serum folate fluctuates daily and does not correlate with tissue stores. Red blood cell folate is more reliable than plasma folate because its levels are less affected by short-term fluctuations in intake.

Management

In women of childbearing age with epilepsy daily folate supplement of 0.4 mg is recommended for prophylaxis against neural tube defects. With documented folate deficiency, an oral dose of 1 mg three times a day may be followed by a maintenance dose of 1 mg a day. Daily doses as high as 20 mg may be needed in patients with malabsorption. Acutely ill patients may need parenteral administration in a dose of 1–5 mg. Coexisting B_{12} deficiency should be ruled out before instituting folate therapy. Plasma homocysteine is likely the best biochemical tool for monitoring response to therapy. Since folate deficiency is generally seen in the context of a broader dietary inadequacy, the associated comorbidities need to be addressed.

Niacin

Niacin [1, 3, 4] in humans is an end product of tryptophan metabolism. Niacin is converted in the body to nicotinamide adenine dinucleotide and nicotinamide adenine dinucleotide phosphate, two coenzymes that have a role in carbohydrate metabolism.

Causes of Deficiency
Pellagra is rare in developed countries. Niacin deficiency is predominantly seen in populations dependent on corn as the primary carbohydrate source. Corn lacks niacin and tryptophan. Nonendemic pellagra may rarely be seen with alcoholism and malabsorption. Pellagra may be seen in the carcinoid syndrome since tryptophan is converted to serotonin instead of being used in niacin synthesis. Biotransformation of tryptophan to nicotinic acid requires several vitamins and minerals like B_2, B_6, iron, and copper. Since tryptophan is necessary for niacin synthesis, vitamin B_6 deficiency can result in secondary niacin deficiency. Isonicotinic acid hydrazide (isoniazid) depletes B_6 and can trigger pellagra. An excess of neutral amino acids in the diet, such as leucine, can compete with tryptophan for uptake and predispose the individual towards niacin deficiency by impairing its synthesis from tryptophan. Hartnup syndrome is an autosomal recessive disorder characterized by impaired synthesis of niacin from tryptophan and results in pellagra-like symptoms. Bacterial colonization of the small intestines can lead to conversion of dietary tryptophan to indoles.

Clinical Significance
Pellagra affects the gastrointestinal tract, skin, and nervous system. The classical clinical hallmarks of pellagra have been alluded to by mnemonic dermatitis, diarrhea, and dementia. The dermatologic and gastrointestinal manifestations are frequently absent, particularly so in nonendemic pellagra. Unexplained progressive encephalopathy in alcoholics that is not responsive to thiamine should raise the possibility of pellagra. The peripheral neuropathy seen in pellagra is indistinguishable from the peripheral neuropathy seen with thiamine deficiency.

Investigations
There are no sensitive and specific blood measures of niacin status. It has been suggested that measures of erythrocyte nicotinamide adenine dinucleotide and plasma metabolites of niacin may serve as indirect markers.

Management
Oral or intramuscular nicotinic acid is used for treatment of symptomatic patients. Advanced stages of pellagra can be cured with intramuscular nicotinamide given in doses of 50–100 mg three times a day for 3–4 days followed by similar quantities orally.

Vitamin B_6

Pyridoxal phosphate [1, 3, 4] serves as a coenzyme in many reactions involved in the metabolism of amino acids, lipids, nucleic acid, one-carbon units, and in the pathways of gluconeogenesis, and neurotransmitter and heme biosynthesis. The interconversion and metabolism of B_6 is dependent on riboflavin, niacin, and zinc. Niacin, carnitine, and folate require B_6 for their metabolism. Humans and other mammals cannot synthesize B_6 and thus must obtain this micronutrient from exogenous sources via intestinal absorption.

Causes of Deficiency
Most diets are adequate in B_6. Its deficiency is seen with B_6 antagonists like isonicotinic acid hydrazide, cycloserine, hydralazine, and penicillamine. Individuals at risk of developing B_6 deficiency include pregnant and lactating women, elderly individuals, alcoholics, and patients with gastrointestinal disease.

Clinical Significance
Dietary deficiency of pyridoxine or congenital dependency on pyridoxine may manifest as infantile seizures. Adults are much more tolerant of pyridoxine deficiency. Up to 50% of slow activators may develop a dose-related peripheral neuropathy when treated with isonicotinic acid

hydrazide. Chronic B_6 deficiency results in a microcytic hypochromic anemia. A form of sideroblastic anemia can be treated with pyridoxine supplementation. Chronic vitamin B_6-deficient patients may develop secondary hyperoxaluria and thus are at higher risk for nephrolithiasis. As with other B vitamin deficiencies, glossitis, stomatitis, cheilosis, and dermatitis may be seen.

Excess consumption of B_6 has been associated with a pure sensory peripheral neuropathy or ganglionopathy. It is characterized by sensory ataxia, areflexia, impaired cutaneous and deep sensations, and positive Romberg's sign.

Investigations

Vitamin B_6 status can be assessed by measuring its levels in the blood or urine. The most commonly used measure is plasma pyridoxal phosphate. Functional indicators of vitamin B_6 status are based on pyridoxal phosphate-dependent reactions.

Management

Isonicotinic acid hydrazide-induced neuropathy is reversible by drug discontinuation or B_6 supplementation. Vitamin B_6 may be supplemented in a dose of 50–100 mg/day to prevent development of the neuropathy.

Copper

Copper [3, 4, 6] is a component of enzymes that have a critical role in maintaining the structure and function of the nervous system. Copper permits electron transfer in key enzymatic pathways. These copper-associated enzymes include cytochrome-c-oxidase for electron transport and oxidative phosphorylation, copper/zinc superoxide dismutase for antioxidant defense, tyrosinase for melanin synthesis, dopamine β-hydroxylase for catecholamine biosynthesis, lysyl oxidase for crosslinking of collagen and elastin, peptidylglycine α-amidating monooxygenase for neuropeptide and peptide hormone processing, monoamine oxidase for serotonin synthesis, and ceruloplasmin for brain iron homeostasis.

Causes of Deficiency

The most common identified cause of copper deficiency in reported patients with a copper deficiency myelopathy has been a prior history of gastric surgery. The duration between gastric surgery and onset of neurological symptoms is generally years. Excessive zinc ingestion is another cause of copper deficiency. Unusual sources of excess zinc have included patients who consumed excessive amounts of denture cream for long periods and patients swallowing zinc-containing coins. Because of copper's ubiquitous distribution and low daily requirement, acquired dietary copper deficiency is rare. Copper deficiency may occur in premature or low-birthweight infants and in malnourished infants. Copper deficiency may be a complication of total parenteral or enteral nutrition. Other causes of copper deficiency include nephrotic syndrome, glomerulonephritis, and enteropathies associated with malabsorption such as celiac disease, cystic fibrosis, Crohn's disease, sprue, and bacterial overgrowth.

Clinical Significance

Menkes disease is a copper deficiency-related disease in humans and is due to congenital copper deficiency. Impaired biliary copper excretion underlies copper toxicity in Wilson disease. Copper deficiency-associated myelopathy has been described in ruminants and other animal species and has been called swayback or enzootic ataxia. The well-recognized hematological manifestations of copper deficiency in humans include anemia and neutropenia. Thrombocytopenia and resulting pancytopenia are relatively rare. Typical bone marrow findings include a left shift in granulocytic and erythroid maturation with cytoplasmic vacuolization in erythroid and myeloid precursors. Ringed sideroblasts and hemosiderin-containing plasma cells may be present. Erythroid hyperplasia with decreased myeloid to erythroid ratio and dyserythropoiesis including megaloblastic changes may be seen. Patients may be given a diagnosis of sideroblastic anemia or myelodysplastic syndrome or aplastic anemia.

The neurological syndrome due to acquired copper deficiency may be present without the hematological manifestations. The most common manifestation is that of a myelopathy or myeloneuropathy that resembles the subacute combined degeneration seen with B_{12} deficiency. Copper and B_{12} deficiency may coexist. It presents with a spastic gait and prominent sensory ataxia. The sensory ataxia is primarily due to dorsal column dysfunction. Clinical or electrophysiological evidence of an associated axonal peripheral neuropathy is common.

Investigations

Laboratory indicators of copper deficiency include reduced serum copper or ceruloplasmin, and reduced urinary copper excretion. Changes in serum copper usually parallel the ceruloplasmin concentration. Ceruloplasmin is an acute-phase reactant. Copper deficiency could be masked under conditions that increase ceruloplasmin levels. Serum zinc elevation should prompt an aggressive search for possible exogenous zinc ingestion. The most common abnormality on the spine MRI is increased T2 signal involving the dorsal columns (fig. 1). The cervical cord is most commonly involved. Somatosensory evoked potential and nerve conduction studies suggest impaired central conduction and varying degrees of peripheral neuropathy, respectively.

Management

In patients with copper deficiency due to excess zinc ingestion, stopping zinc supplementation may suffice. Despite a suspected absorption defect, oral copper is generally the preferred route of supplementation. Periodic assessment of serum copper is essential to determine adequacy of replacement. Because of the need for long-term replacement, parenteral therapy is not preferred and generally not required. If oral therapy does not result in improvement or if there is rapid deterioration or significant hematological derangement, then 2 mg of elemental copper may be administered intravenously daily for 5 days and periodically thereafter. Response of the hematological parameters (including bone marrow findings) is prompt and often complete. Recovery of neurological signs and symptoms is variable. Improvement when present is often subjective and is more so for sensory manifestations. Prevention of progression is often seen.

Vitamin D

Vitamin D [3, 4] exists in two forms: vitamin D_2 (ergocalciferol, produced by plants) and vitamin D_3 (cholecalciferol, produced with exposure to ultraviolet light in the skin). Vitamin D functions more like a hormone than a vitamin. Orally ingested vitamin D is absorbed and hydroxylated in the liver to 25(OH) vitamin D. Further hydroxylation occurs in the kidney to 1,25(OH) vitamin D which is the active form.

Causes of Deficiency

Inadequate sun exposure may cause vitamin D deficiency in chronically ill, institutionalized, or housebound individuals. Vitamin D deficiency can also result from dietary insufficiency or malabsorption. Advanced liver or kidney disease can decrease the active form of vitamin D. The antiepileptic drugs phenobarbital and phenytoin inhibit vitamin D hydroxylation in the liver and inhibit calcium absorption in the intestines.

Clinical Significance

Vitamin D deficiency results in defective mineralization of newly formed bone. Vitamin D deficiency results in hypocalcemia with secondary hyperparathyroidism which further impairs normal bone mineralization. This causes rickets in children and osteomalacia in adults. Vitamin D deficiency can cause a proximal myopathy which often exists in association with osteomalacia, pathological fractures, and bone pain. Severe hypocalcemia may result in tetany. Hypovitaminosis D has been associated with persistent, nonspecific musculoskeletal pain in some studies. Studies have also noted an inverse association between vitamin D (both dietary intake and blood levels) and the risk of developing multiple sclerosis.

Investigations
Since 25(OH) vitamin D is hydroxylated to the active form, the level of 1,25(OH) vitamin D may be normal, while levels of its immediate precursor may be very low. Hence, vitamin D status is best assessed by measuring 25(OH) vitamin D levels. Other laboratory abnormalities may include raised alkaline phosphatase of bone origin, hypocalcemia, hypophosphatemia, raised parathormone, and reduced urinary calcium excretion. Radiological changes of rickets or osteopenia may be present.

Management
Vitamin D can be given orally as vitamin D_2 or vitamin D_3. 400 IU of vitamin D per day is adequate to prevent deficiency in individuals with minimal sun exposure. With clinical deficiency, 50,000 IU weekly may be required. Larger oral doses or parenteral administration may be required in the presence of malabsorption. Laboratory monitoring is required with doses of 50,000 IU three times a week. Toxicity includes hypercalcemia, hypercalciuria, and renal failure. Serum and urine calcium and serum 25 (OH) vitamin D should be monitored and when urinary calcium excretion exceeds 100 mg/24 h, the vitamin D dose should be reduced. Associated secondary hyperparathyroidism can cause hypercalcemia, hypercalciuria, and nephrolithiasis. This can be prevented by ensuring that there is adequate calcium repletion and thus avoiding parathyroid stimulation. An inappropriately high phosphate level suggests secondary hyperparathyroidism.

Vitamin E

In humans, α-tocopherol is the active and most important biologic form of vitamin E [1, 3, 4]. Vitamin E serves as an antioxidant and prevents the formation of toxic free radical products. It appears to protect cellular membranes from oxidative stress, and inhibits the peroxidation of polyunsaturated fatty acids of membrane phospholipids.

Causes of Deficiency
Due to the ubiquitous distribution of tocopherols in foods, vitamin E deficiency is virtually never the consequence of a dietary inadequacy. Vitamin E absorption requires biliary and pancreatic secretions. Hence, vitamin E deficiency is seen with chronic cholestasis and pancreatic insufficiency. Vitamin E deficiency is also seen in other conditions associated with malabsorption. Vitamin E deficiency may be seen due to genetic conditions like ataxia with vitamin E deficiency, hypobetalipoproteinemia, abetalipoproteinemia, and chylomicron retention disease. Vitamin E supplementation in total parenteral nutrition may be inadequate to maintain vitamin E stores.

Clinical Significance
Development of neurological symptoms in adults with acquired fat malabsorption syndromes takes decades. Many years of malabsorption are required to deplete vitamin E stores. The neurological manifestations of vitamin E deficiency include a spinocerebellar syndrome with variable peripheral nerve involvement. The phenotype is similar to that of Friedreich's ataxia. The clinical features include cerebellar ataxia, hyporeflexia, proprioceptive, and vibratory loss, and an extensor plantar response. Cutaneous sensations may be affected to a lesser degree. Ophthalmoplegia, ptosis, and pigmentary retinopathy may be seen. An associated myopathy, at times with inflammatory infiltrates and rimmed vacuoles, has been described. The neuropathy associated with vitamin E deficiency preferentially involves centrally directed fibers of large myelinated neurons.

Investigations
Hyperlipidemia or hypolipidemia can independently increase or decrease serum vitamin E without reflecting similar alterations in tissue levels of the vitamin. Effective serum α-tocopherol concentrations are calculated by dividing the serum α-tocopherol by the sum of serum cholesterol and triglycerides. In patients with neurological manifestations due to vitamin E deficiency, the serum vitamin E levels are frequently undetectable. Additional markers of fat malabsorption such as increased stool fat and decreased serum carotene levels may be present.

Somatosensory evoked potential studies may show evidence of central delay, and nerve conduction studies may show evidence of an axonal neuropathy. Spinal MRI in patients with vitamin E deficiency-related myeloneuropathy may show increased signal in the cervical cord dorsal column.

Management
With cholestatic liver disease, treatment with standard doses of fat-soluble vitamin E may be ineffective because of fat malabsorption. Larger oral doses or intramuscular administration or a water-miscible product (d-α-tocopherol glycol) may be required. An empiric approach is to start with a lower dose, increase it gradually, and based on the clinical and laboratory response consider a higher dose or parenteral formulation. Supplements of bile salts may be of value in some patients. The free radical scavenger and antioxidant properties of vitamin E have led to its use in conditions like Alzheimer disease and amyotrophic lateral sclerosis. The use of vitamin E in these conditions is unproven.

Conclusions

- Optimal functioning of the nervous system is dependent on a constant supply of essential nutrients.
- Particularly important for optimal functioning of the nervous system are the B-group vitamins (B_{12}, thiamine, folate, niacin, pyridoxine), copper, vitamin D, and vitamin E.
- Not infrequently multiple nutritional deficiencies coexist.
- The presence of multiple causes for a nutrient deficiency increases the chances of the development of clinical manifestations related to that particular nutrient deficiency.
- The preventable and potentially treatable nature of these disorders makes this an important subject.
- Prognosis depends on prompt recognition and institution of appropriate therapy.

References

1 Chaudhry V, Umapathi T, Ravich WJ: Neuromuscular diseases and disorders of the alimentary system. Muscle Nerve 2002;25:768–784.
2 Carmel R, Green R, Rosenblatt DS, Watkins D: Update on cobalamin, folate, and homocysteine. Hematology Am Soc Hematol Educ Program 2003:62–81.
3 Kumar N: Nutritional neuropathies. Neurol Clin 2007;25:209–255.
4 Kumar N: Neurologic presentations of nutritional deficiencies. Neurol Clin 2010;28:107–170.
5 Sechi G, Serra A: Wernicke's encephalopathy: new clinical settings and recent advances in diagnosis and management. Lancet Neurol 2007;6:442–455.
6 Kumar N: Copper deficiency myelopathy: human swayback. Mayo Clin Proc 2006;81:1371–1384.

Bier D, et al. (eds): Nutrition for the Primary Care Provider. World Rev Nutr Diet. Basel, Karger, 2015, vol 111, pp 164–168
DOI: 10.1159/000362319

Anemias due to Essential Nutrient Deficiencies

Sally P. Stabler

Division of Hematology, School of Medicine, University of Colorado, Aurora, Colo., USA

Key Words

Anemia · Iron deficiency · Vitamin B_{12} · Folate

Key Messages

- Iron deficiency results from decreased intake in the setting of increased loss due to menstruation, childbirth or gastrointestinal bleeding.
- Diets low in animal source foods are deficient in both iron and vitamin B_{12}.
- Atrophic gastritis (pernicious anemia) and other malabsorption syndromes are the major cause of vitamin B_{12} deficiency megaloblastic anemia.
- Folate deficiency megaloblastic anemia is often the result of alcoholism, drug therapy or malabsorption syndromes.
- Vitamin B_{12} deficiency causes elevated methylmalonic acid levels, and both B_{12} deficiency and folate deficiency cause elevated homocysteine levels.

Introduction

Anemia is defined as hemoglobin (Hgb) less than 13 g/dl for males and 12 g/dl for females. There are many factors influencing Hgb such as sex, age, race, altitude of residence and presence of common hemoglobinopathies such as thalassemia minor and Hgb E which also affect a population's normal values. Anemia may be accompanied by other cytopenias such as leukopenia and thrombocytopenia. Anemia impacts many aspects of health such as growth and development, perinatal health and even survival in seniors with chronic conditions. Anemias due to nutritional deficiencies are easily treated; thus, prompt diagnosis is important. Often, such anemias are a sign of other medical conditions that require investigation.

Iron deficiency is the most common cause of anemia worldwide, especially in women due to the difficulty of replacing iron lost from menstruation and childbearing [1]. Iron is most readily absorbed when bound to heme, as found in animal foods; thus, nutritional iron deficiency is common in populations who do not eat meat. Iron deficiency anemia arises in occult bleeding of the gastrointestinal tract, and thus can be an early sign of malignancy or a consequence of aspirin and/or anticoagulant drug therapy. Both vitamin B_{12} (cobalamin) and folate deficiency cause megaloblastic anemia, and the former also causes a demyelinating disorder of the nervous system. Mixed nutrient deficiencies frequently coexist because diets containing little animal protein are also deficient in both iron and B_{12}, and gastrointestinal disorders may cause malabsorption of all three nutrients as well as occult blood loss.

Iron Deficiency

The largest quantity of iron is bound to Hgb in red blood cells. Absorbed iron is bound to serum transferrin and is delivered to all tissues including the bone marrow. The percent saturation of transferrin is a useful test in the diagnosis of iron deficiency. Iron that is not needed for heme synthesis is stored in ferritin, another useful measurement of iron status. Daily losses of iron are approximately 1 mg in men, which is compensated by absorption of 1 mg of iron per day in males who store about 800 mg of iron in Western countries. Menstruating women have higher iron requirements, needing to absorb 1.5–2 mg of iron daily. A total of 1,000 mg of iron may be required during pregnancy and childbirth.

The bioavailability of dietary iron is much lower from plant foods as compared to the heme iron found in animal foods. Small intestinal gastrointestinal diseases cause iron malabsorption. In developed countries, however, the major cause of iron deficiency is bleeding. Besides peptic disease and cancer, the widespread use of aspirin and warfarin is associated with recurrent episodes of iron deficiency anemia.

Diagnosis of Iron Deficiency

After depletion of stored iron, there is iron-deficient erythropoiesis and eventually microcytic (mean cell volume, MCV <80 fl) and hypochromic anemia with occasional thrombocytosis. A fall in MCV levels in a patient known to be at risk for iron deficiency is a sign that iron supplementation should begin.

Laboratory Testing in Iron Deficiency

Serum ferritin <12 ng/ml is indicative of decreased iron stores (table 1). Unfortunately, ferritin is an acute-phase reactant and may be in the normal range or actually high in patients with iron deficiency and inflammation. Seniors may have absent iron stores with ferritin values as high as 50 ng/ml [2]. Serum iron, the saturation of transferrin, and total iron-binding capacity are also useful tests, best obtained in the fasting state. A low serum iron (<50 μg/dl) and a high total iron-binding capacity (>450 μg/dl) translates into a low transferrin saturation level, i.e. <15%. If malabsorption of iron supplements is suspected, the patient may have the serum iron measured before and after ingestion, where a rise in serum iron of 100 μg/dl after 2 h should be expected.

Treatment of Iron Deficiency

One ml unit of packed red blood cells contains 1 mg of iron; thus, 1 unit of transfused blood contains 250 mg of iron, which will raise Hgb levels by 1 g/dl. Therefore, a patient with 7 g/dl of Hgb will require 1,500 mg of absorbed iron. Iron salts such as ferrous sulfate, gluconate, and fumerate are used for oral supplementation; they contain between 30 and 60 mg of elemental iron, although only about 15 mg is usually absorbed (table 1). Continue supplements for 2–3 months after resolution of the anemia in order to replace stores. In patients with ongoing bleeding, the final maximum Hgb and MCV values should be noted and used to guide retreatment.

There are excellent, safe, intravenous preparations of iron that should be used in intolerant patients, especially when bleeding is brisk, and it is unlikely that oral supplementation will be adequate [3]. The reformulated iron dextran can be used in large doses, up to 1,000 mg administered i.v. over 4 h. There are also three new i.v. iron preparations: iron gluconate, iron sucrose and ferumoxytol. Iron sucrose is dosed at 200–300 mg, iron gluconate at 125 mg/dose and ferumoxytol as high as 500 mg i.v. over 90 s, but the latter only has approval in the United States for dialysis patients.

Iron deficiency anemia is undertreated. Regular monitoring for a fall in red cell MCV and aggressive replacement with oral or i.v. iron will prevent needless blood transfusion and hospitalization for acute anemia as well as maintain quality of life and productivity [1].

Table 1. Iron deficiency anemia

Causes
Bleeding, lack of animal-based food products
Laboratory tests
(1) Hypochromic, microcytic anemia or fall in MCV
(2) Serum ferritin <12 ng/ml (<50 in seniors)
(3) Serum iron <50 μg/dl; TIBC >450 μg/dl; saturation <15%
Treatment
(1) Iron salts, 30–60 mg tablets 1–3/day
(2) i.v. iron dextran, iron sucrose or iron gluconate, 1,000, 300 or 125 mg/session, respectively
(3) Correct bleeding problem

Megaloblastic Anemia due to Vitamin B_{12} or Folate Deficiency

Megaloblastic anemia is caused by a defect in DNA synthesis which leads to the production of larger cells than usual (macrocytosis and hypersegmented neutrophils) and apoptosis and destruction of red blood cells in the bone marrow (ineffective erythropoiesis). Both vitamin B_{12} and folate deficiency cause identical megaloblastic anemia, which can be confused with acute leukemia or hemolytic syndromes when severe [4].

Table 2. Clinical abnormalities in vitamin B_{12} or folate deficiency

Megaloblastic anemia in B_{12} or folate deficiency
Macrocytic red blood cells, high MCV
Hypersegmentated granulocytes
High lactate dehydrogenase
High indirect bilirubin
Low haptoglobin
Hypercellular bone marrow with increased erythroblasts
Neurologic disease in vitamin B_{12} deficiency
Paresthesia, ataxia, loss of position sense
Spongy degeneration of spinal cord or brain
Inverse relationship with anemia

Causes of Vitamin B_{12} Deficiency

Plants do not require vitamin B_{12}; thus, the sources of B_{12} in the human diet are all animal-based including meats, dairy products and seafood, and especially shellfish. Low meat consumers and vegetarians are at risk for vitamin B_{12} deficiency [4, 5]. Although the RDA for vitamin B_{12} is 2.4 μg/day, diets containing 4–6 μg show improved status over lower quantities [5]. The most severe vitamin B_{12} deficiency is seen in pernicious anemia which is caused by a lack of intrinsic factor secreted by gastric parietal cells due to autoimmune attack. Intrinsic factor normally carries bound B_{12} to the ileum, where it is absorbed. Thus, surgical removal or bypass of the stomach or the distal ileum will also cause severe B_{12} deficiency. The breastfed infant of a B_{12}-deficient mother may develop severe B_{12} deficiency with failure to thrive and severe developmental disability.

Diagnosis of Vitamin B_{12} Deficiency

Vitamin B_{12} deficiency should be suspected in patients with anemia or pancytopenia of unclear etiology, especially with macrocytosis and other autoimmune diseases such as autoimmune thyroid disease or vitiligo (table 2).

Table 3. Vitamin B_{12} deficiency vs. folate deficiency

Vitamin B_{12} deficiency	Folate deficiency
Causes	
Diet poor in meat	Diet poor in vegetables
Pernicious anemia	Alcoholism, drugs, small bowel
Gastric or ileal surgery or bypass	disease or hemolysis
Lack of gastric acid	
Diagnosis	
Low serum B_{12}, positive intrinsic factor antibodies	Low serum folate
High methylmalonic acid and homocysteine	High homocysteine
	Normal methylmalonic acid
Treatment	
CN-cobalamin 1 mg/month i.m.	Folic acid 1 mg/day oral
or 1–2 mg/day oral	Correct the underlying cause

Values of serum B_{12} <100 or >400 pg/ml are usually diagnostic. However, the vitamin B_{12} level has poor specificity and sensitivity in the intermediate ranges. Assays of methylmalonic acid and/or total homocysteine prior to treatment with vitamin B_{12} will confirm or eliminate the diagnosis of vitamin B_{12} deficiency [6]. Intrinsic factor blocking antibodies will confirm pernicious anemia; however, they are present in only 50% of cases.

About 30% of patients with pernicious anemia will present with predominant neurologic signs and symptoms, especially paresthesia, loss of proprioception, and ataxic gait. The severity of the neurologic findings is inversely related to the severity of the megaloblastic anemia, leading to delay in diagnosis [7]. Treatment with vitamin B_{12} will halt the progression of these lesions but often recovery is incomplete.

Treatment of Vitamin B_{12} Deficiency

Dietary deficiency can be treated with multivitamin supplements, which contain between 6 and 100 μg of vitamin B_{12}. However, since most patients have malabsorption of vitamin B_{12}, either parenteral administration or high-dose (1–2 mg) oral tablets must be used. One can inject 1 mg cyanocobalamin i.m. daily for several days in cases of severe deficiency, followed by weekly administration for the next 4–8 doses, then monthly for life [5]. A randomized trial showed that serum vitamin B_{12} levels were higher and methylmalonic acid levels were lower at 2 months with high-dose oral supplementation as compared to injections [8]. The most common problem in pernicious anemia is that treatment is discontinued; thus, patient education is an essential part of the management of this disorder.

Causes of Folate Deficiency

In contrast to vitamin B_{12}, a diet rich in fruits, vegetables and organ meats will supply an adequate amount of folate. Folates are absorbed in the jejunum, and some drugs and alcohol as well as diseases of the small intestine will interfere with absorption. Alcoholics have a higher than normal requirement for folate. Persons with hemolysis also require more folate. Table 3 provides an overview of the causes, diagnosis, and treatment of folate deficiency versus vitamin B_{12} deficiency.

Folates appear to play a role in preventing neural tube defects. Thus, the United States, Canada and many other countries mandated folate fortification of grain products as early as 1998 in order to prevent these tragic birth defects. As a result, folate deficiency has become rare with the exception of patients in the above-mentioned groups. There have been population-wide increases in the levels of serum folate and decreases in serum total homocysteine [9].

Diagnosis and Treatment of Folate Deficiency

Low serum folate (<3 ng/ml) indicates folate deficiency with the following caveats: serum folate can be depressed in vitamin B_{12} deficiency and after a short period of poor dietary intake. Red blood cell folate assays are not recommended. There are strong inverse correlations between serum folate levels and serum total homocysteine [9]. Elevated total homocysteine levels can be used to diagnose folate deficiency prior to treatment [6]. Most patients can be treated with an oral folate supplement of 1 mg. Women of child-bearing age are recommended to take a supplement of at least 400 μg/day and/or prenatal vitamins, since neural tube formation occurs prior to knowledge of the pregnancy. It is essential to avoid treating the vitamin B_{12}-deficient patient with folic acid alone. The megaloblastic anemia in vitamin B_{12} deficiency may respond to folate treatment, but any other neurologic disease will remain untreated and may progress.

Conclusions

- Iron deficiency is common and suspected when red blood cells are microcytic and hypochromic.
- Either oral or i.v. iron replacement is safe and effective.
- Vitamin B_{12} deficiency causes both megaloblastic anemia and demyelinating neurologic disease curable with replacement.
- High-dose oral B_{12} (1–2 mg/day) is as effective as parenteral treatment.
- Food folate fortification has improved population folate status and decreased neural tube birth defects in many countries.

References

1 Boccio JR, Iyengar V: Iron deficiency: causes, consequences, and strategies to overcome this nutritional problem. Biol Trace Elem Res 2003;94:1–32.

2 Joosten E, Pelemans W, Hiele M, et al: Prevalence and causes of anaemia in a geriatric hospitalized population. Gerontology 1992;38:111–117.

3 Auerbach M, Ballard H: Clinical use of intravenous iron: administration, efficacy, and safety. Hematology Am Soc Hematol Educ Program 2010;2010:338–347.

4 Stabler SP: Vitamin B_{12} deficiency. N Engl J Med 2013;368:149–160.

5 Bor MV, von Castel-Roberts KM, Kauwell GP, et al: Daily intake of 4 to 7 microg dietary vitamin B-12 is associated with steady concentrations of vitamin B-12-related biomarkers in a healthy young population. Am J Clin Nutr 2010; 91:571–577.

6 Savage DG, Lindenbaum J, Stabler SP, Allen RH: Sensitivity of serum methylmalonic acid and total homocysteine determinations for diagnosing cobalamin and folate deficiencies. Am J Med 1994;96:239–246.

7 Healton EB, Savage DG, Brust JC, et al: Neurologic aspects of cobalamin deficiency. Medicine 1991;70:229–245.

8 Kuzminski AM, Del Giacco EJ, Allen RH, et al: Effective treatment of cobalamin deficiency with oral cobalamin. Blood 1998;92:1191–1198.

9 Pfeiffer CM, Caudill SP, Gunter EW, et al: Biochemical indicators of B vitamin status in the US population after folic acid fortification: results from the National Health and Nutrition Examination Survey 1999–2000. Am J Clin Nutr 2005;82:442–450.

Bier D, et al. (eds): Nutrition for the Primary Care Provider. World Rev Nutr Diet. Basel, Karger, 2015, vol 111, pp 169–173
DOI: 10.1159/000362320

Anorexia Nervosa

Enrica Marzola[a] Walter H. Kaye[b]

[a]Section of Psychiatry, Department of Neuroscience, University of Turin, Turin, Italy;
[b]Department of Psychiatry, University of California at San Diego, San Diego, Calif., USA

Key Words

Anorexia nervosa · Weight restoration · Weight maintenance · Macronutrient · Micronutrient · Nutrient restoration

Key Messages

- There are two subtypes of eating behaviors in anorexia nervosa (AN): the restricting type and the binge eating/purging type.
- In addition to effectively treating mood and cognitive disturbances, weight restoration is a central element of AN treatment.
- Weight restoration can be divided into two phases: acute stabilization and weight maintenance.
- During hospitalization, AN patients tend to require escalating caloric intake in order to maintain a 1–1.5 kg/week weight gain. The caloric intake needs to be increased stepwise over time, to around 60–100 kcal/kg/day, to achieve weight gain.
- After returning to a healthy body weight, AN individuals are still energy inefficient and need at least 50–60 kcal/kg/day for weight maintenance (compared to approx. 30 kcal/kg/day for healthy women).
- A major long-term goal is to increase the variety of foods consumed. Daily essential macronutrient requirements to maintain weight are 110–140 g of carbohydrates, 15–20 g of essential fatty acids and 1 g of protein per kilogram of body weight in adults and adolescents.

Introduction

Anorexia nervosa (AN) is a complex and difficult to treat illness that in a number of cases becomes chronic and disabling. It is a disorder of unknown etiology that most commonly occurs in adolescent girls. AN individuals exhibit an egosyntonic resistance to eating leading to a significantly low body weight, intense fear of gaining weight, body image distortions, and severe weight loss due to a relentless pursuit of thinness and restrictive eating.

Improvements in the understanding and treatment of AN are of particular importance given its chronic and relapsing course, often entailing costly and severe medical morbidity. Importantly, AN has the highest death rate of any psychiatric illness [1], also because there are no proven effective treatments to reverse the symptoms [2].

Individuals with AN, particularly those with the restricting type (R-AN), show altered neural mechanisms and avoid eating because its results are anxiogenic and not rewarding [3, 4]. From a clinical standpoint, individuals with AN appear to become hypermetabolic during weight restoration [5], and they need an increased caloric intake to maintain a safe weight after recovery.

The continuous restrictive eating and malnutrition results in pervasive disturbances of most organ systems. Nutrition restoration is a core element in treatment since weight restoration is fundamental to avoid severe physical complications and to improve cognitive function in order to render therapeutic interventions effective [6].

Etiology

The exact AN etiology is unknown, but it is influenced by biological, developmental, and social processes with cultural attitudes toward physical attractiveness being relevant though not preeminent. AN stereotypic clinical presentation, genetics, sex distribution, and age of onset support the role of intrinsic biological vulnerabilities.

Epidemiology

The onset of AN is common in adolescent females, and up to 0.7% of this age group may be affected [7], while the current lifetime prevalence estimate of this illness is 0.9% in women and 0.3% in men [8]. AN is usually a protracted illness; approximately 50–70% of affected individuals improve or recover, around 20% become chronically ill, and 5–10% die [8].

Clinical Presentation

Two subtypes of eating-related behaviors in AN are typically described. First, R-AN lose weight purely by dieting and exercising without binge eating or purging. Second, binge eating/purging type anorexics (BP-AN) also restrict their food intake and exercise to lose weight, but periodically engage in binge eating and/or purging.

The egosyntonic nature of this syndrome often prevents the evaluation of AN before the illness becomes severe, also promoting dropout from treatments [9]. An accurate differential diagnosis with medical conditions (i.e. endocrine and gastrointestinal disorders) should be carefully performed.

AN Eating Behavior

AN individuals tend to eat significantly fewer calories by restricting caloric intake and avoiding calorie-dense foods. AN patients show unusual eating behaviors like slow and irregular eating, vegetarianism, and choosing a narrow range of foods.

Both adolescents and adults with AN, when compared with healthy individuals, tend to show macronutrient and micronutrient deficiencies with lower intake of all types of fat, higher fiber intake, and usually normal protein and carbohydrate consumption.

Interestingly, these eating behaviors persist during short-term recovery and are related to outcome; in fact, low-energy foods and limited variety are associated with poor outcome [10].

In terms of caloric intake, it should be noted that healthy young adult women tend to eat about 30 kcal/kg/day (range: 20–40) [11]. For a 50-kg woman, this means eating 1,500 kcal/day, with the normal range falling between 1,000 and 2,000 kcal/day. In our experience, individuals with AN tend to find it difficult to eat more than 10–20 kcal/kg/day (30 kg = 300–600 kcal/day).

Treatment

The treatment of AN presents unique challenges; there are currently no FDA-approved medications, and few psychotherapies are evidence based [for review, see 12]. In addition to effectively treating mood and cognitive disturbances, it is critical to provide weight restoration.

Weight Restoration

Given the high caloric needs during the process of weight restoration, many AN individuals are treated in specialized inpatient, residential or day treatment programs. NICE [2] and APA [6] guidelines specify clearly that the first goal of treatment is weight restoration, but both guidelines lack specificity regarding this topic.

During weight restoration, R-AN need more calories than BP-AN to gain the same weight [5]. In our experience, during hospitalization, AN patients tend to require escalating caloric intake in order to maintain a 1–1.5 kg/week weight gain. Healthy women usually require about 30 kcal/kg/day to maintain their weight (range: 20–40). If we start a patient with AN on that amount of calories, however, the patient tends not to gain weight. Rather, we have to increase their caloric intake stepwise over time, usually to somewhere between 60–100 kcal/kg/day to achieve weight gain.

Role of Exercise and Metabolism

People with AN tend to become hypermetabolic. That is, they easily lose weight, and need to eat large amounts of food to gain weight [5], also because in these patients caloric intake shows less efficiency in terms of being converted into tissue.

In AN, excessive exercise (pacing, jogging, making restless motions) is a common symptom even in the face of severe emaciation, contributing to increased caloric requirements [5]. AN people who exercise need almost a 3-fold higher range of calories to gain 1 kg [13]; people who do little exercise only need an excess of 4,000 calories to gain 1 kg of weight, whilst those who engage in extreme exercise need up to 12,000 additional calories to gain 1 kg of weight.

Another issue in AN is that energy intake may be converted into heat, rather than used to build tissue. AN people often complain of becoming hot and sweaty during nutritional restoration. In fact, individuals become hyperthermic since the thermic effect of food in AN patients during renutrition is high, representing up to the 30% of energy expenditure instead of the 14–16% in healthy controls, mostly at the beginning of refeeding [14]. This can be explained by the higher energy intake during refeeding and the low efficiency in the initial phases of renutrition due to changes in hormones or autonomic functions.

Medical Consequences

Emaciation in AN is commonly associated with medical complications (compromised cardiovascular status, hypoalbuminemia, anemia). At high risk are those with body mass index <12, BP-AN individuals, and those with physical comorbidity [2].

Refeeding syndrome is a rare but crucial side effect to be considered at the beginning of renutrition. It is caused by rapid refeeding of someone in a state of starvation, mainly if the patient is chronically ill. Refeeding syndrome is characterized by hypophosphatemia, hypomagnesemia, hypokalemia, glucose intolerance, fluid overload, and thiamine deficiency. This syndrome can lead to cardiac arrhythmias, congestive heart failure, hypotension, encephalopathy, respiratory failure, metabolic acidosis, rhabdomyolysis, coma, seizures, and skeletal-muscle weakness. To avoid refeeding syndrome, electrolyte levels should be determined for the first 5 days and every other day for several weeks, in addition to performing EKG assessments [6]. If indicated, during the first days of refeeding, multivitamins and minerals should be provided under strict monitoring to prevent toxicity in case of excessive supplementation [2].

Phases of Weight Restoration

Treatment approaches can be subdivided into two phases based on the patient's therapeutic needs: acute stabilization and weight maintenance.

Acute Stabilization

At the start of weight gain, the caloric intake should be of 30–40 kcal/kg/day for inpatients to achieve a safe clinical stabilization before beginning weight gain and 20 kcal/kg/day for outpatients [6].

AN patients need 5,000–10,000 excess calories to gain a kg of weight, so a 35-kg patient needs about a 1,000 kcal/day (30 kcal/kg) to maintain her weight and a minimum of 2,000 kcal/day to gain weight.

Later in refeeding, it is possible to gain about 1–1.5 kg/week for inpatients and 0.5 kg/week for outpatients [6]. Studies suggest that AN patients need a higher amount of calories – about 3,400 kcal – to gain 0.5 kg/week above the calories needed just to maintain weight. Over the course of 7 days, this amounts to approximately an extra 500 kcal/day in addition to the calories required for weight maintenance. For example, in the case of a 40-kg woman, if weight maintenance requires 30 kcal/kg/day = 1,200 kcal/day to gain weight, an extra 500 kcal/kg/day should be added (total caloric intake = 1,700 kcal/day).

The maintenance amount of calories needs to be increased at intervals to continue weight gain. According to our experience, if there are plateaus in weight gain, a progressive increase of 10 kcal/kg/day every 5–7 days may be necessary to maintain the rate of weight gain at 0.5 kg/week.

Weight Maintenance

Immediately after getting back to a healthy body weight, AN individuals are still energy inefficient [5]. In fact, they need at least 50–60 kcal/kg/day for weight maintenance, whilst healthy women need 30 kcal/kg/day (range: 20–40). Without this substantial amount of food, rapid weight loss and high rates of relapse occur [5]. Eating attitudes at hospital discharge represent a reliable predictor of outcome, with the presence of psychological and organic causes being a hindrance to long-term recovery. These increased caloric needs tend to normalize with time since over 3–6 months AN people show a normalization of their metabolism needing between 20 and 40 kcal/kg/day to maintain weight as healthy women [5].

Nutrients

From a nutrition standpoint, increasing the variety of foods consumed is a major goal, although this represents a great difficulty for patients [10]. Importantly, no specific recommendations for macronutrient distribution have been developed in AN. According to the Institute of Medicine, daily essential macronutrient requirements (in adolescents and adults) to maintain weight are 110–140 g of carbohydrates, 15–20 g of essential fatty acids and 1 g of protein per kilogram of body weight [15].

Protein intake should be highly encouraged. Consuming small amounts of protein of high biological value, in conjunction with the AN patient's preferred protein source foods (mostly vegetable) can provide a faster restoration of nutrient status even if still underweight.

Fat intake is a critical issue since AN patients tend to avoid consuming fats, resulting in severe lipid depletion entailing the risk of impaired neuronal activity. Thus, AN patients particularly need to replenish lipids during treatment, with a focus on essential fatty acids. A variety of carbohydrates can be offered, both complex (bread, rice and potatoes) and simple (fruits, fruit juices and vegetables).

Medical foods are a useful tool to reduce the stomach and gastrointestinal discomfort that refeeding tends to aggravate; they should be considered when patients have difficulties in achieving weight restoration or as a useful addition in case of unstable weight maintenance.

Conclusions

- AN is a puzzling psychiatric illness with unpredictable outcome and high mortality rates. Renourishment and weight restoration play a pivotal role in AN treatment since – in addition to life-threatening risks – a severely emaciated status is likely to frustrate both psychological and pharmacological therapeutic interventions.
- Weight restoration in AN should start slowly, accelerating as tolerated. Nutrient intake should be reinforced, as opposed to caloric intake, coupled with psychotherapy to encourage increasing amount and diversity in food selection and preferences, and eventual further restoration of body weight to the individual's normal range. Dietary diversity should be encouraged since it is predictive of weight maintenance in AN patients.
- Caloric requirements in AN are high and vary between 30 and 40 kcal/kg/day (up to 70–100 kcal/kg/day) for inpatients and 20 kcal/kg/day for outpatients; after the first phase of treatment, it is possible to achieve a weight gain of 1–1.5 kg/week in the inpatient setting and of 0.5 kg/week in the outpatient setting. Compared to the general population, AN patients also need higher caloric amounts – around 50–60 kcal/kg/day – for weight maintenance.
- When severely malnourished, hospitalization may be required; to avoid refeeding syndrome, a strict monitoring of vital functions, electrolyte levels and cardiac functions should be performed.

References

1 Sullivan PF: Mortality in anorexia nervosa. Am J Psychiatry 1995;152:1073–1074.

2 National Institute for Health and Clinical Excellence: Core interventions in the treatment and management of anorexia nervosa, bulimia nervosa and related eating disorders (Clinical Guideline 9). London, National Collaborating Centre for Medical Health, 2004.

3 Wagner A, Aizenstein H, Venkatraman VK, et al: Altered reward processing in women recovered from anorexia nervosa. Am J Psychiatry 2007;164:1842–1849.

4 Kaye WH, Fudge JL, Paulus M: New insights into symptoms and neurocircuit function of anorexia nervosa. Nat Rev Neurosci 2009;10:573–584.

5 Kaye WH, Gwirtsman HE, Obarzanek E, et al: Caloric intake necessary for weight maintenance in anorexia nervosa: nonbulimics require greater caloric intake than bulimics. Am J Clin Nutr 1986;44:435–443.

6 American Psychiatric Association: Treatment of patients with eating disorders, third ed. Am J Psychiatry 2006;163(suppl):4–54.

7 Fitzpatrick KK, Lock J: Anorexia nervosa. Clin Evid 2011;11.

8 Hudson JI, Hiripi E, Pope HG Jr, Kessler RC: The prevalence and correlates of eating disorders in the National Comorbidity Survey Replication. Biol Psychiatry 2007;61:348–358.

9 Fassino S, Pierò A, Tomba E, Abbate-Daga G: Factors associated with dropout from treatment for eating disorders: a comprehensive literature review. BMC Psychiatry 2009;9:67.

10 Schebendach JE, Mayer LE, Devlin MJ, et al: Dietary energy density and diet variety as predictors of outcome in anorexia nervosa. Am J Clin Nutr 2008;87:810–816.

11 Petersen R, Kaye W, Gwirtsman H: Comparison of calculated estimates and laboratory analysis of food offered to hospitalized eating disorder patients. J Am Diet Assoc 1986;86:490–492.

12 Marzola E, Trunko ME, Grenesko-Stevens E, Kaye WH: Anorexia and bulimia nervosa; in Nemeroff CB: Management of Treatment-Resistant Major Psychiatric Disorders. New York, Oxford University Press, 2012.

13 Kaye WH, Gwirtsman HE, Obarzanek E, George DT: Relative importance of calorie intake needed to gain weight and level of physical activity in anorexia nervosa. Am J Clin Nutr 1988;47:989–994.

14 Moukaddem M, Boulier A, Apfelbaum M, Rigaud D: Increase in diet-induced thermogenesis at the start of refeeding in severely malnourished anorexia nervosa patients. Am J Clin Nutr 1997;66:133–140.

15 Otten J, Hellwig JP, Meyers LD (eds): DRI: Dietary Reference Intakes: The Essential Guide to Nutrient Requirements. Washington, National Academies Press, 2006.

Bier D, et al. (eds): Nutrition for the Primary Care Provider. World Rev Nutr Diet. Basel, Karger, 2015, vol 111, pp 174–178
DOI: 10.1159/000362321

Global Food Policy and Sustainability

Adam Drewnowski

Center for Public Health Nutrition, University of Washington, Seattle, Wash., USA

Key Words

Sustainable diet · Animal foods · Plant foods · Greenhouse gas emissions · Climate change

Key Messages

- Agriculture is the foundation of human nutrition and health. However, global agriculture is vulnerable to the depletion of natural resources and to climate change.
- Human diets need to be sustainable, affordable, acceptable, and nutrient rich.
- Greenhouse gas emissions (GHGEs) are one way to measure the carbon footprint of foods. Animal products, including meat and dairy, have a higher carbon footprint than do sugar or grains but can be of higher nutritional value.
- Paradoxically, some healthier diets may not be environmentally sustainable. Plant-based diets have higher carbon costs per calorie than do diets that include dairy and meat. Conversely, diets high in sweets and snacks were associated with lower GHGE values.
- The competing demands of diet quality and sustainability will be compounded by climate change and the pressure to increase the yields of low-cost, energy-dense crops.
- Global food policies should review the complex interplay between diet quality, sustainability, and monetary costs in relation to children's health.

Introduction

The aims of global food policy are to ensure population access to nutritious and safe food, in quantities sufficient to support healthy, active lives [1–3]. Implementing global food policy requires the development of sustainable agriculture and the widespread adoption of healthy diets that are sustainable in the long term.

Agriculture is the foundation of human nutrition and health. However, global agriculture is highly vulnerable to the depletion of natural resources, land, water, and energy that may result from global warming. Feeding the world in the face of population growth, poverty, and climate change poses new challenges to agro-food industries. Among the many problems are land degradation, scarcity of water resources, limited biodiversity, diversion of food crops to biofuels, spiking food prices and price volatility, and higher greenhouse gas emissions (GHGEs).

International agencies are beginning to recognize that feeding an estimated 9 billion people by the year 2050 will be a major challenge. A drop in global food production may lead to food insecurity, social unrest, poverty, and malnutrition. That can cause irreversible nutritional damage, especially for children.

Measures of Sustainable Agriculture

Agricultural production has an impact on soil, water, air, agro-ecosystem biodiversity, wildlife habitats, and landscape. Among the many indicators of sustainable farming are soil quality and soil protection, fertilizer and pesticide use, land conservation, and other aspects of land management. Other measures have included water quality and resources, fertilizer runoff, air pollution, and GHGEs associated with farming and food production.

The US legal definition of sustainable agriculture is based on the 1990 Farm Bill. It is sufficiently broad to encompass the ecological, economic, and social components of sustainable agriculture, referring not only to food production, but also to economic viability, and quality of life. Sustainable farms need to be viable businesses, contributing to rural economy in terms of employment and incomes. This concept holds for both developed and developing countries.

According to US Code Title 7, Section 3103, sustainable agriculture will, in the long term:

- Satisfy human food needs
- Enhance natural resources and the environment
- Use nonrenewable resources in the most efficient manner
- Make farming economically viable
- Enhance the quality of life for farmers and society as a whole.

Of these many indicators of agricultural production, GHGEs have captured the popular imagination [4]. GHGEs, otherwise known as carbon footprint or carbon costs, are associated with agricultural production, but also with food processing, packaging, transport, distribution and retail. Some life cycle analyses have been even more comprehensive, calculating carbon cost through the postpurchase life of the food product, including preparation, cold storage, disposal, and waste.

GHGEs (mostly methane gas) are often calculated in carbon dioxide equivalents: grams of CO_2 expressed per package, can, or bottle of the food product. Carbon footprint logos have been featured on food packaging in such supermarkets as Tesco (UK) and Casino (France). While their impact on consumer purchases may have been mixed, GHGEs are a powerful tool for calculating the quality and sustainability of individual and population diets.

Definition of Sustainable Diets

By common consensus, sustainable diets are those with low environmental impact on land, water and energy resources. The Food and Agriculture Organization has further defined sustainable diets as nutritionally adequate, economically affordable, culturally acceptable, accessible, healthy, and safe [1, 3]. Furthermore, such diets are sparing of both human and natural resources. These multiple criteria demand the development of new metrics to address nutrient density, affordability, cultural acceptability, and the carbon footprint of individual foods and total diets.

It is important to note that the concept of dietary sustainability, as formulated by the Food and Agriculture Organization, does include both diet quality and population health. Low environmental impact is one aspect of diet sustainability; nutrient density of the diet is another.

Nutrient Density Metrics

Nutrient density of foods can be assessed using a technique known as nutrient profiling. Nutrient profile models assign ratings to foods based on their nutrient composition. Key nutrients include protein, fiber, and selected vitamins and minerals, as well as nutrients of public health concern: saturated fat, added (or free) sugars, and sodium. Their content in foods is calculated per 100 g, 100 kcal, or per serving.

The Nutrient Rich Foods (NRF) index is a formal metric of nutrient density [5]. The positive nutrients are protein, fiber, vitamins A, C, and E, calcium, iron, potassium and magnesium, whereas nutrients to limit are saturated fat, added sugar, and sodium. The NRF algorithm is the sum of percentage daily values (DVs) for the 9 positive nutrients, minus the sum of %DVs for 3 nutrients to limit, each calculated per 100 kcal and capped at 100% DV. The NRF score has been validated against the Healthy Eating Index, an independent measure of a healthy diet.

The French SAIN,LIM score is the mean of %DVs for 5 positive nutrients (protein, fiber, vitamin C, calcium and iron) minus the mean of %DV for the 3 nutrients to limit (saturated fat, added sugar, sodium). Unlike the continuous NRF score, SAIN,LIM assigns foods into 1 of 4 categories. The SAIN,LIM model has been validated using linear programming.

These nutrient profiling models, designed to capture nutrient quality of individual foods, can also be applied to meals and menus, and can be used to capture the overall nutrient density of the habitual diet. Nutrient profiling models can also be used by the food industry to screen the nutritional quality of their product portfolio. Importantly, having a global measure of nutrient density permits the subsequent calculations of nutrients per unit cost – where cost refers to monetary cost as well as carbon cost.

Food Affordability Metrics

Measures of food affordability, designed to address hunger and calorie deprivation in developing countries, are often based on price per calorie or calories per unit cost [5]. The Food and Agriculture Organization and the International Food Policy Research Institute have used the food price-per-calorie metric in evaluating food and agriculture policies for developing nations. The World Bank uses the price of a 2,100-kcal basket of reference foods to set the food poverty line. Studies on poverty in rural India calculated the cost of food commodities in rupees per 1,000 kcal, showing that cereals and sugar provided calories at far lower cost than did meat, dairy, or vegetables and fruit.

Hidden hunger is the term used to describe micronutrient malnutrition that can occur in both developed and developing countries. Here, the appropriate measure would not be calories, but rather nutrients per unit cost. In the US, grains, added sugars and saturated fats are associated with lower per-calorie diet cost, whereas protein, fiber, vitamin C, potassium and other nutrients are associated with higher diet costs. The cost gradient may vary depending on population eating habits, agricultural subsidies, or the use of fortified or supplemented foods. For example, calcium and folate intakes in the US are not associated with sharply higher diet costs, an important point in the nutrition of children and pregnant women.

Are High-Quality Diets Environmentally Sustainable?

Animal food products, meat and dairy, are said to consume land and water resources to excess and contribute to GHGEs more than other foods. On the other hand, transport of out-of-season fresh produce by air has its own very considerable carbon costs.

The question whether healthy diets are also good for the planet would benefit from a more extended debate. Some potential paradoxes were recently explored by Vieux et al. [6, 7] in France and Macdiarmid et al. [8, 9] in the UK. In general, healthy diets are supposed to be more environmentally friendly because plant-based foods have lower GHGEs per unit weight than do animal-based foods. The relation between low-energy-density plant foods and their carbon footprint changes, however, when carbon costs are calculated per calorie.

Vieux et al. [7] estimated diet quality and carbon costs of the diets of 1,918 French adults by attaching GHGEs for 391 foods to dietary intake data. These techniques were analogous to those used to estimate the monetary cost of different quality diets. The most nutrient-dense diets were defined as those of lower energy density, higher mean nutrient adequacy ratio, and lower intakes of nutrients to limit. As expected, the best diets contained more plant-based foods, fruit and vegetables, and fewer sweets and salted snacks than did lower-quality diets. However, on a per calorie basis, higher-quality diets were associated with significantly higher GHGEs. Whereas the consumption of sweets and grains was associated with lower GHGEs, diets higher in fruits, vegetables and animal products were associated with higher GHGEs. The researchers were forced to come to the conclusion that the best diets were not those with lower GHGEs, even if they did contain large amounts of vegetables and fruit.

Similarly, Macdiarmid et al. [8, 9] have now questioned whether healthy diets were environmentally the most sustainable. In that study, linear programming, based on GHGE data for 82 foods, was used to create optimized food patterns for women (aged 19–50 years) that reduced GHGE while meeting dietary requirements for health. Consumption constraints were added to ensure that the food choices were socially and culturally acceptable.

In the model, GHGEs could be reduced by as much as 90%, provided that the diet was restricted to only 7 items in unacceptable amounts. Imposing consumption constraints yielded more varied food patterns (52 foods), but GHGEs were reduced by only 36%. The estimated retail cost of the diet was not increased. The authors concluded that a healthy and more environmentally sustainable diet could be achieved without eliminating meat or dairy products or increasing the cost to the consumer.

Food Prices and Climate Change

Sugars and grains are generally cheaper per calorie than are the more nutrient-rich foods [10]. Cereal and oilseed crops, not meat or dairy, account for most of the calories in the global food supply. Corn, wheat, rice, soy, and sugar cane are all staples that yield inexpensive dietary energy and provide fat, refined carbohydrates, and protein. Energy, land, and water resources for many other crops are becoming scarce, leading to justifiable concerns about hunger and food security worldwide.

Extreme weather events, including severe drought conditions that damage crops, generally lead to sharp price increases, especially for dairy, eggs, and meat. The global food price crises of 2007–2008 and 2010–2011 contributed to political turmoil and social unrest and led to economic difficulties for the global poor. The crops affected by price spikes and price volatility were rice, maize, wheat, and soybeans.

A rise in food prices caused by climate change will lead to higher, not lower, obesity rates in the United States and likely worldwide. As food prices increase or incomes drop, refined grains, sweets, and fats become the best way to provide daily calories at a manageable cost [10]. Added sugars and fats can be inexpensive, flavorful, satisfying, readily accessible, and convenient. As economic pressures mount, they are likely to displace healthier option in the diets of children, first for the poor and later for the middle class. Food prices are a mechanism that links obesity and poverty [10]. One consequence of rising global food prices may be a parallel rise in childhood obesity and diabetes.

Conclusions

- The current dilemma is that, simply put, not all healthy diets are sustainable and not all sustainable diets are particularly healthy.

- On one hand, sugars and grain-based snacks have lower GHGEs than meat and dairy, which consume more agricultural resources. On the other hand, some animal-based products are more calorie dense and more nutrient rich, so that their higher GHGEs are offset by their higher nutritional value.
- In model systems, replacing meat with equicaloric amounts of vegetables actually increased carbon costs [6]. Replacing meat, milk and milk products with sugar may reduce carbon costs, but these lower GHGE diets may not be optimal for population health.
- The hoped-for convergence between diets that are good for people and simultaneously good for the planet is slow in coming. What we need is a better harmonization between dietary guidelines and agricultural production.
- In future analyses of healthy sustainable diets, diet quality, food prices, carbon costs, and likely health outcomes will all need to be taken into account.

References

1 Food and Agriculture Organization of the United Nations: Sustainable diets: what it means, why it matters and what can we do about it. http://www.fao.org/food/sustainable-diets-and-biodiversity/en/.

2 Department for Environment Food and Rural Affairs: Food 2030. London, HM Government, 2010. archive.defra.gov.uk/foodfarm/food/pdf/food2030strategy.pdf (accessed March 17, 2013).

3 Burlingame B, Dernini S (eds): Sustainable diets and biodiversity: directions and solutions for policy, research and action. http://www.fao.org/docrep/016/i3004e/i3004e.pdf (accessed October 1, 2012).

4 Kim B, Neff R: Measurement and communication of greenhouse gas emissions from US food consumption via carbon calculators. Ecol Econ 2009;69:186–196.

5 Drewnowski A: The Nutrient Rich Foods Index helps to identify healthy, affordable foods. Am J Clin Nutr 2010;91: 1095S–1101S.

6 Vieux F, Darmon N, Touazi D, Soler LG: Greenhouse gas emissions of self-selected individual diets in France: changing the diet structure or consuming less? Ecol Econ 2012:75:91–101.

7 Vieux F, Soler L-G, Touazi D, Darmon N: High nutritional quality is not associated with low greenhouse gas emissions in self-selected diets of French adults. Am J Clin Nutr 2013:97:569–583.

8 Macdiarmid JI, Kye J, Horgan GW, Loe J, et al: Sustainable diets for the future: can we contribute to reducing greenhouse gas emissions by eating a healthy diet? Am J Clin Nutr 2012:96:632–639.

9 Macdiarmid JI: Is a healthy diet an environmentally sustainable diet? Proc Nutr Soc 2013;72:13–20.

10 Drewnowski A, Specter SE: Poverty and obesity: diet quality, energy density and energy costs. Am J Clin Nutr 2004;79: 6–16.

Bier D, et al. (eds): Nutrition for the Primary Care Provider. World Rev Nutr Diet. Basel, Karger, 2015, vol 111, pp 179–185
DOI: 10.1159/000362322

Undernutrition in the Developing World

H.H. Vorster

Centre of Excellence for Nutrition, North-West University, Potchefstroom Campus, Potchefstroom, South Africa

Key Words

Undernutrition · Developing countries · Poverty · Human capital · Food and nutrition insecurity

Key Messages

- Undernutrition is an outcome of many interlinked disadvantages rooted in poverty.
- It is also a major cause of poverty. There is a vicious cycle between undernutrition, low human capital, underdevelopment, and poverty.
- Under- and overnutrition often coexist, resulting in a double burden of nutrition-related diseases in the developing world.
- On the population level, undernutrition is a public health problem in low-income countries, and on the individual level, a serious clinical health problem in all countries.
- Health professionals should understand the causes and consequences of undernutrition to support, educate and empower patients to follow healthier diets when they are discharged from clinical settings into unfavorable food and nutrition environments.

Introduction

Undernutrition in developing or low-income countries (LICs) is a major barrier to eradicating poverty and to timeously reach the Millennium Development Goals [1]. Undernutrition leads to arrested physical and mental development of individuals [2], to low human capital (LHC) [3], and therefore has a detrimental impact on social and economic development. Persistent undernutrition in LICs is unacceptable in the light of global overnutrition, with associated obesity and related noncommunicable diseases (NCDs). The latter are major causes of disability and death, also in LICs. This coexistence of under- and overnutrition (malnutrition) is a consequence of food and nutrition insecurity, exacerbated by the nutrition transition in LICs. It places a huge burden on the fragile health economies and services in LICs.

Health professionals (HPs) can help to prevent and treat undernutrition in all settings.

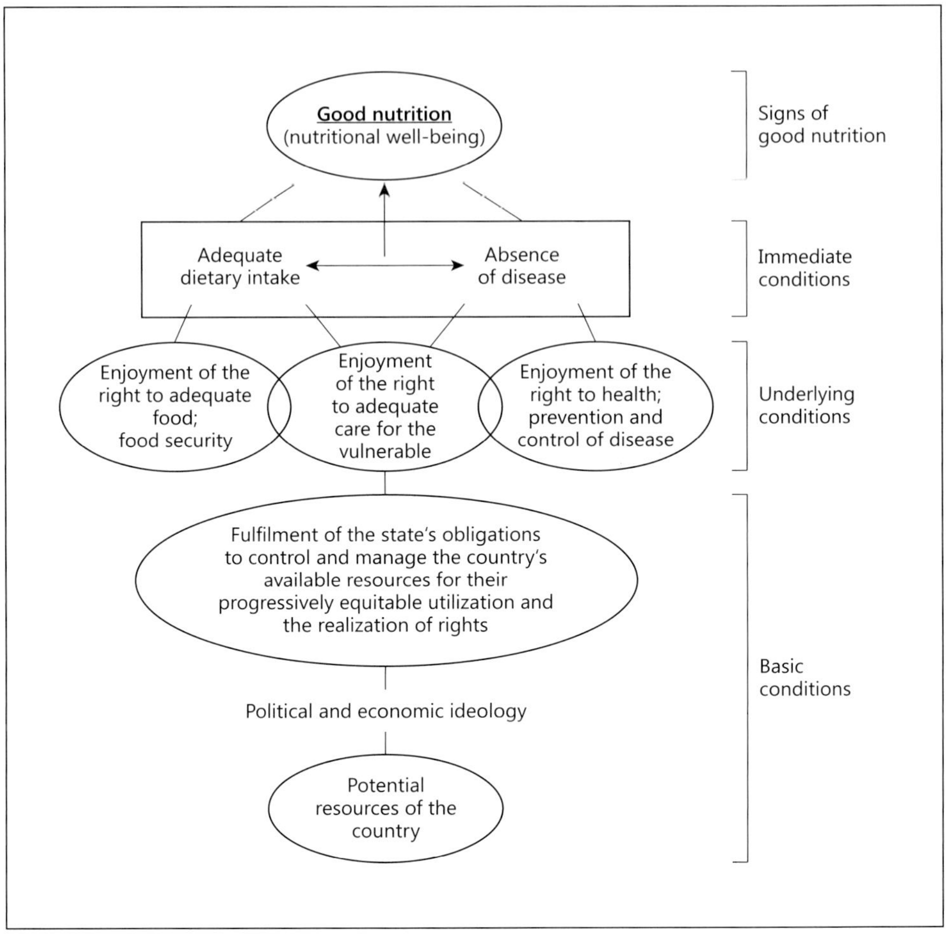

Fig. 1. Adapted UNICEF framework [4] to illustrate the necessary conditions for good nutrition.

However, to do so, they need to understand the immediate, underlying and basic causes, as well as the far-reaching intergenerational biological and social consequences of both under- and overnutrition (malnutrition). They should also be familiar with the concept of the coexistence of under- and overnutrition, and how this problem could be addressed in LICs. Moreover, to support patients that are discharged after optimal nutrition has been restored, they should understand the usual food environment of these individuals and how to educate them to make healthier food choices.

The Causes of Undernutrition

The causes of undernutrition have been conceptualized and classified in the UNICEF framework [4]. Figure 1 shows a positive adaptation of this framework, to illustrate the conditions necessary to obtain nutrient adequacy, security, and optimal (good) nutrition. The conditions are multisectorial, embracing food, health and caring practices, and are classified as immediate, underlying, and basic to incorporate factors influencing food and nutrition security. Many of these factors are rooted in poverty, bad governance

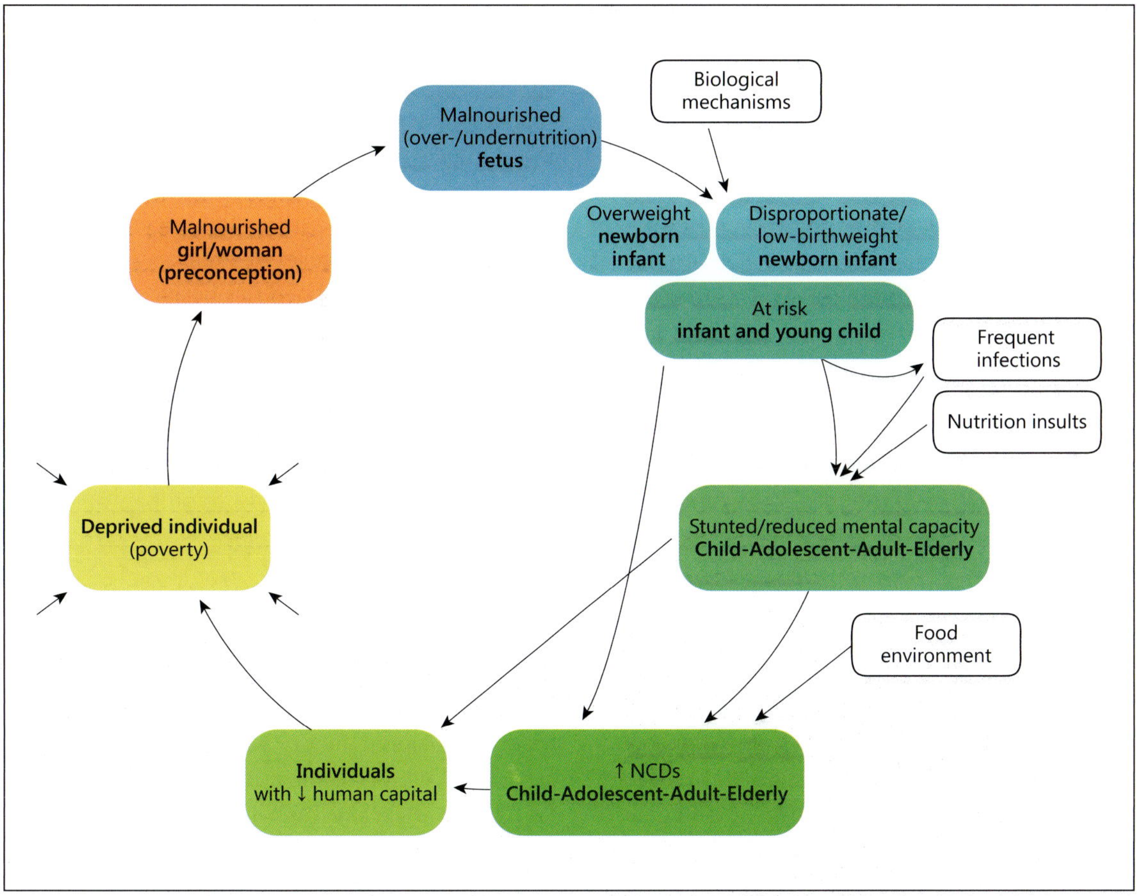

Fig. 2. The vicious cycle of poverty, malnutrition and LHC, also showing the coexistence of under- and overnutrition (malnutrition). With permission from JB Consultancy, RSA.

and natural disasters. The framework is used as a guide for assessing and analyzing the causes of the nutrition problem and to help in identifying the most appropriate strategies and actions for interventions.

The Intergenerational Vicious Cycle of Poverty, LHC and Malnutrition

Developments in the genetic and epigenetic arena [5] provided new insights into the biological links between under- and overnutrition and of the importance of fetal nutrition for long-term health. The acknowledgement that malnutrition is a more complex phenomenon because of the coexistence of under- and overnutrition, as well as our inability to effectively address malnutrition on a global level, have resulted in several paradigm shifts in understanding the interlinked causes and consequences of malnutrition. These links are illustrated in figure 2.

The figure shows that malnutrition during fetal life (because of malnourished mothers and under- or overnutrition of the fetus), could result in low-birthweight babies or overweight and disproportionate babies. These babies may be compromised with respect to normal physical and mental development, and especially with further nutritional insults, will be vulnerable to infectious diseases. They may develop into stunted infants and children who cannot fully benefit from education, having difficulty in reaching their full genetic potential. They are, at the same time, metabolically programmed to be more vulnerable for NCDs in later life. Therefore, when these children are exposed to unfavorable, modern, energy-dense, micronutrient-poor food environments, they are at greater risk of becoming overweight and obese and of developing NCDs in adult life. The combination of underdevelopment, infectious diseases and NCDs could lead to adults with LHC, unable to economically care for themselves and their offspring, eventually leading to deprivation and poverty. Human capital is defined [6] as 'well-nourished, healthy, educated, skilled and alert individuals – an improved human condition – resulting in a labor force that could be any country's most productive asset'. Poverty is a cause of malnutrition, and expectant mothers from poor environments are at greater risk to give birth to babies who have been nutritionally compromised in the womb, perpetuating the poverty-malnutrition cycle.

The Dilemma of the Coexistence of Under- and Overnutrition in LICs

The relationship between household food and nutrition insecurity and the overweight status of mothers and children are observed in both LICs and the developed world. However, in low- and middle-income countries, the coexistence of under- and overnutrition resulting in the double burden of high prevalence of both infectious and NCD is a public health problem.

The nutrition status of South Africans, and consequent morbidity and mortality patterns, is an example of the scope and burden of the problem. At present, at least 27% of South African children in rural and 16.7% in urban areas are stunted, up to 17% of men are underweight, while more than 60% of adults are either overweight or obese, reflecting imbalances in energy intake and expenditure. The documented high prevalence of both infectious diseases related to undernutrition and of NCDs related to obesity and overnutrition [7] illustrates the double burden of disease associated with the coexistence of under- and overnutrition. The nutrition transition in developing countries is a principal cause of this situation.

The Nutrition Transition

The epidemiological transition [8], a result of urbanization, modernization, and acculturation, is characterized by a nutrition transition during which traditional dietary patterns change to diets associated with obesity and a high risk of NCDs [9]. These diets are high in fat, animal-derived foods, salt, alcohol and sweetened beverages, and low in whole grains, legumes and dietary fiber. This transition is accompanied by physical inactivity and often happens before the battle against undernutrition has been won. Infants from undernourished mothers are 'mismatched' to cope with this new food environment and are at risk of becoming obese and developing NCDs in later life.

Other factors associated with the nutrition transition that may contribute to the double burden of malnutrition are 'hidden hunger' or micronutrient and dietary antioxidant deficiencies, large serving sizes, a cultural tolerance of obesity (perceptions that obese individuals are more beautiful, happier, more prosperous and free from HIV/AIDS), an unfavorable food environment, and lack of education and knowledge about healthy food choices.

An Integrated Systematic Approach to Optimize the Food and Nutrition Environment

Modernization, economic development and increased buying power in LICs may result in food choices from an unfortunate 'modernized' food environment. This environment offers convenient, very palatable, high-energy-dense but micronutrient-poor foods and snacks at increasingly affordable prices. The aggressive marketing and promotion of these foods, and peer pressure to consume them, especially when knowledge of healthful diets are lacking, contribute to both under- and overnutrition.

To address the problem of optimizing the food environment in order to achieve nutrition security for the whole population, two important actions should be balanced, as shown in figure 3. Firstly, consumers (individuals, households, communities and populations) should be empowered to create a demand for nutritious food at affordable prices. This can be done by implementing appropriate nutrition education programs. Secondly, all the role players (stakeholders) responsible for the food environment should be motivated to develop a common ethical agenda and work in partnerships to supply these nutritious foods at affordable prices. Therefore, a trans-disciplinary, multisectoral, systematic but also integrated approach is advised.

There are many role players or stakeholders that influence the food environment, each with a potential unique contribution to improve this environment:

- Governments can influence the food supply by inter alia controlling what is available: through policies and actions to support agriculture ensuring food security; by imports and exports of food; by providing the infrastructure for marketing of food; by national fortification and supplementation and other nutrition aid programs; by legislation to control labelling and composition of processed foods; by legislation to prevent advertising of obesogenic foods to children.
- The food industry is to a large extent responsible for the safety of our food supply, and can play a positive role. However, the industry is also aggressively marketing and promoting the energy-dense, micronutrient-poor foods and drinks that are associated with childhood and adult obesity and the resultant NCD epidemic. Public health nutritionists have been concerned about this negative role of industry for many years, realizing that the industry is very good in protecting their profits and influencing public opinion. Nutritionists know that where public demand and actions decreased profits in one country (usually high-industrialized developed countries), the industry simply targets other markets, often in LICs [10]. However, some of the multinational companies have tried to develop more healthful and 'functional food' products (low in fat and sugars, fortified or enriched with micronutrients or other plant substances that can lower serum cholesterol, etc.). These products are usually much more expensive than the products they are supposed to replace and confuse customers about healthy choices from available foods. They are not the answer to optimize the food environment.
- There are other role players or stakeholders that may influence the food environment, either by influencing government and political structures such as nongovernmental organizations (NGOs), civil, and public organizations; by supplying food to consumers (from street vendors, spaza shops, fast-food outlets, restaurants and supermarkets); by influencing food choices (media and advertisements), or by empowering people to make healthier choices (HPs, UN agencies and NGOs). Any nutrition strategy should recognize the potential of partnerships between these role players and provide opportunities for them to work together.

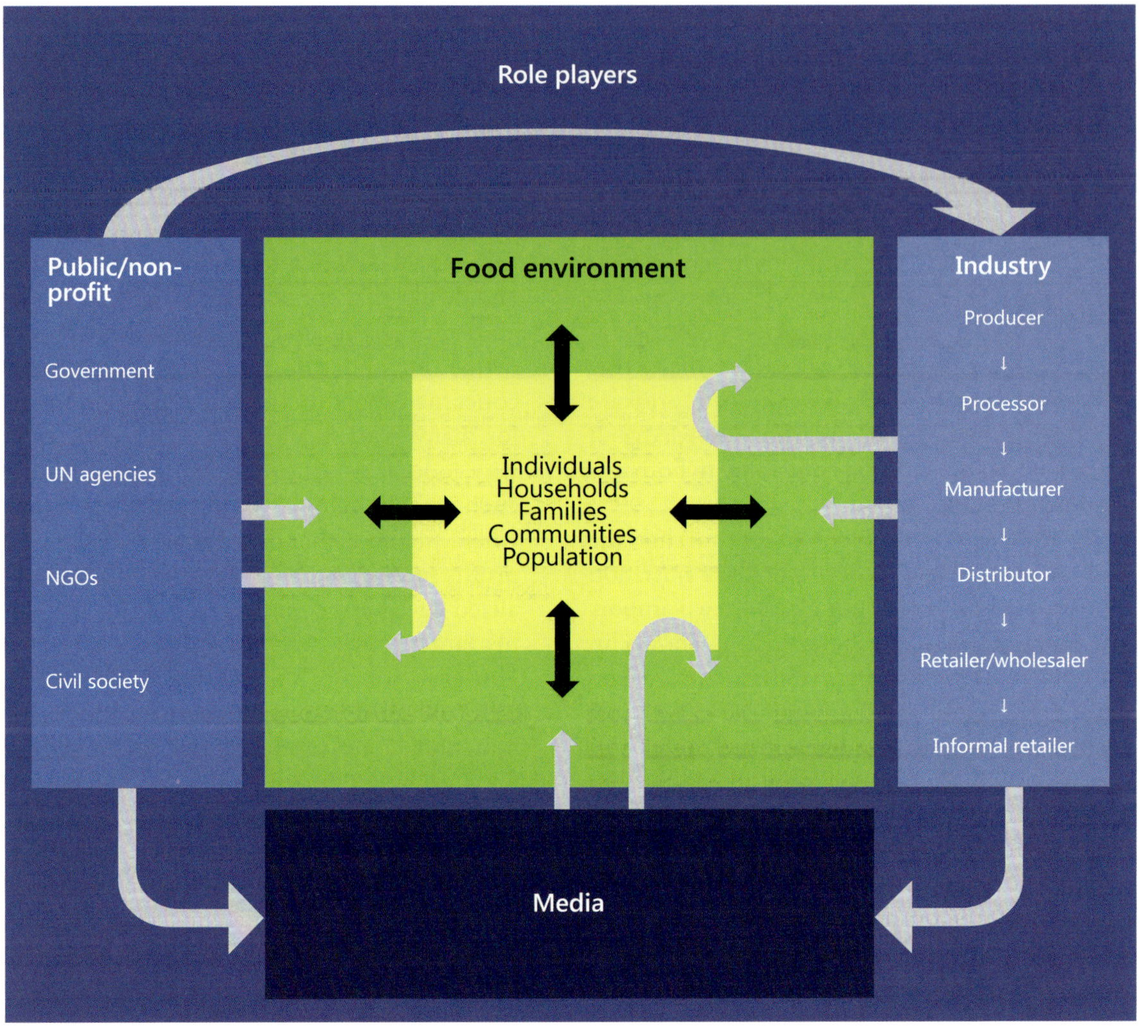

Fig. 3. A framework indicating how several role players determine the food environment. With permission from JB Consultancy, RSA.

Conclusions

- HPs in the developing world should be aware of and understand the food and nutrition environment to support individuals in reaching nutrient adequacy and optimal nutritional status.
- To help them to avoid both undernutrition and overweight, knowledge of the links between poverty, malnutrition and LHC is essential.
- Furthermore, HPs should be able to show individuals how to choose healthier diets, often from unfavorable food environments, indicating a need to understand the many factors influencing these environments.

References

1 Schuftan C: The Millenium Development Goals: who for, and what for? http://www.wphna.org/claudioschuftanoct2010.asp (accessed October, 2010).
2 Grantham-McGregor SM, Fernald LC, Sethuraman K: Effects of health and nutrition on cognitive and behavioural development in children in the first three years of life. Part 1: low birthweight, breastfeeding and protein-energy malnutrition. Part 2: Infections and micronutrient deficiencies: iodine, iron and zinc. Food Nutr Bull 1999;20:53–99.
3 Institute for Fiscal Studies: Human development and poverty reduction in developing countries. www.ips.org.uk (accessed December 28, 2006).
4 UNICEF: Strategy for improved nutrition of children and women in developing countries, policy review paper, E/ICEF/1990/1.6. New York, UNICEF, 1990.
5 Gluckman PD, Hanson MA, Pinal C: The developmental origins of adult disease. Matern Child Nutr 2005;1:130–141.
6 Streeten P: Human development: means and ends. Am Econ Rev 1994;84:232–237.
7 Norman R, Bradshaw D, Schneider M, et al: A comparative risk assessment for South Africa in 2000: towards promoting health and preventing disease. SA Med J 2007;97:637–641.
8 Omran AR: The epidemiologic transition theory. A preliminary update. J Trop Pediatr 1983;29:305–316.
9 Vorster HH, Venter CS, Wissing MP, Margetts BM: The nutrition and health transition in the North-West Province of South Africa: a review of the THUSA (Transition and Health during Urbanisation of South Africans) study. Public Health Nutr 2005;8:480–490.
10 Ynvge A, Haapala I, Hodge A, et al: Making soft drinks the dietary version of the cigarette. Public Health Nutr 2012;15:1329–1330.

Bier D, et al. (eds): Nutrition for the Primary Care Provider. World Rev Nutr Diet. Basel, Karger, 2015, vol 111, pp 186–192
DOI: 10.1159/000362323

The Changing Landscape of Malnutrition: Why It Matters

Rehana A. Salam[a] Zulfiqar A. Bhutta[a, b]

[a]Division of Women and Child Health, Aga Khan University, Karachi, Pakistan; [b]Program for Global Pediatric Research, Hospital for Sick Children, Toronto, Ont., Canada

Key Words

Malnutrition · Nutrition goals · Nutrition interventions · Scale-up · Community-based interventions

Key Messages

- Malnutrition is also dependent upon factors that are not directly related to nutrition, such as growing populations and urbanization, inflation, climate changes and water shortages, political conflicts and natural disasters.
- Alongside nutrition-specific interventions, large-scale programs that address these underlying determinants should also be considered to achieve specific nutrition goals.
- The strategy for combatting malnutrition therefore requires a multipronged approach involving not only interventions directed at the biological causes of suboptimum growth and development, but also large-scale programs that broadly address the social, political and environmental determinants of malnutrition.
- Many countries have achieved success in improving nutrition and health outcomes at the population levels through investments in agriculture, education, and social sector development alongside implementing nutrition-specific interventions.
- The scale-up of selected nutrition interventions through community-based approaches has the greatest impact in the poorest social quintiles, suggesting that community-based delivery platforms have the potential to reach these inaccessible groups and reduce existing disparities in both access and mortality.

Introduction

Despite the global economic growth, there is little evidence of change in the burden of undernutrition in many countries. According to a report by the Food and Agriculture Organization, around 870 million people were undernour-

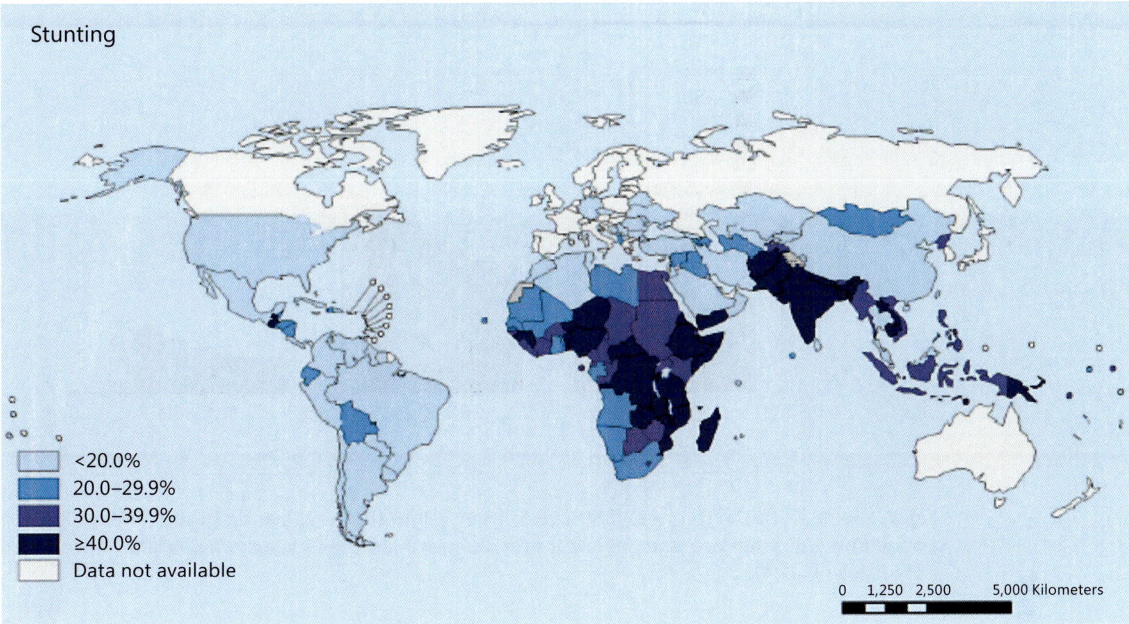

Fig. 1. Latest prevalence estimates for stunting among children under 5 years of age shown by country. Reproduced from UNICEF, WHO, World Bank [6].

ished in the period of 2010–2012, representing 12.5% of the global population with the vast majority, 98% (852 million), from developing countries [1]. Likewise, maternal and child undernutrition rates also remain high in these regions, with prevalence of maternal undernutrition (defined as body mass index, BMI <18.5) as high as over 20% in many countries of Africa, Southeast Asia, Latin America, and the Caribbean [2]. In 2011, one third of the 6.9 million deaths of children under 5 years of age worldwide were attributable to suboptimal breastfeeding and micronutrient deficiencies; particularly vitamin A and zinc [3]. Moreover, around 165 million children under 5 years of age were stunted, 101 million underweight and 52 million wasted globally; 90% of which live in just 36 countries, with the highest prevalence in Southeast Asia and sub-Saharan Africa (fig. 1) [4]. Micronutrient deficiencies are also widespread globally, especially among these vulnerable groups, given their increased nutritional demands. Prevalence of iron deficiency anemia among pregnant women is around 19.2%, while that of vitamin A deficiency is 15.3% [4]. According to the World Health Organization (WHO), globally around 190 million preschool children and 19.1 million pregnant women are vitamin A deficient, approximately 100 million women of reproductive age have iodine deficiency, and an estimated 82% of pregnant women worldwide have inadequate zinc intakes to meet the normal needs of pregnancy [5].

The following discussion in this chapter will revolve around the malnutrition trends over the past decades, emerging challenges and exiting inequities and how best to combat the issue taking into consideration the existing proven interventions and their delivery mechanisms.

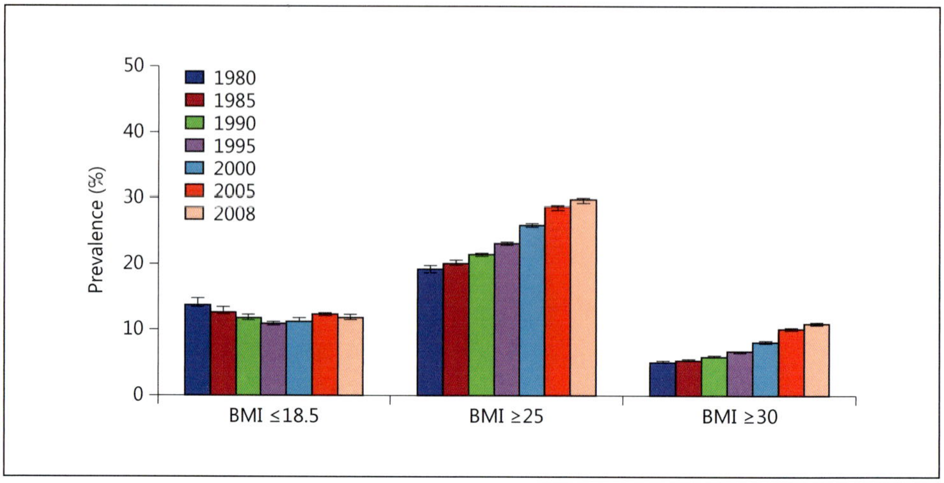

Fig. 2. Global trends in thinness (BMI <18.5), overweight (BMI ≥25), and obesity (BMI ≥30) using population-weighted average prevalence for women aged 20–49 years; 1980–2008. Reproduced from Black et al. [4].

Nutrition Trends

In the last few decades, there has been some improvements in the nutritional indicators; stunting among children under 5 years of age has shown a 35% decline from an estimated 253 million in 1990 to 165 million in 2011, and the prevalence of low BMI in adult women has decreased in Africa and Asia since 1980. Nonetheless, the magnitude of malnutrition and associated detrimental health consequences still remains high. Furthermore, many of the low- and middle-income countries now bear the double burden of malnutrition due to the emerging issues of overweight and obesity along with the existing high rates of stunting and other micronutrient deficiencies. Figure 2 depicts the global trends in thinness (BMI <18.5), overweight (BMI ≥25), and obesity (BMI ≥30) prevalence for women aged 20–49 years, from 1980–2008.

In 2011, an estimated 43 million children under 5 years of age were overweight, marking a 54% increase from an estimated 28 million in 1990. In Africa, the estimated prevalence increased from 4% in 1990 to 7% in 2011, whereas these figures are a little lower in Asia (5% in 2011), though the absolute number of affected children is higher compared to Africa (17 and 12 million, respectively) [6]. These figures are alarming and require immediate attention as childhood overweight is associated with multiple immediate and long-term risks including: raised cholesterol, triglycerides, and glucose; type 2 diabetes; high blood pressure; adult obesity and its associated consequences [7, 8].

Strategies to Combat Malnutrition

Malnutrition is not only dependent upon the direct determinants of nutrition and growth, including diet, behavior and health, but is also greatly affected by certain indirect determinants such as food security, education, environment, economic and social conditions, resources and governance. Hence the agenda for combatting malnutrition requires a multipronged approach involving not only interventions directed at the

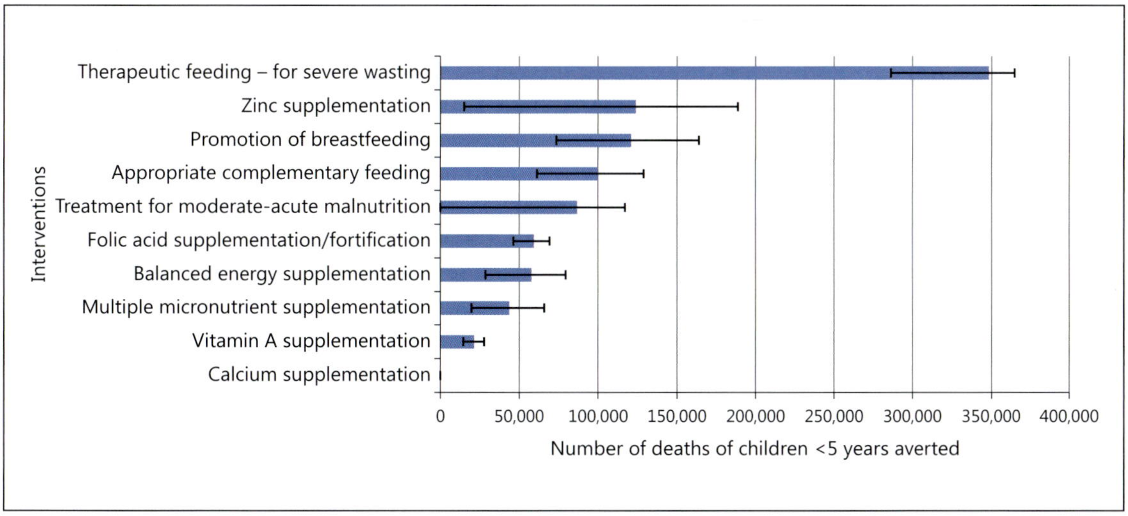

Fig. 3. Deaths averted by scale-up of selected nutrition interventions. Reproduced from Bhutta et al. [9].

more immediate causes of suboptimum growth and development but also the large-scale programs that broadly address the underlying determinants of malnutrition. The recent Lancet Nutrition Series highlights the existing promising interventions to improve maternal nutrition and consequently reduce fetal growth restriction and small-for-gestational-age births and improving child nutrition specifically in developing countries [9]. These include simple interventions like periconceptional folic acid supplementation/fortification, maternal balanced energy protein, vitamin A, multiple micronutrient and calcium supplementation, breastfeeding promotion, appropriate complementary feeding, preventive zinc supplementation and management of acute malnutrition in children. Scaling up of these identified interventions to 90% coverage could potentially reduce nearly 15% of deaths among children under 5 years of age, while also reducing stunting and severe wasting by 20 and 61%, respectively (fig. 3) [9]. Since maternal malnutrition, micronutrient deficiencies and small-for-gestational-age births remain major determinants of stunting in early childhood, malnutrition prevention has undergone a paradigm shift from targeting pregnant women to increased advocacy to target these deficiencies earlier in the life cycle through promoting adolescent health and nutrition, delaying age at first pregnancy and increased birth spacing [9]. An estimated 10 million girls younger than 18 years are married each year, putting them at a higher risk of delaying their own growth, poorer birth outcomes, delivery complications and mortality in mothers and children [10].

As mentioned earlier, malnutrition is also greatly dependent upon factors that are not directly related to nutrition such as growing populations and urbanization, inflation, climate changes and related water shortages, conflicts and emergencies, and natural disasters affecting agriculture production [11]. Hence, along with the nutrition-specific interventions, large-scale programs that address these underlying determinants should also be considered to achieve specific nutrition goals. These programs involve complementary sectors such as agriculture, health, social protection, early child development, education, and water and sanitation to improve the environment and health at the population level [4]. Targeted agricultural programs, early child development and education, and social safety nets have the potential to achieve large scale and high coverage of nutritionally at-risk households and individuals [11]. With the emerging focus on adolescent nutrition, these programs offer a unique opportunity to improve the preconception nutrition status of young girls, consequently improving pregnancy and birth outcomes either through school-based or home-based programs. However, these programs would require specific nutrition goals with targeted nutrition outcomes for the evaluation of effectiveness and to bring about improvements in nutrition indicators. These programs can also serve as delivery platforms for the nutrition-specific interventions and can be effective at reaching poor populations as these are often implemented at a larger scale [11]. Many countries including Brazil, China, Saudi Arabia, Kuwait and Chile have achieved success in improving nutrition and health outcomes at the population levels through investments in agriculture, education, and social sector development alongside implementing nutrition-specific interventions [12].

Challenges and Inequities

Despite the existence of proven interventions and relative improvements in nutrition indicators overall, nutrition data indicate considerable disparity between the developed and developing regions, with South Asia bearing the highest burden [13]. Maternal undernutrition is particularly severe in the South Asian Countdown countries, with a recent Demographic and Health Survey indicating that the median prevalence of low BMI among women of reproductive age is 10.9%, and almost three quarters of all the world's low-birth-weight infants are born in South Asia alone. In the 75 Countdown countries globally, stunting rates are well above the 3% threshold with more than 1 in 3 children being stunted, while the median prevalence of wasting is 7.1%. Within countries, there is a wide disparity between the richest and poorest wealth quintiles as in one fifth of the Countdown countries, more than half of the children in the poorest 20% of all families are stunted. With these existing disparities, another challenge is the high rates of HIV that threaten to reverse all the nutrition gains achieved through large-scale programs.

How Best to Deliver

While individual interventions such as micronutrient supplementation/fortification, exclusive breastfeeding, appropriate complementary feeding and management of childhood undernutrition have shown to be effective, an integrated approach is needed to achieve optimal results. The coverage of various proven interventions discussed above is below the acceptable cutoffs, and delivery of these interventions to the neediest groups has to be ensured [14]. Various delivery strategies have been suggested to increase the uptake of these interventions and at the same time ensure equitable delivery. These include community-based delivery platforms for nutrition education and promotion, food fortification, financial incentives, school-based delivery platforms, Integrated Management of Childhood Illnesses and Child Health Days.

Community-based delivery platforms are increasingly being advocated and have the potential for scaling up coverage of nutrition interventions and reaching poor populations through creating mass awareness and door-to-door service delivery. Community-based interventions delivered by health-care personnel or lay individuals, and implemented locally in homes, villages, or any defined community group, have shown to reduce inequities in maternal child health interventions and can be used as a platform for nutrition intervention delivery. In many low- and middle-income countries, community health service delivery through community health workers already exists and is utilized to deliver a wide range of interventions and hence offer a unique opportunity to engage and reach poor and difficult to access populations through communication and outreach strategies. Equity analysis based on the data from three countries (Bangladesh, Ethiopia and Pakistan) in the recent *Lancet* Nutrition Series has shown that scale-up of the selected nutrition interventions through community-based approaches has the greatest impact in the poorest quintiles, suggesting that the community-based delivery platforms have the potential to reach these inaccessible groups and substantially reduce the existing disparities in both access and mortality [9].

Nutrition interventions could also be potentially integrated with other maternal, newborn, and child health interventions since several countries are investing in programs to address maternal, newborn, and child health [15]. School feeding programs have been introduced in many countries to improve attendance, achievement, growth, and other health outcomes. Child Health Days have been introduced in response to the declining coverage of many essential child survival interventions as a result of weakening health systems. The Integrated Management of Childhood Illnesses strategy developed by the WHO in collaboration with UNICEF and other agencies has been implemented to provide both curative and preventive interventions targeted at improving the health practices at health facilities, home and in the community. Financial incentives including conditional and unconditional cash transfers can also be utilized to counteract poverty, reduce financial barriers and improve population health with a potential to promote increased coverage of several important child health interventions. Besides maternal, newborn, and child health interventions, food fortification is another attractive public health strategy which can reach wider at-risk population groups through existing food delivery systems, and without major changes to existing consumption patterns [5]. All of these strategies can provide scale-up opportunities to reach large segments of the vulnerable population.

Conclusions

- Changing the landscape of global malnutrition will involve health system policies, actions, and advocacy at all levels.
- Investments in the scale-up of large-scale nutrition programs should be prioritized by the policy makers with an effort to maximize the implementation of large-scale nutrition-directed programs.
- Effective coordination between sectors, national and subnational levels, private sector engagement, resource mobilization, and state accountability to its citizens are needed to prioritize political actions.

References

1 Food and Agriculture Organization: The State of Food Insecurity in the World. http://www.fao.org/docrep/016/i3027e/i3027e.pdf.

2 Kothari MT, Abderrahim N, Macro ICF; United States Agency for International Development: Nutrition Update 2010. Washington, United States Agency for International Development, 2010.

3 You D, Jin NR, Wardlaw T: Levels and Trends in Child Mortality: Report 2012. New York, UNICEF, 2012.

4 Black RE, Victora CG, Walker SP, et al: Maternal and child undernutrition and overweight in low-income and middle-income countries. Lancet 2013;382:427–451.

5 Das JK, Salam RA, Kumar R, Bhutta ZA: Micronutrients food fortification and its impact on woman and child health: a systematic review. Syst Rev 2013;2:67.

6 UNICEF, WHO, World Bank: Levels and trends in child malnutrition. Joint child malnutrition estimates. New York, UNICEF; Geneva, WHO; Washington, World Bank, 2012.

7 Koplan JP, Liverman CT, Kraak VI: Preventing childhood obesity: health in the balance: executive summary. J Am Diet Assoc 2005;105:131–138.
8 Lloyd LJ, Langley-Evans SC, McMullen S: Childhood obesity and risk of the adult metabolic syndrome: a systematic review. Int J Obes 2012;36:1–11.
9 Bhutta ZA, Das JK, Rizvi A, et al: Evidence-based interventions for improvement of maternal and child nutrition: what can be done and at what cost? Lancet 2013;382:452–477.
10 Gibbs CM, Wendt A, Peters S, Hogue CJ: The impact of early age at first childbirth on maternal and infant health. Paediatr Perinat Epidemiol 2012; 26(suppl 1):259–284.
11 Ruel MT, Alderman H: Nutrition-sensitive interventions and programmes: how can they help to accelerate progress in improving maternal and child nutrition? Lancet 2013;382:536–551.
12 UNICEF: Improving child nutrition: the increasing imperative for global progress. New York, UNICEF, 2013.
13 Stevens GA, Finucane MM, Paciorek CJ, et al: Trends in mild, moderate, and severe stunting and underweight, and progress towards MDG 1 in 141 developing countries: a systematic analysis of population representative data. Lancet 2012;380:824–834.
14 Bhutta ZA, Chopra M, Axelson H, et al: Countdown to 2015 decade report (2000–10): taking stock of maternal, newborn, and child survival. Lancet 2010;375:2032–2044.
15 Global Health Workforce Alliance: Global experience of community health workers for delivery of health related millennium development goals: a systematic review, country case studies, and recommendations for integration into national health systems. Geneva, Global Health Workforce Alliance, 2010.

Bier D, et al. (eds): Nutrition for the Primary Care Provider. World Rev Nutr Diet. Basel, Karger, 2015, vol 111, pp 193–197
DOI: 10.1159/000362324

Food Preparation, Processing, Labeling and Safety

Susanna Magrietha Hanekom

Center of Excellence for Nutrition, North-West University, Potchefstroom, South Africa

Key Words

Food preparation · Processing · Labeling · Safety

Key Messages

- It is easy to cook healthy food by making small changes to the manner of food preparation.
- Learn how to read and interpret labels to be able to make better and healthier food choices.
- Wash hands regularly when preparing food and be aware of food-borne illnesses.

Introduction

Although most modern consumers do not realize the efforts which go into preparing and serving healthy, safe food at their tables, they still demand safe food products in terms of hygiene and safety, and take for granted that the food they buy is intrinsically safe. Consumers must be aware that the food preparation and processing process is prone to a large number of food safety problems which may arise even before they buy or eat the products. It is important for consumers to buy from reputable producers, thereby ensuring properly and safely prepared food, issued with a label that lists all the food items included as well as other nutritional information, such as allergens, nutrient information and 'use by' date.

Definitions

- Food preparation and processing can be defined as any act or process to get something ready and a series of things that are done in order to achieve a particular result, respectively [1].
- Labeling is defined as 'writing of information on a label and fixing it to something' [1].
- Safety means 'to be safe and protected from danger or harm' [1].
- Allergens are 'substances that cause allergies' [1].

In the next part of the chapter, some of the key issues will be addressed in more detail.

Food Preparation and Processing

Cooking healthy food does not need extra time and effort. Individuals with or without diagnosed illnesses, such as diabetes, hypertension, spastic colon, irritable bowel syndrome, obesity and chronic diseases, can reap the benefits of simple dietary adjustments which may be all that is needed to improve the quality of their diet and lives. Empty calories (energy) in most instances are the easiest to address because decreasing the amount added to food does not decrease the portion size. Other non-nutrient additions will also be addressed.

- Reduce the amount of table sugar added to food and beverages before or after cooking by half, at least for a start, thereby reducing the amount of refined carbohydrates. Later on, sugar can be reduced even further until it is left out of the cooking process completely. The benefit of this is that the actual taste of the food item will become more apparent.
- Any visible hard fat (or animal fat, which is solid at room temperature and high in saturated fatty acids) should be removed from meat before cooking, thereby reducing the energy contributed by fat considerably, without compromising the taste or nutritional value of the food item. Never add additional fat during the cooking process, as this will only add extra energy, without adding volume or other nutritional benefits. Discard any cooked fat still visible after the cooking period, before a sauce is made from leftover fluids. Fats emulsify with thickener when sauces are made and are not visible to the naked eye, leading one to believe that there is no fat in the sauce.
- Processed food items, such as soup powders, sauce powders, ready-to-eat meals, and stock cubes are traditionally high in added salt and should be avoided. Reduce salt intake by decreasing its addition during the preparation and cooking process, using spices and herbs instead for improvement of taste. Remove salt from the dining table and taste before adding additional salt to fresh or cooked food. Use lemon juice and other herbs for seasoning of salads instead of salt.
- Include whole wheat flour and products in any cooking and baking instead of refined flour to increase fiber for gut health and improvement of constipation. Water-soluble fiber (e.g. oat bran) also has the benefit of being able to 'capture' excess fats in the gut and excrete it unabsorbed.
- Cook food in as short a time and using the least amount of fluids as possible. Water-soluble vitamins (vitamin B-complex, vitamin C) are especially vulnerable as they dissolve in water and are heat sensitive. It is always good practice to buy food as fresh as possible (be aware of the 'use by' date on packaging), store it for as little time as possible and cook it for the shortest possible time.

Hints

- Use vegetable oil spray to prevent food from sticking to cooking utensils, instead of oil or animal fat dripping.
- Invest in a non-stick pan, as this will reduce the need for oil or added fat during cooking.
- Remove fat from cooked food and liquids by cooling it and removing the solid fat, which will rise to the top, skimming it off with a spoon/fork.
- Use oils and fats low in saturated fatty acids (read the labels on products), for example olive oil, if affordable.

Food Labeling

The best indicator for consumers to decide when to discard food is the 'use by' date which, according to international laws, should be available on all consumables and perishables. Labels will only help people if they have the knowledge, motivation and education to use the information given on packaging [2]. Ingredients labeled on processed food items are listed in order of most to least used in the product. This may give an idea of what the main ingredient for that product is. In addition, all food products are obliged by law to have a label indicating the literal content of the product. Consumers prefer simplified, easy-to-use labels and nutritional facts panels (e.g. recommended daily values) on the label to make food choices. It is also important to understand any 'claims' which may be indicated on the item label. 'Reduced fat', for example, may mean that the product must contain at least 25% less fat than a comparable product, while 'low fat' means the product must contain less than 3 g fat per serving. When a product indicates that it is 'cholesterol free', consumers may interpret the product to be 'healthier' than another comparable product without this claim. It is, therefore, important that the consumer understands the true meaning of the label. Front-of-pack nutrition logos should be interpreted carefully, using the nutritional fact panels on the back of the product. Not all of these logos use the same criteria when identifying a specific nutrient or groups of nutrients as (non-)preferable (e.g. trans-fatty acids, salt, sugars, etc.) [3].

Food Safety

The greater the distance food travels, the greater the adverse health and environment impact [4]. Fresh food from a production unit is handled a number of times before it reaches the consumer, whether it is in raw form or processed. Food contamination may occur during storage, handling, and cooking food at home or in shops. The prevention of foodborne diseases (FBDs) caused by bacteria such as *Escherichia coli* (minced beef, venison, mutton, goat, horsemeat, unpasteurized milk, fruit juice, raw unwashed vegetables), *Listeria* (unpasteurized cheese, smoked fish, pâté, products conserved in jelly) and *Salmonella* (cattle, poultry, seafood) [5], which can cause life-threatening illnesses, requires favorable hygienic conditions during food preparation, a step in which the food handler plays an important role [6].

Food safety is a nonnegotiable attribute, and a 'rational' consumer would never purchase or consume unsafe food [7]. Prior to purchase, it is therefore important to always inspect the condition of the food for damages and leakages, dents in cans, and torn plastic wrappings. Personal hygiene, best practices, workplace hygiene, hand washing and basic microbiology are the basis for food safety [6].

Definitions

- FBD is usually caused when bacteria/pathogens are carried by a person or item to the food being prepared, causing contamination. Consumers ingest the contaminated food and become ill (FBDs). Cooked food is less prone to FBDs since bacteria are killed by heat.
- Pathogens are defined as 'something that causes disease' [1].

The following safety tips may make shopping, preparing and storing food easier:

- Insulated carry bags are available at all retail suppliers for keeping frozen/chilled foods cold on the way home. Put these foods in the freezer or fridge on arrival at home. Never break the cold chain.
- Keep raw meat, fish and poultry (which will be cooked eventually) separate from any fresh ingredients which will be used in the raw form as salads (and not be cooked). Contamination of raw, uncooked food may be hazardous as contaminants may cause severe FBD. Also store them separately in the fridge [8].

- Wash fruits, vegetables and poultry before cooking or eating, even if the packaging suggests that it has already been pre-washed.
- Always use separate cutting boards, knives and containers for preparation of foods to be cooked and those which will not undergo any heat treatments, and sterilize the equipment with a disinfectant directly after use. Plastic and wooden cutting boards should be washed daily and replaced regularly. Work surfaces should be disinfected directly after use.
- Most FBDs occur after eating raw or undercooked food. Only thorough cooking will kill most of the bacteria carried by foods of animal origin. When the origin of the meat, fish or poultry is not in question, the general cooking time according to a recipe should be enough to kill most of these bacteria. If, on the other hand, the origin is not clear, prolonged cooking times may be needed to kill off harmful bacteria (at least 30 min at 100°C – boiling point).
- Wash hands and utensils every time you handle and prepare food [8].
- Wash hands between tasks, especially when preparing raw foods for cooking, and fresh food which will be served raw.
- Wash hands after smoking, using the telephone, toilet, blowing your nose, sneezing, or any other task which could carry bacteria. If you are ill, try not to prepare food for other people as you may contaminate them. Use a surgical mask to prevent bacteria from spreading.
- Do not wear rings, as food can become stuck in them and contaminate other food items.
- Cool leftover cooked food within 30 min after meals to below 10°C to prevent bacterial growth. Store in a fridge at below 5°C for 3–5 days, depending on the type of food. Cooked fish should not be stored for more than 2 days. Only reheat food once and discard any leftovers [8].
- Never refreeze thawed food.
- Store raw and cooked food separately to prevent contamination. Always store food which spoils first in the coolest part of the fridge.

Proper Hand Washing Technique

- Wet hands using water as warm as possible.
- Soap hands from a dispenser which should be available at the basin.
- Work soap to a lather up to the elbows. Remember to also wash between the fingers. Use a brush to remove any dirt from underneath fingernails.
- Rinse with warm water.
- Repeat the soaping process.
- Rinse hands and dry with a disposable paper towel. Do not use a fabric towel or kitchen drying cloth as these may harbor bacteria [8].

Conclusions

- It is evident that consumer education is an important part of changing food preparation and processing behavior and habits.
- Interventions to improve eating habits of (low-income) individuals should focus on education to improve knowledge, skills and attitudes related to healthy eating and food preparation [9].
- Nutrition labels are potentially a major instrument for enabling and educating consumers to make healthier food choices, but current insight into how nutrition labels are used by consumers in real-world setting situations is limited, making the science-based formulation of new labeling policies and the evaluation of existing ones difficult [10].

References

1 Hornby AS, Ashby M, Wehmeier S: Oxford Advanced Learner's Dictionary, ed 7. New York, Oxford University Press, 2005, pp 1143, 1157, 823, 37.

2 Hieke S, Taulor R: A critical review of the literature on labeling. J Consum Affairs 2012;46:120–156.

3 Vyth EL, Steenhuis IHM, Vlot JA, et al: Actual use of a front-of-pack nutrition logo in the supermarket: consumers' motives in food choice. Pub Health Nutr 2010;13:1882–1889.

4 Calverley D: Keeping food local. Nurs Standard 2007;21:18–19.

5 Srianta I, Kusumawati N, Nugerahani I, et al: The presence of *Salmonella* in food: a challenge to detect it and to improve food safety continuously in a global scale. Int J Food Safety Nutr Pub Health Tech 2009;1:6–10.

6 Medeiros CO, Cavalli SB, Salay E, et al: Assessment of the methodological strategies adopted by food safety training programmes for food service workers: a systematic review. Food Control 2011; 22:1136–1144.

7 Tsakiridou E, Mattas K, Tsakiridou H, et al: Purchasing fresh produce on the basis of food safety, origin, and traceability labels. J Food Prod Mark 2011;17:211–226.

8 Payne-Palacio J, Theis M: Foodservice Management: Principles and Practices. New York, Prentice Hall, 2012, p 600.

9 Mello JA, Gans KM, Risica PM, et al: How is food insecurity associated with dietary behaviours? J Am Diet Assoc 2010;110:1906–1911.

10 Bonsmann SS, Celemín LF, Grunert KG: Food labeling to advance better education for life. Eur J Clin Nutr 2010; 64:S14–S19.

Bier D, et al. (eds): Nutrition for the Primary Care Provider. World Rev Nutr Diet. Basel, Karger, 2015, vol 111, pp 198–204
DOI: 10.1159/000362325

The Food Industry and Consumer Nutrition and Health

Denis Barclay[a] Ferdinand Haschke[b]

[a]Nestec SA, Vevey, Switzerland; [b]Department of Pediatrics, Paracelsus Medical University, Salzburg, Austria

Key Words

Malnutrition · Micronutrient malnutrition · Overweight/obesity · Medical foods · Functional foods · Food industry

Key Messages

- The food industry is facing important challenges as it endeavors to help address over- and undernutrition against a background of major demographic trends of population ageing and rural-to-urban migration.
- To help prevent and manage overweight/obesity, the most effective approaches combine nutritionally balanced and portioned foods with regular counselling from health-care professionals.
- An important approach to reducing micronutrient malnutrition is through fortification of staple and packaged foods, which must be accessible, affordable and nutritionally and culturally relevant to the target population.
- Medical foods and oral nutrition supplements are designed for patient groups, such as the elderly and those with specific diseases.
- Collaboration between the food industry and other public and private stakeholders is essential for improving the nutritional value of food products and to ensure the sustainability of the food supply, in addition to the safety and sensory aspects of food.

Introduction

Food processing dates back to prehistoric times as our hunter-gatherer ancestors began to domesticate plants and animals, and food preservation and storage became necessary [1]. Traditional processing methods such as fermentation, sun drying, salt preservation and various types of cooking (e.g. roasting, smoking, baking) preceded modern methods such as bottling, canning, pasteurization and ultra-high temperature treatment. The second half of the 20th century witnessed increasing need for convenience foods, and companies marketed foods especially to middle-class working wives and mothers; these included instant soups and beverages, breakfast cereals and prepared meals.

Today, the food industry is facing major challenges as it endeavors to feed the planet. As the world population grows beyond 7 billion, 50% live in urban settings; by 2050, this will rise to two thirds. While this can improve dietary diversity for some population groups, it can also favor less nutritionally balanced diets and sedentary lifestyles, resulting in overnutrition and related noncommunicable diseases (NCDs), as well as undernutrition including micronutrient deficiencies [2]. The population over 60 years old is growing faster than other age groups through increasing longevity and decreasing fertility [3]. In this chapter, we focus on food industry efforts to address the wide variety of nutritional and health needs of consumers against the background of evolving demographic trends.

Malnutrition at the Population Level

Malnutrition, encompassing both under- and overnutrition, affects the health, livelihood and well-being of nearly half of the people in the world, causing irreversible impairment to the physical and cognitive development of infants and children, increased morbidity and mortality of all age groups, as well as decreased productivity, both for individuals and for nations. Populations in many developing countries are often affected by a triple burden of malnutrition, with protein-energy malnutrition, micronutrient malnutrition, and overweight/obesity occurring together. In general, lower-income populations in all countries are at higher risk of suffering from malnutrition in any form.

Overnutrition

Over 1.4 billion people suffer from overnutrition, with nearly 1 billion overweight and 0.5 billion obese globally [4]. The industry is responding to this challenge by improving the nutritional value of packaged foods though decreasing the levels of public health-sensitive nutrients (sugar, salt, saturated fat, trans-fatty acids) and increasing those of essential nutrients (fiber, micronutrients, etc.), as well providing appropriate portion guidance (labelling, portion size and consumption frequency).

Diet-Related NCDs

Poor diet is a major risk factor for overweight and obesity, and related NCDs such as cardiovascular diseases, cancers and type II diabetes, the health costs of which are enormous [5]. Although the prevalence of overnutrition and related NCDs are higher in industrialized regions, the absolute numbers of affected people are considerably higher in developing countries. The ageing trend is increasingly important for NCDs; by midlife and in the later years, NCDs are responsible for the vast majority of deaths and diseases, as well as for decreased quality of life and independence during the latter decades of life.

The industry is increasingly providing foods and services for weight management; the most effective approaches combine nutritionally balanced and portioned foods with regular counselling and monitoring from specialized nutrition professionals. Low-calorie (1,000–1,500 kcal/day), low-carbohydrate and low-fat diets are offered. In the case of an intended rapid weight loss, patients can be prescribed commercially available very-low-calorie diets (VLCD; 800 kcal or 3,300 kJ/day). They are formulated, nutritionally complete, liquid meals containing the recommended daily requirements for vitamins, minerals, trace elements, fatty acids and protein. Carbohydrate may be entirely absent, or substituted for a portion of the protein. Commercially available VLCD products are usually powders which are mixed with water or another low-food-energy liquid. The VLCD is prescribed on a case-by-case basis for rapid weight loss (about 1.5–2.5 kg or 3–5 lb per week) in patients with BMI of 30 and above. The health care provider can also recommend the diet to a patient with BMI between 27 and 30 if the patient's medical complications due to overweight present a serious health risk. This choice has important metabolic effects and medical supervision is highly recommended.

Undernutrition

Although agriculture has made enormous advances in increasing food productivity several-fold in the past half century [6], one form of undernutrition, protein-energy malnutrition, affects almost 1 billion people globally, principally small-holder farming and fishing families in developing regions [7]. Since packaged foods are often inaccessible for undernourished populations, the food industry cannot address their needs directly, but can contribute by supporting governmental and NGO efforts though farmer development programs, as well as technology and knowledge sharing.

Micronutrient Malnutrition
The less visible form of undernutrition is micronutrient malnutrition or vitamin and mineral deficiencies, sometimes referred to as 'hidden hunger'. Deficiencies in one or more micronutrients affect 2 billion people globally [8]. The food industry contributes significantly through fortification of staple and packaged foods, which must be affordable, accessible, nutritionally and culturally relevant to the target population, consumed on a regular basis and provide nutritionally relevant and safe amounts of bioavailable micronutrients without negatively impacting taste and stability [9].

Medical Foods

Individuals at risk for malnutrition also include the elderly, patients recovering from acute incident/illness, patients with cancer, stroke, gastrointestinal, respiratory, or neurological disease. Disease-related malnutrition increases hospital costs by 30–70%, average length of hospital stay by 40–70%, and results in substantial economic costs, e.g. USD 140 billion/year in the EU [10]. Screening and a rapid diagnosis of malnutrition is necessary to identify those patients who need nutritional support. A widely accepted and scientifically validated method for screening and diagnosis is the Mini-Nutrition-Assessment (MNA®; www.mna-elderly.com). The industry needs to provide adequate medical nutrition products/foods for special medical purposes (Codex Alimentarius), which promote recovery and in the case of the elderly, maintain strength, functional ability and independence. Specialized products with claims on promotion of musculoskeletal strength, support of the immune system, and reduction of inflammatory response are already marketed.

Whenever possible, oral nutrition supplements should be used. If this is not possible or does not result in sustainable improvement of nutritional status, feeding via nasogastric or percutaneous endoscopic gastrostomy tubes needs to be considered. Industrial products include complete (all nutrients according to daily requirements) and incomplete (key nutrients only) oral nutrition products. Tube feeding products have to be complete and are continuously or intermittently administered using medical devices (pumps, tubes, giving sets, and accessories), which must meet international standards [e.g. ISO 18485, US Food and Drug Authority (FDA) approval].

Young Women

With the realization of the importance of nutrition in young women of childbearing age and especially during the first 1,000 days of life (i.e. from conception until the child has reached 2 years of age), nutritional science is increasingly focusing on their nutritional needs, not only during pregnancy and lactation, but also prior to pregnancy. Maternal over- or undernutrition before and during pregnancy can have long-term negative effects on the health of the offspring ('metabolic programming' hypothesis). The fuel-mediated 'in utero' hypothesis suggests that intrauterine exposure to an excess of fuels causes permanent changes in fetal metabolism that lead to obesity and related NCD in postnatal life; the accelerated postnatal weight gain hypothesis proposes an association between rapid weight gain in infancy and an increased risk of later obesity and adverse outcomes; and the mismatch hypothesis suggests that experiencing a developmental 'mismatch' between a suboptimal pre- and perinatal and an 'obesogenic' childhood environment is related to a particular predisposition to obesity and corresponding comorbidities [11]. Therefore, before pregnancy, undernourished young women should have access to affordable, micronutrient-fortified food or supplements [12], while obese women should reduce weight by eating safe, low-calorie diets or VLCDs whilst changing their lifestyle.

Nutrition and Health Research and Technology

In order to offer safe, good-tasting, nutritious and affordable foods to people across the globe, closer collaboration between nutrition and food scientists is essential [13]; indeed food companies are increasingly investing not only in food processing research, but also in food science, nutrition, and in understanding consumer behavior. Some of the world's largest food and nutrition research centers are found within the food industry. Food industry research is ever more carried out in collaboration with leading food and nutrition universities and institutes, each research partner bringing to the table specific competencies in order to better identify and implement solutions to address the specific nutritional needs of different population groups. One such example is the micronutrient fortification of appropriate food vectors to effectively bring missing nutrients to target consumer groups. The university partner may provide knowledge concerning the extent, severity and geographical location of deficiencies in a population, as well as appropriate methodologies to assess nutrient status, whereas the food industry partner can provide the fortification technology and quality assurance for appropriate delivery vehicles, as well as consumer research on how to communicate the associated health message in the most compelling way.

Nutritional Value of Foods (Nutritional Profiling)

Nutrient profiling of foods, described as the science of ranking foods based on their nutrient content, is fast becoming the basis for regulating nutrition labels, health claims, and marketing and advertising to children [14]. A number of nutrient profiling models have now been developed by research scientists and regulatory agencies. Whereas some of these models have focused on nutrients to limit, others have emphasized nutrients known to be beneficial to health, or combinations of both. For example, The Nutrient Rich Foods index ranks foods based on their nutrient content; combined with food prices, it can help identify foods that are both nutritious and affordable [15].

In anticipation of and in response to consumer demand for nutritionally superior foods, companies are increasingly using such nutritional profiling systems during development and renovation of food products. Many major food companies base nutritional improvement pledges on such systems, either voluntarily or in response to international or national nutritional guidelines related to food advertising, in particular towards children.

Food Industry and Health-Care Professionals

Health-care professionals (HCP) such as family doctors, nurses and dieticians are primary sources of nutritional information for consumers to reduce risk of, or manage chronic diet-related conditions, as well as nondiet-related disorders. Since many such HCP do not have access to appropriate nutritional training, the food industry is increasingly making available independent, science-based nutrition information to HCP encompassing all life stages, geographies and cultures. In this context, the information provided must be noncommercial and provided by independent scientists with no conflict of interest. For example, the Nestlé Nutrition Institute (www.nestlenutrition-institute.org) and the Danone Institute (www.danoneinstitute.org/) provide independent science-based nutritional information and training to HCP. Table 1 lists a number of health conditions and situations for which nutritional guidance from HCP is necessary for efficient management.

HCP may sometimes receive invitations from the food industry to attend seminars which focus on the health benefits of food products. Some may even be invited to participate in clinical trials designed to determine the efficacy of a functional food in the prevention or treatment of a health condition. In such cases, the manufacturers should provide to the HCP all the relevant literature and in the case of clinical trials, the full study protocol as well as the full protocol assessment and approval by the relevant ethical committee. If a product is already launched and an HCP is invited to participate in a post-launch survey or 'phase 4 study', it is highly recommended to contact independent health agencies (e.g. FDA) to determine whether such an offer is ethical and for the benefit of the consumer. HCP may also encounter reports of food industry practices apparently infringing environmental (e.g. genetically modified organisms), social (e.g. child labor), and other regulations. In such cases, the HCP may need to contact a government or company contact point to request full information relative to the reported infringement.

Table 1. Conditions and situations requiring HCP counselling

Overweight and obesity
Metabolic disorders (e.g. diabetes)
Cardiovascular diseases
Osteoporosis
Inflammatory bowel disease
Lactose intolerance
Gluten intolerance (celiac disease)
Allergy
Micronutrient deficiencies
Sports nutrition

Table 2. EFSA favorable claim evaluations

Vitamins and minerals
Specific dietary fibers related to blood glucose control, blood cholesterol, or weight management
Live yoghurt cultures and lactose digestion
Antioxidant effects of polyphenols
Meal replacement and weight control
Fatty acids and function of the heart
The role of a range of sugar replacers (such as xylitol and sorbitol) in maintaining tooth mineralization or lowering the increase of blood glucose levels after meals
Carbohydrate-electrolyte drinks/creatine and sports performance

Functional Foods

Over the last 10 years, the food industry has developed numerous functional foods targeting common nutrition-related NCD; for example, foods such as milks and spreads are enriched with plant sterols for lowering blood cholesterol, and dairy products are enriched with probiotic bacteria or prebiotic carbohydrates for gastrointestinal health. In order to ensure that the health claims on such foods are factual and not misleading consumers, regulatory authorities have established systems that assess their level of scientific substantiation based on objective evaluation. The FDA has published a summary of qualified health claims [16], and the European Food Safety Authority [17] developed and implemented a rigorous system used to assess nearly 3,000 submitted claims, of which approximately 20% were approved, relating to a limited number of areas (table 2).

HCP may encounter product health claims with which they are not familiar, e.g. for imported products. In order to be able to appropriately advise patients on the validity of such claims, they may consult local regulatory authorities; in countries where there are no health claim regulations, HCP may need to consult the opinions of the European Food Safety Authority or FDA on such claims.

Consumer Awareness

The food industry has a responsibility to help consumers make informed, healthier choices. Many food companies have introduced self-regulation regarding product information and advertising to consumers. On-pack nutritional information systems such as Guideline Daily Amounts and nutrition tables (e.g. Nestlé Nutritional Compass™) have been designed for this purpose. As above, nutrition claims and health claims are increasingly controlled by regulatory authorities, allowing only claims with adequate scientific substantiation. This helps to reduce confusion amongst consumers and HCP about the nutritional and health benefits of foods.

Sustainable Food Supply

Another major challenge facing the agricultural and food sectors is that of sustainability encompassing the entire food chain from farm to fork [6, 18]. In addition to the essential aspects of safety, taste, nutrition and affordability, ensuring food supply sustainability necessitates reduction of its impact on the environment, including water and fuel usage and long-distance transportation of raw materials and finished products, improved farmer livelihood through production of high-quality and high-yielding raw materials, increased use of local raw materials and reinforcement of local food cultures. Many food companies are already undertaking research and implementing programs addressing these issues in order to ensure sustainability.

Conclusions

- The food industry is addressing a number of important challenges as it endeavors to provide tasty and nutritious foods to a growing global population which is also ageing, increasingly urbanized and affected by overnutrition and related NCDs, while undernutrition and micronutrient malnutrition remain widespread.
- The food industry has a key role to play in concert with the other public and private stakeholders, and is amplifying its efforts to improve the nutritional value of food products and related communication to consumers and to ensure the sustainability of the food supply, in addition to the safety and sensory aspects of food.
- Consumers today are increasingly basing food purchases on these aspects, creating intense competition within the food industry, which will ultimately improve the food supply with respect to these criteria.
- The future of the food industry will thus increasingly depend on creation of shared value for all the players along the food chain.

References

1 Henry CJK: New food processing technologies: from foraging to farming and food technology. Proc Nutr Soc 1997;56: 855–863.

2 WHO: Diet, nutrition and the prevention of chronic diseases. World Health Organ Tech Rep Ser 2003;916:i-viii, 1–149, backcover.

3 WHO: 10 facts on ageing and the life course. http://www.who.int/features/factfiles/ageing/en/index.html (accessed August 2012).

4 WHO: Obesity and overweight. Fact sheet No 311. http://www.who.int/mediacentre/factsheets/fs311/en/ (accessed April 2014).

5 WHO: Non-Communicable Diseases (NCD). http://www.who.int/gho/ncd/en/index.html (accessed August 2012).

6 International Food Policy Research Institute: Leveraging agriculture for improving nutrition and health. Highlights from an international conference. New Delhi, International Food Policy Research Institute, 2011. http://www.ifpri.org/sites/default/files/publications/oc66.pdf.

7 FAO: The State of Food Insecurity in the World. Rome, FAO, 2011. http://www.fao.org/docrep/014/i2330e/i2330e.pdf.

8 WHO: Micronutrients. http://www.who.int/nutrition/topics/ida/en/index.html (accessed August 2012).

9 WHO/FAO: Guidelines on food fortification with micronutrients. Geneva/Rome, WHO/FAO, 2006. http://www.who.int/nutrition/publications/micronutrients/9241594012/en/.

10 European Medical Nutrition Industry, 2012. www.medicalnutritionindustry.com.

11 Koletzko B, Brands B, Poston L, et al: Early nutrition programming of long-term health. Proc Nutr Soc 2012;71: 371–378.

12 Bhutta ZA, Ahmed T, Black RE, et al: What works? Interventions for maternal and child undernutrition and survival. Lancet 2008;371:417–440.

13 Dwyer JT, Fulgoni VL, Clemens RA, et al: Is 'processed' a four-letter word? The role of processed foods in achieving dietary guidelines and nutrient recommendations. Adv Nutr 2012;3:536–548.

14 Drewnowski A, Fulgoni V: Comparing the nutrient rich foods index with 'Go', 'Slow', and 'Whoa', foods. J Am Diet Assoc 2011;111:280–284.

15 Drewnowski A: The Nutrient Rich Foods Index helps to identify healthy, affordable foods. Am J Clin Nutr 2010; 91:1095S–1101S.

16 Food and Drug Administration: Label claims. http://www.fda.gov/food/labelingnutrition/labelclaims/default.htm (accessed August 2012).

17 European Food Safety Authority: EFSA finalises the assessment of 'general function' health claims. Press release, 28 July 2011. http://www.efsa.europa.eu/en/press/news/110728.htm.

18 FAO: Sustainable diets and biodiversity: directions and solutions for policy, research and action. Proceedings of the International Scientific Symposium Biodiversity and Sustainable Diets United against Hunger, 2010. Rome, FAO, 2012.

Author Index

Subject Index